Military Medical Ethics in Contemporary Armed Conflict

Military Medical Ethics in Contemporary Armed Conflict

*Mobilizing Medicine in the
Pursuit of Just War*

MICHAEL L. GROSS

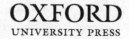

OXFORD

UNIVERSITY PRESS

OXFORD
UNIVERSITY PRESS

Oxford University Press is a department of the University of Oxford. It furthers the University's objective of excellence in research, scholarship, and education by publishing worldwide. Oxford is a registered trade mark of Oxford University Press in the UK and certain other countries.

Published in the United States of America by Oxford University Press
198 Madison Avenue, New York, NY 10016, United States of America.

Library of Congress Cataloging-in-Publication Data
Names: Gross, Michael L., 1954- author.
Title: Military medical ethics in contemporary armed conflict :
mobilizing medicine in the pursuit of just war / Michael L. Gross.
Description: New York : Oxford University Press, 2021. |
Includes bibliographical references and index.
Identifiers: LCCN 2020056006 (print) | LCCN 2020056007 (ebook) |
ISBN 9780190694944 (paperback) | ISBN 9780190694968 (epub) |
ISBN 9780190694975 (online)
Subjects: MESH: Military Medicine—ethics
Classification: LCC R725.5 (print) | LCC R725.5 (ebook) |
NLM WD 921 | DDC 174.2/9698023—dc23
LC record available at https://lccn.loc.gov/2020056006
LC ebook record available at https://lccn.loc.gov/2020056007

DOI: 10.1093/med/9780190694944.001.0001

1 3 5 7 9 8 6 4 2

Printed by LSC Communications, United States of America

To my grandparents
Becky and Harry; Yetta and Moshe Labe
Who had the good sense to leave Eastern Europe when they did
And to my father, Phil, who made his most of it.

Contents

PART IV. AFTERWAR: POSTWAR JUSTICE
AND THE RESPONSIBILITY TO REBUILD

Preface

There is no compelling experience that offers one some privileged vantage point to write about medicine and war. I once thought there was. In *Bioethics and Armed Conflict* (2006), I wanted readers to know that I was neither a physician nor a professional soldier, but, like others, merely a one-time conscript, incidental reserve officer, and part-time patient. It seemed important to establish some bona fides. Maybe those experiences do that.

Then there is door-step history, a local pastime. The plains of Armageddon sit just outside my gate. It's a real place that extends from the foot of Mt. Carmel, through the Jezreel Valley, and as far as Megiddo, hence, Armageddon or (h)ar Megiddo (Mt. Megiddo). Not the most dangerous place on Earth today, but surely the only one with its own eschatology. And although threats always percolate in and around, the sorriest story is Syria, 145 kilometers from Haifa, as close to me now as my childhood home in Chicago was to Milwaukee. More than 500,000 people have lost their lives there, while millions of refugees pile up at the Jordanian border. But it shocks us none and moves us little. So experiences of war and proximity to violence offer no unique insights into its tragedy or resolution but often bring complacency. We call this habituation or, better yet, resilience. I think this is how many cope with war.

Still, writing about catastrophically injured combat soldiers, maimed civilians, desperate refugees, and debilitated veterans is as humbling as it is harrowing. One cannot go it alone but requires support and assistance from clinicians, professional soldiers, and philosopher friends. Over the years, I have had the good fortune to participate in the annual military medical ethics workshops hosted by the International Committee of Military Medicine (ICMM) under the direction of Daniel Messelken and David Winkler. These sessions offered me the opportunity to present work-in-progress and proved a source of unending inspiration. Participants provided rich material for case studies together with keen philosophical insights that led to writes and rewrites. My sincere thanks to the many participants who joined the workshop over the years and aided my research. Chatham House rules govern ICMM workshops so that readers will encounter one or two un-attributed cases. They may contact me for additional details.

As the title suggests, this book marries military and medical ethics. That means more than one workshop! The ICMM meets in Ermatingen, Switzerland in May. As luck would have it, many of my medical ethics colleagues gather in June in Paris for an annual International Bioethics Retreat. Tomi Kushner organizes this retreat with a keen eye for controversial issues and a firm hand to keep things moving. Here, I benefited from a different kind of feedback. If the ICMM offers a military viewpoint, the International Retreat is decidedly, shall we say, more civilian. The clash of ideas has been stimulating.

Additionally, of course, are the many colleagues who offered their time to read through various chapters or supply data and comments as they developed. Some are longtime friends; others are those gracious enough to respond to an out-of-blue e-mail asking about their research. My sincere thanks to Y. Michael Barilan, Yitzhak Benbaji, David Bennahum, Elizabeth Bernthal, Matthew Borgman, Martin Bricknell, Alan Brockie, Nikki Coleman, Jacob Collen, Neta Crawford, Heather Draper, Sheena Eagan, Neil Eisenstein, Eric Elster, Cécile Fabre, Nizan Feldman, Sara Goldkind, Paul Gilbert, Randy Howe, George Lucas, Stephen Latham, Rain Liivoja, Kristina Lundberg, Jon Moreno, Ali Okhowat, James Pattison, Rees Porta, Todd Rasmussen, Rosamond Rhodes, David Rodin, and Daniel Statman. Finally, I am grateful to the *American Journal of Bioethics* and *The Journal of Royal Army Medical Corps* for permission to use portions of previously published articles in Chapters 5 and 8.

Abbreviations

AR	Army Regulation (US)
COIN	Counterinsurgency
CSH	Combat Support Hospital
DNR	Do Not Resuscitate
DoD	Department of Defense (US)
FDA	Food and Drug Administration (US)
FM	Field Manual (US)
FOB	Forward Operating Base
FST	Forward Surgical Team
ICRC	International Committee of the Red Cross
ICU	Intensive Care Unit
IED	Improvised Explosive Device
IRA	Irish Republican Army
ISAF	International Security Assistance Force
LRMC	Landstuhl Regional Medical Center (Germany)
MEDCAP	Medical Civic Action Program
MoD	Ministry of Defence (UK)
MoH	Ministry of Health
MRoE	Medical Rules of Eligibility (Engagement)
NHS	National Health Service (UK)
POW	Prisoner of War
PRT	Provincial Reconstruction Team
SIGAR	Special Inspector General for Afghanistan Reconstruction
SIGIR	Special Inspector General for Iraq Reconstruction
SSCI	Senate Select Committee on Intelligence of the CIA's Detention and Interrogation Program (US)
TBI	Traumatic Brain Injury
USAID	United States Agency for International Development
WHO	World Health Organization
WMA	World Medical Association

Introduction

In an age of Twitter brevity, Introductions are vital but dangerous. If they summarize the arguments too well, they might deter all but the most intrepid from reading on. If they don't summarize the argument well enough, even the intrepid may balk. The trick is to pique the reader's curiosity without giving away the show.

Let's start with this: Anyone searching "military medical ethics" in the decade or more following revelations of torture and abuse at Abu Ghraib prison in Iraq (2003–2004) will be overwhelmed by such harrowing titles as *A Stain on Medical Ethics* (Wilks, 2005); *Unspeakably Cruel* (Annas 2005); *Oath Betrayed* (Miles 2006); *Science in Dachau's Shadow* (McCoy 2007); *The Hippocratic Myth* (Bloch 2011); and *Ethics Abandoned* (Rubenstein & Thomson 2013). Comments such as "Military medicine has always remained on the borderline of ethics . . ." (Fox 2013: 275) or "The post-9/11 'war on terror' has deformed military medical ethics in the US" (Annas & Crosby 2019: 303) are not uncommon. The upshot is clear: Military medical ethics is hardly deserving of its name; it is ethics more honored in the breach than the observance.

This book repudiates that notion entirely. Medical ethics must certainly address things that must not be done and it should suffer rebuke when it does not. But Abu Ghraib and Guantanamo Bay are not the only provinces of moral inquiry. Military medical ethics also tackles a perplexing mix of things that must be done but may not, things that can be done but need not, and things that should be done but are not.

Things that Must be Done but May Not

Consider war injuries first—over three million American and international troops deployed to Iraq and Afghanistan since 2003. There, medical workers faced devastating multisystem injuries unencountered in any previous war. Improvised explosive devices (IEDs), not the gunshot wounds or booby traps of Vietnam, were the chief cause. Hemorrhage, exsanguination, and traumatic brain injury were the primary causes of death among the more than 8,500 Coalition soldiers who lost their lives. These numbers are low. And in a time where Americans and Europeans see pandemic deaths multiply into the tens and hundreds of thousands, the numbers of dead and injured warfighters in Iraq and Afghanistan risk becoming a footnote. But these numbers are low for a reason. Despite the ferocity of the fighting and the severity of the injuries, fewer service personnel died of wounds than during any other war in history. Dedicated, innovative medicine, speedy evacuation, body and vehicle armor, and technological development combined to conserve fighting strength and enhance mission success.

But isn't this claim tone deaf? Since when are force conservation and mission success the metrics of good medicine? What about lives saved or lost? Certainly, the devastation of war reached far beyond the relatively low casualties of allied forces. Many tens of thousands of contractors, local allies, police, enemy combatants, and civilians suffered violent death, injury, accident, and disease. These numbers are very far from low. Yet, military medical facilities are often the only provider as wars ramp up. Military planners do not look past what is required to attend to their own needs. Their perspective is not unusual. In war, medical resources are scarce by design, and local nationals clamoring for care may soon overwhelm the system. Here, then, is the first and most tenacious of ethical dilemmas: Who gets what, when, and where?

The challenge of allocating scarce resources is not new to medical ethics. For civilian or peacetime medical ethics, the "what" is medical attention, the "when" is as medical need dictates, and the "where" is in the facility best able to meet a patient's need. In military medical ethics, things immediately go awry precisely because force conservation and mission success are its metrics. Still, the answer starts the same. The "what" is medical attention, but the "when" is as *military* necessity dictates and the "where" can be an in-theater combat support hospital, a poorly equipped and understaffed Iraqi or Afghan facility, or, if you happen to wear the uniform of a Coalition soldier, a first-class hospital in Bethesda, Maryland; Landstuhl, Germany; or Birmingham, England. Military necessity usurps medical need as the fundamental criterion of allocating treatment in wartime. As a result, a patient's identity or affiliation rather than a patient's medical need determines the extent and kind of care he or she will receive.

A pediatrician deployed to a war zone tells me the following story. But before I continue, ask yourself this: Who takes pediatricians to war? Anyway, he winds up managing admissions in a combat support hospital. Every day, mothers mob the front gate hoping someone will care for their children. Some were caught in the crossfire; others were just sick and injured in the way kids are. Most are turned away; there is only room for military casualties. But one of the hospital staff asks: What about the kids *we* hurt? What about our "collateral" damage? Shouldn't we at least tend them? So the doctor asks: How many of you were hurt by our gunfire, missiles, or bombs? They all raise a hand. So a few get in, but not many. The rest, despondent, just leave. Telling the story back home, people wonder: What kind of pediatrician sends away sick children? "But we needed the beds for our own," comes the answer. "Our own?" comes the response. "Our own are grown men and women." Showing no patience for the bald demands of military necessity, civilian medicine embraces impartiality and vigorously repudiates any notion of treating the sick and wounded based on the uniform they do, or don't, wear. So he stops telling his story. People want to hear M*A*S*H, but it's not that at all.

Military medical ethics, then, has considerable work to do. Establishing the permissible criteria of *differential* medical care across patients who are combatants, detainees, and civilians is the subject of *Caring for the Wounded of War* (Part II).

Caring for the Wounded of War opens with a road map of military medicine during nearly two decades of post 9/11 warfare in Iraq and Afghanistan. In Chapter 4 and those following, these two conflicts provide much of this study's raw material. Here, we see how multinational forces, led by the United States and Great Britain, rapidly ended a conventional war against Taliban and Iraqi regular forces with medical assets to spare. In short order, however, a protracted insurgency soon engulfed Coalition forces. With less than 300 beds to service nearly 200,000 troops in Iraq, there is precious little for anyone else. Multinational forces receive the best care, detainees the second best, and local nationals the dregs. Complicating things further, scarce medical resources prove useful for other reasons. Highly prized, medical attention lends itself to gathering actionable intelligence and gaining, as the Swedes put it, "force protection." Pediatric care, in particular, delivers some of the most valuable information and the best force protection. Saving kids generates enormous goodwill and some handy side benefits too. A *quid pro quo*? Maybe. Something that must be done but may not be? Maybe not.

More Things that Must be Done but May Not; One that Can be Done but Need Not

Now, think about weaponizing medicine to serve the aims of war. This is the theme of Part III: *Medicine as a Weapon of War*. Civilian health care serves only the ends of medicine: saving lives and improving their quality. During armed conflict, medicine serves the ends of war: saving lives and improving their quality. They sound identical but are not. To save lives in peacetime, one must prevent death and cure. To save lives in war, one must pursue death and kill. Military medicine, no less than any other military means, serves war by ensuring warfighters are fit to kill.

There are many ways to kill in war and many ways for doctors to participate. The most obvious is their strenuous efforts to patch up wounded soldiers so they can fight another day. This duty requires some thought but is not overly disturbing unless troops run riot and kill gratuitously once they have recovered. But when troops do their job as they should, there is good reason to nurse them to health. When doctors, nurses, and medics fail, there is good reason to look for new ways to help. Medical experimentation is one answer. Although a staple of medical science, "experimentation" carries considerable baggage owing to Nazi and Japanese pseudoresearch that brutalized civilians and prisoners of war. In fits and starts since then, medical research has trod carefully in wartime. Perhaps too carefully, with the result of inhibiting lifesaving research on the battlefield (Chapter 8).

For all its challenges, healing remains the goal of experimentation. Sometimes, however, physicians experiment to help build bombs. Bomb building is less than therapeutic and prompted modest soul searching when the United States and Britain recruited medical doctors into their fledgling biological and chemical warfare (BCW) programs after World War II. But international laws put the brakes on BCW and most programs closed by 2000. In their place, some clinicians abandoned their therapeutic vocation to partner with military scientists to reinforce the human fighting machine with chemical, biological, and neurological enhancements. The moral context is not quite the same as weapons development but raises some compelling similarities. In each case, medicine serves war directly.

Lost in the debate is another crucial question: Does anyone need a neural interface implant? More generally, do enhanced warfighters meaningfully enhance warfighting? Many people think they do. Think of modern-day gladiators fortified by an exoskeleton and hard wired into a computer interface embedded in their brains, cyborg-like. Strong, ever alert, super decisive, and exceptionally lethal, they're the perfect Special Forces operative. Right? Not really. Most gladiators went the way of Spartacus. To get their job done, what Special Forces really need today is quick language acquisition. Enhancement can help, but it is not sexy. The sexy stuff is often a complicated and sometimes dangerous medical procedure we can do but may not need. A more thorough answer to these questions occupies Chapter 9.

Nonlethal, but no less benign, weaponization finds its mark in medical diplomacy. Successful diplomacy is to convince others of one's purpose. Diplomacy is a vital wartime enterprise when civilian loyalties are torn between insurgents and government forces. What better way to bring civilians over than to offer them timely and sophisticated medical care? Intuitively, this sounds like mercenary medicine, something that medical ethics should forbid. Trading favors for medical attention is corrupt. And, in peacetime, it may be. But in wartime, one asks different questions: Can medical diplomacy get the job done, offer greater military benefits than costs, and avoid egregiously violating anyone's fundamental human right to health care? For the answer, see Chapter 10.

Things that Should be Done but Are Not

War fatigue plagues every conflict. Countries run out of men, materiel, money, ideological fervor, and patience. They just want to go home. When they do, postwar justice suffers. The first thing victorious armies neglect is their obligation to rebuild a war-torn nation's essential infrastructures. Chief among them is health care. Attention falls aside because postwar reconstruction is not a constant duty. These duties occupy Part IV: *Postwar Justice and the Responsibility to Rebuild*. Typically, a victorious defensive army has no obligation to rebuild the nations it traverses and tramples. But humanitarian armies do. Defensive armies go to war to protect their compatriots while humanitarian armies go to war to protect others. So it would be exceptionally counterproductive for humanitarians to leave for home before their job is finished. But the cost is high, so high that everyone looks for a way out (Chapter 11).

Finding the way out of foreign entanglements does not offer a way out of domestic entanglements. What do we do with all those veterans who fill Chapter 12? They did their duty but, then, they do not always reintegrate well. Others are just sick, injured, or otherwise damaged. Still, others fall into poverty, suicide, divorce, and alcoholism. How a nation treats its veterans is the final reckoning of war. Often, the solution is to forget them once the bands die down and the confetti is swept away. As veterans, too, are swept aside, postwar justice fails at home as badly as it fails abroad. These things should not be done. But the cost of postwar justice is enormous, so much so that the inability to allocate sufficient funds for postwar reconstruction and veteran care *before* commencing war may proscribe war from the get-go. The projected cost of veteran health care and disability payments in the United States exceeds $700,000,000,000. Add to that the many billions of reconstruction, and pretty soon you're talking real money.

What about Theory?

Books about theory and practice, like this one, begin with theory even though some people skip these sections. I end here with some remarks about theory to disabuse readers of that temptation. Applied ethics is dynamic. Moral discourse works from ethical principles to medical practice and back again. *Back again* is to think more carefully and, when necessary, amend or abandon first principles. The back again peeps out of each chapter and settles in the conclusion of this book. Part I, *Theoretical Foundations,* digs into the principles of military medical ethics and just war that frame this book. Chapters 1 and 2 spotlight the moral terms and ethical principles used throughout this book as they pertain to the rights and duties that military and medical ethics accord soldiers, civilians, detainees, and patients. But not all the theory chapters are theoretical. Chapter 3 is a how-to chapter and explains how to implement the principles of military medical ethics and to disentangle its conundrums and dilemmas. The upshot of these three chapters is to place military medical ethics squarely in the ambit of just war.

As a weapon of war, military medicine enjoys no forbearance unless the war it supports is just. To prosecute a just war, one must kill permissibly. Now we are beginning to see how radically military medical ethics differs from civilian medical ethics and how intimately military medical ethics is tied to the conduct of war. Absent just war, military medicine loses its ethical moorings. Absent morally informed medical practice, just war is similarly cast adrift. Military medical ethics, then, is not just about repudiating torture and vivisection. Rather, military medical ethics is about ensuring fair and equitable treatment when resources are scarce, maintaining mission readiness while respecting every patient's rights, weaponizing medicine while preserving its therapeutic function, and, ultimately, saving lives so others may take them.

Crossing and combining military and medical disciplines to address these questions, some of the accompanying terms may be unfamiliar to single-minded readers of medical or military ethics (spoiler alert!). *Associative duties*, for example, refer to special obligations of care that friends, family, and, as I will argue, soldiers owe one another. The distinction between *impartiality* and *neutrality* may be fuzzy for some. I try to clarify each before I torpedo both. Readers of medical ethics may be less than familiar with some basic principles of just war and international humanitarian law (IHL). These include the principles of *necessity* (adopting the least harmful means to accomplish a mission expeditiously), *distinction* (the obligation to distinguish among military and civilian targets), *proportionality* (the duty to avoid excessive civilian casualties), and *collateral harm* (unintentional, incidental civilian death or injury).

Other concepts are unique constructions. These include *military-medical necessity* and *broad beneficence*. Each is similar but not identical to its roots. *Military-medical necessity* refers to the medical means required to achieve military goals. *Broad beneficence* invokes the collective good, that is, the best interests of an entire political commonwealth. In contrast, narrow beneficence turns on an individual patient's best interest.

If Part I integrates military medical ethics and the principles of just war, it does not mean that I think the wars in Iraq and Afghanistan are necessarily just. Just wars are either defensive or humanitarian. A defensive war turns against an aggressor who invades, subjugates, or plunders a peace-loving nation. Germany's invasion of Poland in 1939 is the classic example, but most others offer less certitude. Who defended and who invaded in the Falklands/Malvinas (1982), Iraq–Iran (1980), or Israel–Lebanon (2006)? A humanitarian war confronts a regime that brutalizes its people who, in one form or another, invite foreign forces to rescue them. Humanitarian wars and the accompanying responsibility-to-protect and responsibility-to-rebuild are new phenomena. Examples are sparse, effective interventions more so. NATO's demolition of the Kaddafi regime in Libya (2011), and United Nations and African Union troop deployments to save Darfur (2007) are two examples. The best example is probably the one that wasn't: Western intervention in Syria (2011 ongoing). Whether defensive or humanitarian, each archetype of war provides the context for the theory and practice of military medical ethics.

A Brief Methodological Note

Before moving on, a brief methodological note is appropriate. I noted that Chapter 3 explains how applied ethics confronts theoretical ethical principles with real-life military medical practice. Each chapter is an exercise in applied ethics. The normative principles outlined in Chapters 1 and 2 draw from moral philosophy and international law. The practice of military medicine that occupies the rest of the book emerges from varied and voluminous literature by doctors, nurses, lawyers, military commanders, politicians, and policymakers since the turn of the 21st century.

During recent wars, healthcare professionals and scientists published substantial research, surveys, clinical guidelines, and case studies in military and nonmilitary medical journals that engaged the fundamental question of medical care in an austere environment. An overview of this publication activity appears in Chapter 8. The United States, Britain, NATO, and the defense departments of other multinational forces circulated handbooks, policy papers, legal opinions, and lessons-learned reports about military and health doctrine, strategy, equipment, and protocols across their services. Special Inspectors General for Iraq and Afghanistan Reconstruction audited Coalition operations regularly since the early years of these wars. International organizations were equally energetic. The United Nations, World Health Organization, International Committee of the Red Cross, and numerous health and human rights nongovernmental organizations (NGOs) did their best to keep an eye on belligerents and offer guidance and reproach as needed.

The result is a panoply of independent actors, sometimes cooperating and other times working at odds with, or ignorant of, one another. The data are not always consistent. Agencies report their findings in different ways, and the numbers do not always reconcile. Later versions of military and field manuals replace the earlier editions, leaving guidelines of the war years to sometimes vanish into irretrievable archives. Rarely did anyone engage their moral qualms directly. But the material for ethical discourse is there if you look closely.

Despite the range of sources enlivening the following chapters, this book is neither an empirical nor exhaustive study of military medicine or just war since 2000. Rather, this book uses the data that military, governmental, and nongovernmental sources supply to exemplify medical practice, illustrates the shortcomings and strengths of military medical ethics, and suggests modest resolutions as necessary. Before beginning in earnest, one more story.

During World War II, doctors bandage up a soldier named Yossarian to masquerade as another who recently died of his wounds. It's a gesture to the family coming a long way to see their dying son. After a few Helleresque interlocutories, a brother wants to know:

"Did you have a priest?"

"Yes," Yossarian lied, wincing again.

"That's good," the brother decided. "Just as long as you're getting everything you've got coming to you. We came all the way from New York. We were afraid we wouldn't get here in time."

"In time for what?"

"In time to see you before you died."

"What difference would it make?"

"We didn't want you to die by yourself."

"What difference would it make?" (Heller 1955: 177)

In real life, insurgents ambush a French military convoy in Afghanistan. Fighting off gunfire, the French squad weaves a ring around two catastrophically burned soldiers to afford the medic room to work. Medical attention is futile; the wounded men have no chance of survival. Nevertheless, the medic depletes his stock of medicinals, leaving precious little if attacked again. But their goal is closely focused: to send the two soldiers home before they die. What difference would it make?

Indeed.

PART I
THEORETICAL FOUNDATIONS

1

Military Medical Ethics and Just War

Haphazard throughout much of history, sound wartime medical management, and with it, military medical ethics is a recent phenomenon. The Geneva Conventions first introduced the term *medical ethics* into the law of armed conflict in 1977:

> Persons engaged in medical activities shall not be compelled to perform acts or to carry out work contrary to the rules of medical ethics or to other medical rules designed for the benefit of the wounded and sick. (ICRC 1977a: Art 16 (2); 1977b: Art. 10)

"What is the essential maxim of these principles [of medical ethics]?" ask the commentators. The answer is terse:

> It is never to act in conflict with the wounded person's interests, to help him to the fullest extent of the means available, whoever he is (principle of non-discrimination), to be discreet regarding his condition and never to abuse his sense of dependence on the person administering care, particularly not with a view to gaining an advantage from him (ICRC 1987: §658).

There is nothing in this maxim or international law more generally to suggest that war appreciably alters the principles of medical ethics. The World Medical Association (WMA) follows suit. Emphasizing respect for dignity, confidentiality, impartial treatment, and the duty to treat any sick or injured person solely according to medical need and the urgency of care, the WMA (2017) declares: "medical ethics in times of armed conflict is identical to medical ethics in times of peace."

The *practice* of military medicine, however, puts paid to such a hasty conclusion. Consider impartiality on the battlefield. Antedating the WMA declaration, the First Geneva Convention (ICRC 1949a: Art. 12) instructs belligerents to provide medical treatment "without any adverse distinction founded on sex, race, nationality, religion or any other similar criteria" and declares "... Only urgent medical reasons will authorize priority in the order of treatment to be administered." Faced with scarce resources and the overwhelming need to minister to compatriot troops, military organizations struggle to implement this directive. The US Army Medical Department (AMEDD) *Emergency War Surgery* (2018), for example, reminds personnel: "the ultimate goals of combat medicine are the return of the greatest possible number of warfighters to combat and the preservation of life, limb, and eyesight ... Commitment of resources should be decided *first* based on the mission and immediate tactical situation *and then* by medical necessity, irrespective of a casualty's national or combatant status" (Cubano 2018: 24, emphasis added; also JP 4-02 2001: II-1; 2006:ix).

Do guidelines backtrack or not? In practice, military necessity, not medical necessity, often prevails. In contrast to peacetime, civilian medical ethics, military medical ethics infringes on soldiers' rights to refuse medical treatment, sets aside impartiality to attend to compatriots first, medically enhances warfighters when there are no therapeutic benefits, and utilizes medicine to gain civilian support. Medical ethics in war is not identical to medical ethics in peace.

Military medical ethics embraces the ethical principles that govern the provision of military medicine in times of war, on the battlefield and off. During armed conflict and on the battlefield, medical staff treats warfighters, detainees, local civilians, and host-nation allies. Off the battlefield, medicine is a weapon of war as practitioners and policymakers experiment with new technology and politicize medical care to win the support of the local population. Postwar, states rebuild war-torn nations while healing the accumulated mental and physical injuries of veterans.

In contrast, *civilian medical ethics* governs the provision of care by non-military medical organizations, whether state or private, to a nation's civilian population at home. Civilian medical ethics is largely apolitical. The doctor-patient relationship and the duties to "do no harm" and respect autonomy do not require a political relationship. Military medical ethics, on the other hand, is heavily invested in politics and war. Without wars or the standing armies that feed them, there is no military medicine. One cannot justify the practices of medicine during war without justifying killing in war.

Permissible killing marks war off from any other human endeavor, and it places inordinate weight on the means required to kill (or, more accurately, "disable") enemies effectively. This is the principle of military necessity, and it dominates every ethical dilemma in wartime, whether medical or military.

Military medical ethicists spend inordinate time confounded by dual loyalty: Are military surgeons officers first or doctors first? Do they serve the mission or the patient? Does military necessity trump medical necessity? This is not a narrow question for medical ethics but part of a much larger puzzle that pits national sovereignty against human rights. It is not a problem of medicine; it is the problem of war. Killing violates the most basic human right. Justify killing in war, and you defuse the alleged antagonism between military and medical ethics that plagues many discussions of military medical ethics today.

Paramount concern for the ethics of war was apparent to physicians early on. According to legend, the king of Persia, Artaxerxes I, asked Hippocrates to cure his soldiers of the plague. Hippocrates refused, telling the supplicants, "Honor will not permit me to succor the enemies of Greece." Victor Sidel and Barry Levy (2003: 294) use the parable to make a point about dual loyalty, describing how it "illustrates the tension between dedication by a physician to patriotism . . . and the dedication to medical ethics." But does it? Hippocrates offered the fledgling practice of medicine the nobility of profession and firm guiding principles that resonate to this day. But Hippocrates also knew something of war. Born in 460 BC and only 20 years after Xerxes nearly subjugated Greece, Hippocrates understood the Persian threat intimately. There is no tension, conflict, or dual loyalty here. He simply would not succor his enemies. With this judgment, Hippocrates readily discerned that medical ethics does not exist alongside military ethics or patriotism but is subsumed by war and transformed into "military medical ethics" in the process.

As the subsequent discussions demonstrate, military medical ethics differs markedly from its civilian counterpart. Military medical ethics is a political phenomenon, unintelligible apart from military ethics and just war theory. As a result, its theory and practice differ from civilian medical ethics. With this distinction in mind, the central question is, "What is morally permissible military medical practice?" To answer, this chapter outlines two central principles mostly absent from civilian medical ethics: military-medical necessity and broad beneficence.

War, Just War, and Military Medical Ethics

Entering what may be uncharted waters for medical ethicists, the foundations of military medical ethics lie not only in the well-known principles of biomedical ethics such as respect for patient autonomy or nonmaleficence (do no harm), but in two fundamental norms of international politics: national sovereignty and human rights. National sovereignty and human rights lay the ground for defensive and humanitarian wars, respectively. Despite their disparate genesis, each type of war demands the same rules of fighting (*jus in bello*): proportionality, utility, distinction, noncombatant immunity, and humane treatment. In this context, two fundamental principles of military medicine follow: military-medical necessity and broad beneficence.

The Nature of National Sovereignty

National sovereignty reflects the ascendant value of the territorial nation-state as the optimal vehicle for developing human capabilities and unpacks to include the principles of collective self-determination and national security. Political communities are at the core of the modern nation-state. More than the aggregation of individual interests, the political community embraces what Michael Walzer (1970: 92) calls, "our common life": the ethnic, cultural, linguistic, national, religious, and people-specific norms, ideals, and beliefs that we hope will endure across generations and leave a mark on the world. There is no human life outside the political community and, for the most part, no political community outside the nation-state.

Modern notions of sovereignty emerged following the cataclysmic events of the Thirty Years War. They afforded a political framework to regulate the early modern international order of territorial monarchies and upstart revolutionary states. Sovereignty provided states and kingdoms with the moral status and authority necessary to mobilize their people and resources for industrialization, urbanization, and economic development. To safeguard national sovereignty, international law slowly codified laws of armed conflict—first in the 1899 and 1907 Hague Conventions and later in the Geneva and related conventions. These are the laws of defensive war wherein the right of self-defense, a fundamental feature of state sovereignty, remains tightly constrained by human rights nonetheless.

Conceptually, human rights antedate the state and political community. The United Nations Universal Declaration of Human Rights, for example, confers individuals with moral and legal standing by virtue of their humanity. Digging deeper, contract theory delineates a compendium of rights that political authorities must respect to gain free peoples' consent. Visions vary. Whether to gain security (Hobbes), efficient management (Locke), or a well-ordered, rights-protecting commonwealth (Rawls), individuals willingly give up their absolute freedom insofar as the state safeguards freedom, liberty, autonomy, and self-determination. History, however, is messier than the theory that tries to schematize it. Human history knows of no primordial state of nature or prepolitical "original position" comprising autonomous, self-legislating individuals. Instead, norms develop as human society does. In time, emerging perceptions of nationhood and the Enlightenment's underlying individualism charged the modern state with protecting the welfare of the people under its jurisdiction. In this way, norms of sovereignty and human rights reinforce one another. To secure their hallowed place in the international community, many nations, even authoritarian regimes, understand how they must proclaim respect for human rights (Katzenstein 1996a; Reus-Smit 2001).

The Nature of Human Rights

Human rights coalesce around a dignified life that delivers more than subsistence and satisfies more than basic needs. A dignified life is characterized by a level of self-worth, fulfillment, and, in Hugo Bedau's (1969: 567) elegant words, "the opportunity for the release of productive energy." Such opportunities allow people and their communities to exercise self-determination and to formulate, pursue, and realize a life plan that develops their intellectual, physical, emotional, and social capabilities (Alkire 2002 for review; Nussbaum 2007; Sen 2000, 2005). A dignified life is active and participatory; it is not only about attaining capabilities but *using* them to push at the limits of oneself and one's community. To reach its goals, a dignified life requires human rights to protect individuals from murder, rape, servitude, torture, and cruelty. Human rights embrace material rights to forestall crushing poverty, illness, and ignorance; cultural rights to preserve a people's community and heritage; and civil rights that safeguard personal autonomy through political representation, employment opportunities, property ownership, freedom of press and assembly, and so forth.

Following World War II, an uneasy tension emerged between sovereignty and human rights. Just as World War I did, World War II and its aftermath reinforced the norm of sovereignty, collective security, and national self-determination. But Nazi atrocities and the wholesale slaughter of civilians also turned the world's attention to human rights. The victorious allies fought to protect their populations *and* their civilized, liberal way of life. Norms of sovereignty infused the UN Charter while the 1949 Geneva Conventions and 1977 Additional Protocols I and II protected human rights during armed conflict by codifying international humanitarian law (IHL) (ICRC 1949a; 1949b; 1977a; 1977b).

Human rights translate into claims against the state when any people or persons face grievous harm at its hands. In defensive wars, human rights protect belligerents and civilians. More recently, the international community recognized its responsibility to protect those beyond one's parochial political community. The 2005 Responsibility to Protect (R2P) doctrine permits the international community to deploy armed force against sovereign nations perpetrating systematic murder, rape, plunder, forced population transfer, and ethnic cleansing against their citizens (World Summit 2005: §138-140). When diplomatic or economic measures fail to remedy human rights abuses abroad, victims turn to the world community to demand humanitarian war on their behalf. Today, the international community repudiates aggressive wars of conquest but recognizes two kinds of just war: defensive war and humanitarian war. The first draws on *self*-defense, the latter on *other*-defense.

Defensive wars preserve the vital interests of the commonwealth and the peace of the international community of which each nation is part. Sometimes, as in World War II, the threat is existential. Often, commonwealths face lesser threats: territorial infringement (Falklands/ Malvinas War), theft of resources (First Gulf War), terrorism (Global War on Terror), civil war (Sri Lanka), or occupation (Palestine, Eritrea). While broad national security interests drive defensive wars, grave human rights violations alone justify armed humanitarian intervention. Sovereignty, security, and human and civil rights vie during defensive war, leaving democratic polities to seek balance and compromise when catastrophe threatens the political community. In a humanitarian war, on the other hand, the defense of fundamental human rights replaces national self-defense as its just cause. If defensive wars prize national sovereignty, humanitarian wars ride roughshod over states' rights to rescue a brutalized people from grievous abuse.

The intricacies of defensive and humanitarian war reflect a tension between collective and individual rights, sovereign and human rights, reason-of-state, and cosmopolitan values. Thus, what military medical ethics sometimes characterizes as competing or "dual" loyalties that compel one to choose between the military mission and broader norms of conduct, more accurately reflect friction built into the nature of armed conflict. At stake is not loyalty, but the relative value of collective and individual interests hit hard by the exigencies of war.

Military medical ethics is, therefore, incoherent without the broader envelope of just war theory, international humanitarian law, and their subsidiary principles of military necessity, proportionality, distinction, and noncombatant immunity. These principles afford the normative framework for military medical ethics and the unique principles that guide it. Military medical ethics is not a fusion of military ethics and medical ethics but a discipline in its own right. During war, the norm of permissible killing colors every military action, including the practice of medicine.

Military Medical Ethics and the Ethics of Just War

Military medicine conserves and enhances a fighting force. Maintaining fighting strength entails unit readiness (JP 4-02 2006: xi; also, NATO 2019 AJP-4.10: LEX-5). For this purpose, two measures assess quantity and quality:

> *Personnel*: The number and type of required personnel available to the unit for the execution of the wartime or primary mission.
> *Training*: The commander's assessment of the unit's training proficiency on mission-essential tasks (AR 220-1 2007: 1-1b(2); 4.1; 7.1(a)).

Medical care is crucially important to maintain sufficient numbers of personnel to execute military missions. In this way, military medicine is therapeutic and curative. And while these are the traditional roles of medicine, military medicine preserves patient health to maintain unit readiness. Properly maintained, the fighting force kills. The first rule of military medical ethics then is: *conserve a fighting force to kill justly*. "Killing justly" means to kill in a war that is just and in a manner that is just.

In principle, defensive and humanitarian wars are just when they defend one's own people or nation, or another's, against aggression. "Aggression" signifies rights-violating conduct. An aggressor violates a country or people's rights by significantly threatening their political community. Invading deep into another nation's territory by armed force, imposing a strangling blockade, or employing terrorism to viciously deny a people self-determination and a dignified life are common examples. Absent successful attempts to rectify rights-violating behavior by other means, each violation permits recourse to armed force.

Assigning just cause, however, can be exceptionally complex. Some cases seem clear: Poland's defensive war against Nazi Germany and Algeria's war of independence against France are two examples. But many cases are far less clear. Consider, for example, the Falklands/Malvinas conflict, American intervention in Somalia, UN intervention in Sudan, and the many national struggles in places like Israel/Palestine, Turkey/Kurdistan, East Timor, South Sudan, Northern Ireland, or Tibet that have rattled the world for the last half-century and more. Wars of national liberation are often posters for just war, but not every aggrieved people requires statehood to lead a dignified life. When autonomy satisfies self-determination, the cause for just war disappears (Gross 2015: 21–36).

Determining just war is not only about identifying a just cause but demands convincing answers to related questions about alternatives to armed force, the probability of success, the costs and benefits of war, and the prospect of postwar reconstruction. Reconstruction is particularly important when alleviating the plight of another people is the sole justification for war. A humanitarian war must look to the future of the people it hopes to save. Saving a people is a long-term, exorbitantly expensive project that a nation must understand before it goes to war.

Answering some of these questions about the recent wars in Iraq and Afghanistan helps portray the idea of just war. These wars were both defensive and humanitarian, first to protect the political communities of the Coalition nations against weapons of mass destruction (WMDs) and global terror, and then to save the Iraqi and Afghan people from ruthless regimes. Despite the dubious claims about WMDs, fighting terrorism and protecting human rights are admirable goals of war. But was success feasible? Were the costs reasonable? At one point, perhaps, but later events proved otherwise. Twenty years on, the war on terror has done little to reduce terrorism, and human rights in that part of the world are not much improved. On the contrary, the rise of ISIS, the genocidal war in Syria, the mass migration of refugees to Europe, and the growing strength of Western political populism find their roots in the prolonged war in Iraq and Afghanistan. But these events were not immediately foreseeable, and despite the deliberate dissemination of misinformation about WMDs, it would be difficult to judge the decision to go to war as entirely unjust or misguided.

Alternatively, none of this may be true. The lies about WMDs did not just skew the public debate but undermined it fatally. The US and British governments erred grievously by failing to recognize the interminable cost and ultimate futility of trying to wage and win a counterinsurgency. Enhanced interrogation indelibly stained any attempt to paint the Coalition as the guarantor of human rights. Reconstruction has stalled, leaving Iraq and Afghanistan little better off, if at all. Stalemate should not have surprised anyone; the writing was on the wall for a long time. Not only was each war unjustified, it also brought horrors and hardship that condemn its injustice in the strongest terms.

This brief exposition exemplifies some of the difficulties of clearly identifying aggression to classify war as just or unjust. So rather than formulate the first rule of military medical ethics to *conserve a fighting force to kill justly*, it is more useful to reformulate the rule to *conserve a fighting force that does not kill unjustly*. More specifically: *does not kill in a manifestly unjust way*. This formulation turns the inquiry around. Rather than look for wars that are just, it is only necessary to identify wars that are not manifestly unjust to satisfy the demands of just war.

Manifestly Unjust War

Obeying a superior order does not relieve a subordinate of criminal responsibility if the subordinate knew that the act ordered was unlawful or should have known because of the manifestly unlawful nature of the act ordered (ICRC 2020: Rule 155).

Emphasizing a positive duty, American practice obligates service members to follow superior orders unless they demand the performance of a military duty that "a person of ordinary sense and understanding would know to be illegal" (ICRC 2020: Rule 155, USA Practice). Concise definitions of "know to be illegal" are elusive. An Israeli military court underscores how a "black flag flies over a manifestly unlawful order as a warning sign" and how "the unlawfulness of the order . . . is *absolutely certain* to anyone looking at the order." "Its illegality pierces the eyes and revolts the heart," declared the presiding judge (IDF 1958: 92, §9). *Manifest*, these citations suggest, means obvious, plainly apparent, or self-evident. But despite the prevalent reference to *unlawfulness*, manifest illegality is a fusion of legal and moral injunctions synonymous with injustice. On the one hand, a manifestly unlawful order violates a public statute. On the other hand, the same order also "stands in evident contradiction to all human morality," is "contrary to the highest ethical principles," or "outrages fundamental concepts of justice . . . accepted by civilized nations generally" (Green 1985: 268–269). Moral proscriptions weigh heavily.

Wars then are generally just unless they violate fundamental moral principles. A war to exterminate or subjugate another people is one example. Another is a kleptocratic war of personal enrichment at the expense of one's people or another's. These wars egregiously violate universal human rights and the abiding rights of a political community. Understanding just wars as those not manifestly unjust leaves medical personnel to tend the sick and injured in most conflicts but cannot warrant medical care for those who take part in manifestly unjust wars. This conclusion is unsettling, perhaps, because any reservation, even manifest injustice, rankles against the duty of medical professionals to treat any wounded person, anywhere. But it is not entirely counterintuitive or morally misplaced: no one, whether a medical professional or layperson, should contribute to a manifestly unjust war in any way, much less maintain its fighting strength. This caveat, however, does deny medical attention to captured unjust belligerents or criminals. No longer a threat, detainees and prisoners of war enjoy the same rights as any noncombatant (Chapter 6).

The principle of manifest injustice sets the bar for permissible combat relatively low. Many wars are not manifestly unjust. Some conflicts adhere clearly to defensive and humanitarian aims. But others are muddied. When reasonable ambiguity obscures the designs of war, ethics must weigh conduct more than cause. Apart from repudiating wars of noxious aims, "not killing unjustly" also means to fight well. Perhaps Germany fought chivalrously in North Africa, but its objectives were odious. Perhaps Russia had good cause to subdue Chechnya, but its conduct was often detestable. Fighting well shifts the focus from ends to means. Regardless of how one settles the question of just cause, assuming one can, each side must fight justly. Attentive to the ways of war, military ethics confers moral equality on each belligerent, whether friend or foe. Every soldier who fights by the rules merits respect. What, then, are the relevant rules of war that infuse military medical ethics?

Jus in Bello: The Rules of Just War

Two rules govern permissible killing in war:

1. Combatants may kill one another but not cause superfluous injury and unnecessary suffering.
2. Combatants may **not** kill noncombatants (a) directly or (b) disproportionately.

The first rule turns on the threat an enemy combatant poses to individual soldiers, their army, or political community. Self-defense only permits the force necessary to remove this threat. For this reason, international instruments speak of "disabling" rather than killing enemy soldiers. Of course, killing is to disable someone permanently. Yet, there are no rules that require soldiers, unlike law enforcement officers, to use minimal force or to kill fewer rather than greater numbers of enemy soldiers. Combatants do not enjoy the forbearance accorded criminal suspects whose liability to harm remains unproven. Uniformed soldiers and irregular combatants are instantly liable to deadly attack. To slaughter them in droves rarely moves the moral compass. Nevertheless, individual soldiers retain certain rights even in the crosshairs. Torture is a gross affront to their dignity, while unspeakable suffering, such as that associated with biological or chemical weapons, goes beyond disabling or death to no purpose. But, the rules are few.

The second rule about civilians has two parts. The first (a) prohibits direct harm and is the bedrock of just war and noncombatant immunity. Noncombatants pose no threat and have, therefore, not forfeited their right to life. They, and their property, enjoy protection from direct harm and destruction. Noncombatant immunity enforces the principle of distinction that requires military organizations to distinguish between military and civilian targets. Despite the firm prohibition of killing civilians, the second part of Rule 2, proportionality, carves out an exception that ignores a civilian's innocence, blurs the imperative of distinction, and turns to military necessity. This exception is the principle of collateral harm. While purposely killing noncombatants *violates* their right to life, collaterally killing noncombatants *infringes* on their right to life when significant military advantages outweigh civilian fatalities. In this case, "infringing a right" means to set it aside for a greater good. "Necessary" entails that no less harmful means are available to attain military aims. "Military advantage" is exceptionally elastic and can mean saving compatriot lives, taking enemy lives, seizing territory, or destroying war materiel. Against military advantage, civilian deaths are permissible if they are incidental, necessary, and proportionate.

The underlying moral principle is the doctrine of double effect (DDE). Medical ethics sometimes invokes the DDE to justify passive or active euthanasia, but it originated with medieval scholars' attempt to justify killing the innocent in war. The logic is the same: (1) The act itself (attacking a military target or treating severe pain) must be morally good; (2) the agent may not positively will the bad effect (the death of a noncombatant or a patient) but may permit it; (3) the beneficial outcome (military or medical advantage) cannot come from the second, bad effect (killing civilians) but must come from the first effect (destroying a military target); (4) the good effect must be sufficiently desirable to compensate for the bad effect (Boyle 1980; McIntyre 2019). Under these conditions, the DDE is exculpatory and justifies the harm accompanying the second effect. The key lies in intention and the contentious argument that unintended bad effects are justifiable if the injurer fulfills the other DDE conditions.

Incidental harm is not unintended harm. One cannot say that bomber pilots do not mean or intend to kill civilians when they strike a military target in their midst. They do so knowingly and willingly. Instead, collateral harm is the necessary and foreseen consequence of an essential military operation. It is incidental because the deaths of noncombatants confer no military benefit. Harm to civilians that offers some benefit, deterrence, or demoralization, for example, is no longer collateral. It is, instead, direct harm and impermissible. Proportionality further restrains incidental harm by designating some undefined limit beyond which civilian casualties are excessive (ICRC 1977a: 51§5b). While the principle of proportionality hopes to limit civilian casualties, it faces the formidable task of assessing military advantage before an assault, comparing civilian deaths to military benefits, and determining when the former are excessive. Except in the rare and obvious case, such as destroying an entire village to disable a single soldier (ICRC 1987: §2213), the principle of proportionality is rarely useful in practice. Instead, closer attention to avoiding unnecessary harm and futile missions affords a better prospect of protecting civilians (Gross 2008a).

Combatants and Noncombatants

The rules of warfighting require clear definitions of combatant and non-combatant but they are elusive. Ordinarily, civilians or more generally "noncombatants" include anyone who is not a combatant. Noncombatants comprise prisoners of war (POWs), as well as sick and wounded soldiers and civilians. Civilians are a subset of noncombatants and include those who do not bear arms and do not belong to any state or nonstate military organization. Medical and religious personnel also enjoy noncombatant immunity. But theirs is of a different sort than other noncombatants. Civilians, POWs, and the wounded enjoy immunity because they pose no threat and, thereby, have not lost their right to life. Conversely, medical staff, like clerics, play an integral role in war but are among those whom the warring sides find it advantageous to immunize from harm. I return to this point in the following chapter.

In contemporary warfare, guerrillas, insurgents, and "participating" civilians muddy a once-firm definition of combatant. Before and during the two World Wars, combatants comprised those openly carrying their arms, wearing a uniform or insignia, and fighting in the service of a state military organization that observes the law of armed conflict (Hague Convention 1907, Annex, Article 1). The law's purpose was to deny combatant privileges to armed criminals, pirates, and insurgents. By 1977, however, irregular soldiers clad only in mufti, but fighting wars of national liberation against colonial regimes, gained combatant status (ICRC 1977a: Art. 44). No longer criminals, guerrillas enjoy POW status on capture, humane treatment, and speedy repatriation at the end of hostilities. Also joining the fray, participating civilians assumed a significant role by providing insurgents with intelligence and other logistical, financial, diplomatic, and technological aid (Gross 2015: 68–71). Their prominent role led the ICRC to propose rules governing the liability of civilians taking active roles in war (Melzer 2009). In practice, US-led forces in Iraq and Afghanistan would target what were hitherto civilian assets: "economic objects of the enemy that indirectly but effectively support and sustain the enemy's warfighting capability" (NWP 1-14M 2007: 8.2.5) and "al Qaeda leaders responsible for propaganda, recruitment, [and] religious affairs" (Bush 2010: 218). The result was a great deal of confusion on the battlefield. Armed persons might be legal combatants, unlawful combatants, criminals, and/or gun-toting farmers. The unarmed may be innocent civilians or civilians in the service of a guerrilla organization.

Table 1.1 describes how each of these actors enjoys disparate military and medical rights during war.

Table 1.1. Battlefield Actors in Contemporary Armed Conflict: Military and Medical Rights

1 Actor	2 Definition	3 Example	4 Belligerent Status	5 Liable to Attack	6 Medical Rights of a . . .
Civilian Noncombatant	Civilian	Civilian population of Iraq and Afghanistan	Not applicable	No	Local national
Humanitarian Force Combatant	Uniformed service member of a humanitarian military force	International Security Assistance Force (ISAF) in Afghanistan (Coalition Forces)	Yes	Killing	Multinational soldier
Host-Nation Combatant	Uniformed service member of a host-nation-state army	Iraqi Security Forces (ISF) Afghan National Security Forces (ANSF)	Yes	Killing	Local national
Lawful Guerrilla Combatant	Armed fighter, in or out of uniform, serving in a recognized national liberation organization	Taliban fighter after 2009[1]	Yes	Killing	Military detainee
Unlawful Guerrilla Combatant	Member of an unrecognized armed group	Taliban before 2009	No	Killing	Military detainee
Participating Civilian	Provides war support to insurgents	Political wing of guerrilla organization	No	Disabling	Local national
Criminal	Violates domestic law	Drug dealers	No	Killing or Disabling	Local national

[1]By 2009, US Code, Title 10, §948a dropped the Taliban from its list of unlawful combatants.

Columns 1 through 3 of Table 1.1 label, define, and exemplify contemporary battlefield actors: civilian noncombatants, combatants, guerrillas, unlawful combatants, participating civilians, and ordinary criminals. Regular combatants (ISAF, multinational forces, Afghan and Iraqi security personnel) and guerrilla soldiers are lawful combatants who qualify for belligerent status (Column 4), including POW status upon capture and repatriation at war's end. Unlawful combatants (such as the Taliban prior to 2009), participating civilians, and ordinary criminals do not qualify. They will stand trial for criminal activity. Liability to attack (Column 5) falls on any actor posing a military threat. When individuals threaten the life, limb, or property of others, they lose their right not to be harmed or killed when their victims defend themselves. At that point, combatants, guerillas, unlawful combatants, and armed criminals are liable to lethal attack or *defensive killing*. Participating civilians and unarmed criminals who do not pose a deadly threat but endanger others nonetheless are liable to less-than-lethal *defensive disabling*.

Once injured in the course of killing or disabling, each actor's right to medical attention (Column 6) varies with his or her status. In Iraq and Afghanistan, for example, multinational forces delivered care to Coalition soldiers, the Iraqi and Afghan security forces who fought at their side (host-nation allies), local nationals, and military detainees. As I describe more thoroughly in Chapter 4, various types of facilities managed medical care. Combat support hospitals provided in-theater care, while advanced medical facilities in Europe and the United States treated the critically injured. As a rule, multinational forces enjoyed prompt in-theater care and evacuation as necessary. Detainees could receive emergency and continuing care at Coalition facilities in Iraq and Afghanistan, but not abroad. Host-nation allies could receive short-term emergency care from multinational forces but had to turn to underequipped and poorly funded indigenous medical facilities for continuing care. Local civilians were the worst off. With few exceptions, they were ineligible for medical attention in multinational hospitals and were left to find the care they required at indigenous facilities.

In stark contrast to civilian medicine, then, military medicine implements differential care based on discrepant medical rights that vary with combatant status and national identity. While military ethics helps us establish each battlefield actor's belligerent status, military medical ethics substantiates their variable rights to health care.

Military Medical Ethics

Absent war, there is no military medicine; absent the ethics of war, there is no military medical ethics. If military medicine serves the broader aims of a defensive or humanitarian war, then its ethical system is considerably thicker than civilian medical ethics. In wartime, the public good or good of the political community supplements and sometimes supplants the individual's best interest. If military medicine serves the war effort, then medical necessity serves military necessity in a significant way, most obviously by maintaining force capabilities and returning soldiers to duty.

The following section introduces the principles of broad beneficence and military-medical necessity, and it reaffirms proportionality to place military medical ethics squarely within the province of just war. These principles significantly affect military medical ethics' traditional concerns: individual autonomy, patient beneficence, and impartiality.

Broad Beneficence

In medical ethics, the principle of beneficence reflects a "moral obligation to act for the benefit of others" (Beauchamp and Childress 2009: 197). "Others" are usually patients, that is, individuals who require medical attention: a drowning swimmer, a kidney donor, or a terminally ill, suicidal patient, to name a few that Tom Beauchamp and James Childress describe (2009: 197–221). In military medicine, however, the locus of concern often moves away from the individual patient and the attendant duty of *narrow* beneficence to consider the collective interests of a political community at war. In contrast to narrow beneficence, *broad* beneficence remains the "moral obligation to act for the benefit of others." "Others," however, speak to the interests of all those affected by war. Benefit, moreover, is not exclusively medical and may reach to the military advantages of medical care as they play out in defensive and humanitarian war. These benefits include defending a political community, ensuring a dignified life for others, and preserving the peace and stability of the international order.

To gain perspective, it is useful to consider the resemblance between military medicine and public health policy. Both military medicine and public health policy serve the common good as defined by the aggregate interests of the body politic. Proposing a framework of public health ethics, James

Childress and Ruth Bernheim (2015) charge public health with preventing harm and maximizing benefits across an entire national population (also Kass 2001). Like war, public health policy may harm some individuals to avoid causing greater harm to many others. To obviate the abuse that might come from an "ends justify the means" doctrine, individual rights constrain utility maximization. These include "autonomous choices, liberty of action, privacy, confidentiality, and truth-telling" (Childress et al. 2002: 171), as well as the fundamental human right to a dignified life I noted earlier.

The tension between the utility maximization and the principles of right that constrain it is an endemic problem for any practical moral theory. To resolve these conflicts, Childress and colleagues (2002: 173) recognize five "justificatory conditions": effectiveness, proportionality, necessity, least infringement, and public justification (also, Benatar and Upshur 2008). These principles require little elaboration. The first three—effectiveness, proportionality, and necessity—track the same-named principles of military ethics. Any policy must be feasible, effective, and necessary while its benefits offset the harm some will suffer as it unfolds. Least infringement further constrains harm. Not only must benefits outweigh harms, but officials also must make as reasonable efforts to minimize harm as practicable. Public justification reflects the critical role of local, national, and international deliberation as the paramount vehicle for well-informed, transparent, and inclusive policy decisions (Callahan and Jennings 2002; Upshur 2002). I will discuss the legitimizing role of public moral discourse in Chapter 3. From the perspective of public health, these principles and conditions help policymakers weigh the collective good against the harm done to individual rights when individuals must vaccinate their children, complete courses of medical treatment, submit to medical screening, or abide by government safety regulations.

Might this framework serve military medical ethics? To answer this question, it is important to note several crucial differences between public health and military medicine. First, public health focuses on aggregate health, the sum of all citizens' health interests. Military medicine, in contrast, focuses on aggregate *and* collective health. Aggregate health sums up all soldiers' health interests as embodied in the fighting force. Collective health is coterminous with broad beneficence and signifies a political community's health and welfare, its ethos, and way of life.

Second, public health is distinct from the practice of medicine; military medicine is not. While the former focuses on the policy necessary to ensure the health of a nation's residents through resource allocation, health programs, and regulation, the practice of military medicine pivots on the dyadic doctor-patient relationship. For reasons of public health, the citizen-government relationship supersedes the doctor-patient relationship when aggregate health interests outweigh an individual's. Compare again the benefits of mandatory vaccinations against the risks they impose on some people. In contrast, the doctor-patient relationship remains at the center of military medical practice. Military medicine is all about doctors, nurses, and medics tending patients. But as medical personnel treat the sick and wounded, broader considerations of aggregate health and collective welfare significantly affect care decisions. Looking to war's ends, military doctors may set aside urgent medical need when tending multinational forces, provide civilian care to win hearts and minds, or offer nontherapeutic "enhancement" to warfighters.

Third, the "public" in "public health" is all-inclusive. Public health reaches out to every national but usually stops at the border. There, it turns into foreign aid and a contentious debate about global justice that asks whether and how states may see to their own before considering aid to developing nations (Risse 2009; Pogge 2009; Singer 1972). Modern military medicine, in contrast, operates in a maelstrom of converging and conflicting medical interests. It is not always all-inclusive. In war, military medicine supports the military mission and its broader goal of prevailing in a just war. This objective generates different classes of patients: soldiers, civilians, and detainees, each enjoying a different set of healthcare rights, a phenomenon unknown in national public health where officials ignore the health of those over the border but attend to compatriots equally, based on medical need.

Defensive and humanitarian wars also generate different obligations toward the local population. In a defensive war, health care for the local community is often an afterthought. At best, defensive armies comply with a vague imperative of international law to maintain existing health care subject to their strategic interests and resources. But in a humanitarian war, local health care is of fundamental concern. If the grounds for humanitarian war are to attain a dignified life for the persecuted minority, then preserving and improving their lives cannot be an afterthought. It must be the goal. Reaching that goal requires a basic level of health care that a dignified life requires. Nevertheless, nations usually go to war with far fewer resources than they need to accomplish this goal. Even in humanitarian wars, medical care for the local population often remains an afterthought.

Finally, the measure of public health is health, while the measure of military medicine is broad beneficence. Indeed, one benchmark of broad beneficence invokes such health measures as combat survival and return to duty rates for military personnel, or infant mortality and infectious disease control for civilian populations. Broad beneficence also includes military advantages: warfighting fitness (from compulsory vaccines) and strength (from enhancement), host-nation loyalty (from military diplomacy), or public order (from force feeding detainees). Each measure points to a different benefit that balances against ensuing harms when medical personnel disregard confidentiality, sidestep informed consent, or deny care to local civilians. The weight of competing costs and benefits impinges directly on calculations of utility and proportionality. If civilian medical ethics weighs individual health costs against private or public health benefits, military medical ethics weighs the same individual costs against broad military and security benefits.

While public health ethics offers a coarse template for balancing public and individual interests, military medicine moves beyond public health to utilize medicine for nonhealth-related benefits in the service of war. Broad beneficence marks the obligation to act for the benefit of others by maintaining individual, aggregate, and collective medical health and political welfare. Broad beneficence is a central goal of military medicine. To satisfy broad beneficence, military medical ethics calls upon *military-medical necessity*.

Military-Medical Necessity and Clinical-Medical Necessity

An action or item is necessary when no other means can attain the designated goal at a lower cost. Medical necessity, therefore, refers to the least costly medical means required to achieve a justified medical goal, whether saving lives or improving their quality. For example, surgery is only necessary when less harmful therapies are ineffective or unavailable. Questions about how to treat those in need turn on the gravity of injury or illness, the patient's express wishes, and healthcare costs. In all cases, however, these decisions reflect the needs of specific individuals or, in the case of a public healthcare system, aggregate individuals. Medical needs do not speak to the less tangible collective interest of a national ethos or way of life.

Military necessity refers to the military means to effectively pursue just war, whether national self-defense or humanitarian intervention.

In contrast to medical necessity, military necessity sanctions the least costly means to protect individual, aggregate, and collective interests. Fusing the ends and means of military and medical necessity, *military-medical necessity* designates the least costly medical means a military force requires to effectively pursue just war. To clearly distinguish military-medical necessity from medical necessity alone, I will refer to the latter as *clinical-medical necessity*. Clinical-medical necessity registers the therapeutic care to satisfy urgent medical needs and the imperative to give priority to dire cases.

In this view, only military-medical necessity justifies the practice and provision of military medicine during armed conflict while clinical-medical necessity pulls in a different direction. Pursuing military advantage in just war defines the required outcomes that military-medical necessity serves by tending the sick and wounded. These outcomes are construed broadly in terms of safeguarding the political community or protecting human rights, or more narrowly in terms of operational success to save compatriot lives, disable enemy assets, support allies, or seize territory. In military medical ethics, proportionality evaluates the cost associated with military medical care against the advantage it seeks. The costs may be military, medical, or moral. Military costs refer to military disadvantages from pursuing a particular medical policy, such as opening a combat hospital to treat local civilians (Chapter 7). Medical costs reflect lives or limbs lost when resources are insufficient to attend to all in need or the reputational harm the medical corps may suffer when armies use medical diplomacy to win hearts and minds (Chapter 10). Moral costs, in the form of rights violations or infringements, may accrue when mandatory vaccinations or medical treatment override patients' wishes.

Military, medical, and moral costs are disproportionate when they exceed expected military advantage. For example, mass casualty triage aims to save first responders at the expense of the more seriously wounded, so police, fire, and medical personnel can attend to the sick or injured of a disaster or attack. In this case, proportionality requires that those ultimately saved outnumber those sacrificed. Calculating proportionality during mass casualties on the battlefield is more complicated. By first working to return the lightly or moderately wounded to battle, it is conceivable that many more warfighters will die from lack of care than return to duty. Nevertheless, this outcome may be proportionate if the military advantage of deterrence or territorial reclamation, for example, outweighs lives lost.

Built into the principle of proportionality is a firm measure of effectiveness. Effectiveness speaks to the realistic probability of successfully attaining a justifiable goal and is the first moral test of any proposed policy or operation. Proportionality is the second test and reserved for operational decisions that admit of a reasonable chance of success but are laden with costs. An ineffective operation is futile, and anyone killed in the process loses his life unnecessarily. When too many civilians die in a bombing attack to successfully destroy a weapons depot, disproportionate casualties result. When intelligence errs or equipment malfunctions, armies are negligent. Disproportionate, unnecessary, and negligent suffering are distinct moral outcomes.

As some of these examples demonstrate, military-medical necessity and proportionality step back from the individual patient to embrace the material good of all soldiers and the intangible good of a national ethos. Ordinarily, and in civilian medical ethics, clinical-medical necessity, proportionality, and beneficence revolve around the patient. Clinical-medical necessity defines the care an individual patient requires, while proportionality weighs the costs and benefits of her treatment. The goal is always the patient's welfare. In contrast, military-medical necessity and proportionality speak to broad beneficence understood as aggregate and/or collective welfare.

Military Medical Ethics: From Principles to Practice

Military medical ethics is inseparable from the practice of war. Therefore, it is impossible to evaluate the morality of military medicine inattentive to the justice of war. Nations and peoples wage just war in defense of a nation-state's right to sovereignty, a people's right to self-determination, and anyone's human rights. To secure these objectives, just war theory and international humanitarian law require armed forces, whether state or guerrilla, to protect combatants from superfluous harm and to protect noncombatants from direct or disproportionate harm. Military necessity, therefore, links the ends and means of just war to permit the measures necessary to attain war's goals while subordinating its means to every participant's human rights (ICRC 1977a: Art. 35). Similarly, military-medical necessity is subject to the moral constraints of armed conflict. War and wartime medicine invoke broad beneficence: collective goods, aggregate welfare, and the well-being of the political community. With these aims in mind, the next chapter turns to patient rights and practitioner duties in military medicine. Both are at the center of military medical ethics but differ in important ways from their civilian counterparts.

2

Patient Rights and Practitioner Duties

Patient rights and practitioner duties are a central theme of medical ethics. Patient rights are claim rights; that is, a right to health care that nations must provide, and a right to informed consent, privacy, and confidentiality that practitioners must fulfill. Practitioner duties are professional obligations to serve patient welfare, deliver health care impartially, and respect patient rights. Very little about these rights and duties is controversial in medical ethics. Dilemmas and questions arise when rights and/or duties conflict. Euthanasia, for example, pits patient self-determination against the obligation to preserve life. Similar end-of-life and beginning-of-life issues have dominated medical law and ethics for more than 50 years.

In military medical ethics, however, the substance of patient rights remains contentious. In general, military medicine acknowledges that mission requirements restrict the scope of a service member's right to refuse treatment or maintain privacy and confidentiality. On the other hand, practitioner duties seem to *transcend* mission requirements and embrace impartiality and neutrality irrespective of military necessity. Something is amiss. It cannot be that military necessity affects patient rights but leaves practitioner duties untouched. There is no compelling reason, however, to regard practitioners any differently from patients. If broad beneficence and military necessity impose unique constraints on patient rights, then they equally influence practitioner duties. Before trying to reconcile patient rights and practitioner duties, the following sections of this chapter drill into each. Patient rights include the right to health care, informed consent (and refusal), privacy, and confidentiality. Practitioners' duties embrace their obligations to patients and compatriots.

Patient Rights

The patient rights of service personnel track those of nonmilitary patients. Among the most central is the right to receive medical care from qualified medical practitioners. Health care is a claim right that anyone in need holds against those capable of tendering appropriate medical aid. Claim rights generate duties. Among medical professionals, beneficence reflects the duty to act for the benefit of others, whether a private individual (narrow beneficence) or the political community at large (broad beneficence). "Benefit" unpacks as net gain so that fulfilling the duty of beneficence should aid relatively large numbers of individuals whether to save their lives or improve their quality.

Health care is essential to achieve a flourishing and dignified life. Together with adequate income and education, good health and longevity are fundamental for developing the human capabilities necessary to implement a rational life plan. The central role of health in human life raises two questions: What level of health care is required to achieve a dignified life and who delivers the requisite resources and infrastructures? The United Nations Universal Declaration of Human Rights (Article 25) demands a standard of living adequate for the health and well-being of oneself and one's family. The United Nations Committee on Economic, Social and Cultural Rights (CESCR 2000) entitles every human being to the "highest attainable standard of health" (Article 12.1) subject to "a State's available resources" (Article 12.9). As such, adequate health care is a moving target that varies with a nation's resources. Citizens of wealthy states will expect a higher standard than residents of poor states. On the other hand, a state must meet a minimum baseline of care for its poorest citizens, recipients of foreign aid, and local civilians it encounters during armed conflict and postwar reconstruction.

If the right to health care is easy to state, the devil is in the details. Subsequent chapters investigate the kind of care, the necessary resources, and the appropriate provider for local nationals and security troops, detainees, and military veterans. International development aid, for example, translates the minimum baseline into a basic package of healthcare services (BPHS) that underlies postwar reconstruction. Veteran care often tracks the benefits of national healthcare systems. Among deployed personnel, medical care is exceptionally sophisticated, a function of concern for the mission and the patient.

Military Medical Patient Rights

Although mission readiness restricts some patient rights, it can broaden health care rights when medical attention is necessary to maintain fighting strength. Facing numerous casualties with only limited resources, the principle of mass casualty triage, for example, curtails the rights of the critically wounded but expands the rights of the injured who can return to duty. Rather than wait, the less critically wounded enjoy immediate attention. As such, the right to military medical care turns on the requirement that warfighters can perform their assigned tasks. In general, subsidiary rights of health care are subordinate to mission readiness and force conservation. Service personnel have limited rights to refuse treatment or sign DNR (Do Not Resuscitate) orders, demand privacy, protect confidentiality, or receive medical attention when they cannot return to duty.

On paper, civilian and military medical facilities formulate the rights to medical care, informed consent, privacy, and confidentiality similarly, but the implications are very different. Table 2.1 compares patient rights at Mayo Clinic and Walter Reed Medical Center, prominent civilian and military medical facilities in the United States.

Table 2.1. Patient Rights in Civilian and Military Medical Facilities

	Civilian Medical Facility (Mayo Clinic 2019)	Military Medical Facility (Walter Reed National Military Medical Center 2019)
Medical Care	You have the right to emergency treatment to stabilize your condition.	You have the right to receive quality medical and dental care and treatment.
Informed Consent	You have the right to reasonable, informed participation in decisions involving your health care.	You have the right to receive the necessary information to make knowledgeable decisions regarding consent or refusal of treatment.
Informed Refusal	You or your legal representative may refuse treatment to the extent permitted by law.	You have the right to refuse treatment to the extent permitted by law and to be informed of the consequences of your refusal.
Privacy/ Confidentiality	You have the right, within the law, to personal and informational privacy.	You have the right, within law and military regulations, to security, personal privacy, and confidentiality of information regarding your medical treatment.

Medical Care

Without universal health care or private insurance, American patients have no claim for medical services beyond the stabilizing emergency care Mayo Clinic describes (Black 2006). In contrast, Walter Reed's declaration of "quality medical and dental care" is far more expansive and compares favorably with patient rights in a national health care system. Britain's National Health Service (NHS 2015: 7), for example, advises patients: "You have the right to receive care and treatment that is appropriate to you, meets your needs and reflects your preferences." Nevertheless, the NHS Constitution enshrines a human right, while Walter Reed highlights a contractual right between employer and employee.

Informed Consent

Informed consent draws from the patient's right to self-determination that permits one to formulate rational life plans without outsiders' interference. Choosing a course of treatment requires that providers meet the informational requirements described in Table 2.1. In each facility, patients are entitled to a concise explanation of their illness, course of therapy, probability of success, side effects, and alternative remedies. To exercise informed consent, patients require the cognitive wherewithal to process data competently and determine their course of action. In some cases, patients are unconscious or mentally incompetent. In these circumstances, the law often allows patients to appoint a proxy decision-maker, whether a family member or legal representative (Chapter 8).

Despite its bumpy evolution (Jonson 1998: 353–358), the norm of informed consent is today a permanent fixture and incontrovertible condition of health care that only emergencies might override. Ordinarily, these are medical emergencies following traumatic injury when neither patient nor proxy can consent to lifesaving care. During war or public emergencies, it also may be infeasible to obtain informed consent for necessary medical treatment. Not only might battlefield conditions make informed consent challenging to secure, there are often fears that soldiers may refuse treatment if asked, thereby imperiling a mission. Such were American concerns as they required service personnel to accept mandatory vaccinations during the 1990 First Gulf War (Chapter 3). All is well until soldiers refuse treatment.

At that point, informed refusal, the flipside of informed consent, brings a myriad of difficulties to the practice of military medicine.

Informed Refusal and the Right to Die

No issue in bioethics has been more contentious than the right to die. The right to die plays off respect for autonomy and patient self-determination against the duty of the medical community and the state to preserve life. Resolved slowly through the courts and legislation, patient self-determination eventually afforded competent, incompetent, and minor patients the right to withhold or withdraw medical care, or request medical assistance to end their lives (Jonson 1998: 233–281; Laurie, Harmon, & Porter 2016: 67–127, 516–567). These rights, so ingrained in public healthcare systems, attenuate in military medicine. Although patient rights statutes in the United Kingdom and the United States allow patients to refuse treatment under the principle of informed consent, military service limits this right when care is necessary to keep service personnel fit for duty.

Refusing Mandatory Medical Care

Table 2.1 describes how civilian and military patients enjoy the right to refuse treatment "to the extent permitted by law." In civilian medicine, the authorities may override the right to refuse treatment when necessary to protect a patient, a community, or healthcare workers (Bingham 2012; Stewart 2009). In addition to these exceptions, military medicine adds one more: service personnel cannot refuse treatment that keeps them fit for duty. This exception has two ramifications. First, refusing treatment violates military law. And although physicians cannot override informed refusal and treat a patient in defiance of his wishes, failure to accept care can result in disciplinary action. Second, DNR orders are uncommon in military medicine.

Military regulations require soldiers to accept standard therapies and may impose sanctions for refusing treatment that keeps them fit to perform their duties. If a patient in the American Army refuses treatment, a medical board assesses the necessity of treatment and the reasonableness of the patient's refusal. Should the board uphold the order for medical treatment, the patient must comply. Further refusal may result in disciplinary action or administrative action to "separate the Soldier from service through retirement, discharge, or other legal means" (AR 600-20 2014: §5-4(f)2; Department of the Navy 2002: §3413, 3–28).

Invoking the collective good inspired by broad beneficence, military-medical necessity can justify coercive measures to ensure fitness for duty when the costs are proportionate. Military patients differ from civilian patients in significant ways. When, for any reason, a civilian patient refuses treatment, there are no consequences for anyone but himself. Nor are the consequences anything but health-related. The situation is much different for service personnel whose refusal may undermine discipline, increase the risk to others, and reduce mission readiness. All told, an individual's refusal may impair force capabilities. Against these collective costs is the punishment an individual soldier must suffer for refusal. Patients refusing treatment are not treated against their will. And although the authorities respect patient autonomy and self-determination, service personnel may lose their jobs. Discharge from service is a proportionate cost assuming that (a) the proposed treatment is reasonably effective and (b) no other remedy or prophylactic measure is available. As a practical matter, however, there are few conflicts between physicians and their patients. Usually, both agree on the same course of treatment. When they do not, military authorities will take disciplinary action and court-martial soldiers who refuse mandatory care (Chapter 3).

Do Not Resuscitate (DNR) Orders

In contrast to the limitations imposed on the right to refuse treatment, restrictions on DNR orders are more difficult to explain because neither military-medical necessity nor broad beneficence is at stake. As part of a competent patient's advance directive, DNR orders require medical personnel to forego lifesaving resuscitation procedures. A DNR order affords the option of avoiding resuscitation following cardiac arrest or a stroke that might only leave a patient worse off. As such, DNR orders are usually the purview of terminally ill or catastrophically injured patients.

In civilian medicine, such regulations as the US *Patient Self-Determination Act* (PSDA) or the EU *Convention on Human Rights and Biomedicine* (1997) strengthen the force of DNR orders. To ensure timeliness, some professional associations recommend a policy of "required reconsideration," which periodically re-evaluates a patient's treatment goals, values, and preferences in light of up-to-date data about operative risks and benefits (American College of Surgeons 2014). For the most part, military regulations track these guidelines. In the US Army, for example, "a patient with decision-making capacity has the legal and moral right to participate in medical care decisions, including the right to refuse medical treatment at any time even if the treatment is lifesaving" (AR 40-3 2013: §2-3). These regulations mirror those for refusing cardiopulmonary resuscitation (CPR) in civilian hospitals when a patient faces imminent death or significant deterioration of quality of life following resuscitation (Brigham Health 2019).

Military regulations, however, also reserve the right to override advance directives when patients are on active duty:

> While active duty (AD) patients usually determine their own care, occasionally the requirements of the Service will override their decision. These situations are unusual but when questions concerning mandatory medical or surgical procedures on AD Soldiers arise, the procedures in AR 600–20 will be followed. Because of the unusual nature of such situations involving AD patients, physicians may wish to additionally consult with their institutional medical ethics committee. (AR 40-3 2013: §2-9)

Army Regulation AR 600-20 (2014: §5-4) permits American military authorities to override informed refusal when necessary to maintain a soldier's fitness for duty or alleviate a health-related threat that she poses to others. When patients are critically ill, DNR orders do not affect a service member's fitness for duty. In principle, there is nothing peculiar about battlefield conditions that would relieve caregivers of the obligation to honor a DNR order assuming they could reasonably assess the likelihood of imminent death or post-resuscitation quality of life. In practice, however, anecdotal evidence suggests that this is rarely the case. First, in-theater care often focuses on urgent lifesaving treatment impelling caregivers to leave the "trickier" healthcare dilemmas to out-of-theater facilities where there is sufficient time to deliberate "in the cold light of day" (Brocke 2017). Second, as the French case outlined in the Introduction describes, field surgeons sometimes fight to keep the critically injured alive so they may return home to their families to die.[1] Each practice may prove beneficial to soldiers' and families' welfare, respectively. However, there is currently insufficient evidence to evaluate the costs and benefits of setting aside DNR orders until the critically injured reach a full-service facility in their home country (Bennet 2016).

Privacy and Confidentiality

Privacy and confidentiality are closely related. Privacy is a subsidiary right of personal self-determination: the right to keep information close and release only what one wants others to know about oneself (Bok 1989: 120). Confidentiality is a duty imposed on others to guard another's private information until that person authorizes its disclosure. The right to privacy and duty of confidentiality ensure self-esteem, job security, and social status that the release of personal information may jeopardize. In medicine, respect for privacy maintains the trust necessary for practitioners to tend patients successfully. Usually, privacy and confidentiality are straightforward. Patients disclose information so medical practitioners can provide proper care. Beyond that, it is nobody's business. In civilian bioethics, confidentiality obligates respect for privacy unless protected information puts the patient or third parties at risk. Common examples include self-inflicted harm, child abuse, or credible threats to murder another (Gross 2006: 118).

During war and among compatriot soldiers, the private sphere shrinks. In contrast, the public sphere expands when broad beneficence offers grounds to divulge information that is otherwise confidential in civilian settings. US Army regulations, for example, prohibit the army from disclosing records (including medical records) without "prior written consent *except* when disclosure is made to officers and employees of DoD who have a need for the record in the performance of their duties" (AR 25-22 2016: §7.1) or is "necessary to ensure the proper execution of the military mission" (DoD 2019: 3–4). The authorized recipient list is long: "unit commanders; inspectors general; officers, civilian attorneys, and military and civilian personnel of the Judge Advocate General's Corps; military personnel officers; and members of the US Army Criminal Investigation Command or military police performing official investigations" (AR 40-66 2008: §5-23e).

Failure to disclose prior treatments, noncompliance with medical care, clinical instability, or personality disorders may, in some circumstances, impair mission performance, upset the discipline and cohesiveness necessary to maintain an efficient fighting force, and harm the patient or third parties (Hoyt 2013; DoDD 2003: §4.6.3.2). Under such circumstances, military-medical necessity affords the moral justification for disclosing confidential information without a service member's explicit consent. Disclosure remains the exception, not the rule. But military-medical necessity also anchors the rule. Just as the right to privacy ensures well-being among civilians, it also ensures warrior well-being. Everyone, and perhaps warfighters even more so, thrive when their secrets remain private. For soldiers, respect for privacy is not only a right that protects their best interests (narrow beneficence). Privacy is also a right that assures collective best interests and mission success (broad beneficence) by contributing to each service member's mental health and stamina. Only rarely does mission success justify the cost of violating a service person's privacy. The 2003 US Army's textbook of *Military Medical Ethics*, for example, explains how it may be ethically permissible to disclose confidential information to commanders if necessary to protect a mission, or to shade the truth about the effects of investigational drugs if full disclosure might undermine morale (Howe 2003b).

In these cases, the benefits that come from disclosing private information must overcome the harm soldiers suffer when military or medical authorities violate or restrict their right to privacy. Otherwise, the cost to the individual soldier is disproportionate. Well into the Iraq and Afghanistan wars, for example, concerns mounted that service personnel were resisting psychotherapy for fear of prosecution should they disclose infractions of military law (Dao and Frosch 2009). Balancing costs and benefits to ensure proportionality might only permit disclosure of personal medical data if protecting confidentiality poses a "serious" risk of harm to individuals (Neuhauser 2010: 1034), third parties, or the mission (Gibbs and Olmsted 2011; Johnson 2008). "Serious" harm evokes the idea of "excessive" harm integral to the general principle of proportionality and will, I suspect, prove equally resistant to any firm definition.

Respect for patient rights is the lynchpin of proper health care. It is clear, however, that military medicine restricts, or rather redefines these rights subject to military-medical necessity and broad beneficence. The result is to bifurcate the rationale of patient care. As service personnel perform their duties, medicine helps maintain fitness and ensure mission capability. However, when soldiers can no longer perform their duties, medical attention turns to narrow beneficence and a patient's best interest. Veteran care, therefore, operates under guidelines different from those described in this chapter. For veterans, the right of informed consent, refusal, and privacy do not, indeed should not, deviate from civilian medicine. Active-duty personnel, on the other hand, enjoy a narrower set of patient rights due to limits imposed by broad beneficence, military-medical necessity, and proportionality. Few contest this. It is perplexing then that this firm grasp of military-medical necessity that animates patient rights does not extend uniformly to practitioner duties.

Practitioner Duties

Practitioner duties are a corollary of patient rights. Active-duty patients enjoy a claim right against practitioners to deliver care consistent with the constraints imposed by broad beneficence and military-medical necessity. To fulfill their correlative duties of care practitioners must offer care subject to the same provisos. Service personnel, for example, have the right to expect priority treatment for those who can return to duty. Similarly, a soldier should expect military doctors to release private health information, whether theirs or another's, if nondisclosure jeopardizes their unit's readiness. Structuring care any differently, by adhering to the demands of impartiality or absolute privacy, for example, violates the obligations that military physicians owe active-duty personnel. There is, then, an apparent contradiction between the patient rights of military medicine and the duties imposed on military medical personnel by international humanitarian law. The result is to generate conflicting duties and "dual loyalties" that only the lens of military-medical necessity and broad beneficence can resolve.

The Duty to Provide Impartial Medical Care

The Geneva Conventions and national military medical guidelines are a tangle of conflicting rules and regulations:

a. The wounded and sick shall receive to the fullest extent practicable and with the least possible delay, the medical care and attention required by their conditions. There shall be no distinction among them on any grounds other than medical ones (ICRC 1977a: Art. 10).

b. To the fullest extent of the means available to it, the Occupying Power has the duty of ensuring the food and medical supplies of the population (ICRC 1949b: Art. 55).

c. Contrary to the ordinary meanings of the terms "wounded" and "sick," persons who continue to engage in hostilities do not qualify as wounded or sick under humanitarian law, no matter how severe their medical condition may be (ICRC 2016: Art. 12, §1345).

d. The ultimate goals of combat medicine are the return of the greatest possible number of warfighters to combat (Cubano 2018: 24).

Paragraph (a) embodies clinical-medical necessity and medical urgency, the gold standards of impartial health care. Initially referring only to enemy combatants in 1949, the Geneva Conventions extended the rule to civilians in 1977 (ICRC 1987: §304, 312). Nevertheless, there are important qualifications to the sweeping duty of impartiality. Paragraph (b) backs away from needs-based care to subordinate an army's healthcare obligations to "important military requirements," as well as to the "material difficulties with which the Occupying Power might be faced in wartime" (ICRC 1949b: Art. 55; ICRC 1958: 310). In other words, medical care for civilians is subject to military necessity and compatriot needs.

Paragraph (c) considers the medical rights of enemy combatants. Only enemy soldiers who no longer pose a threat enjoy the right to medical care. The cases are probably rare but instructive. Consider a field surgeon who might treat and release enemy soldiers because there are no facilities to hold them captive. These soldiers remain an active threat, and paragraph (c) denies them medical care from their enemies, "no matter how severe their medical condition may be." The rationale behind the law is clear: no one has any obligation to abet a threat against one's life or the lives of compatriots. Paragraph (d) reiterates force conservation as military medicine's chief mission and joins paragraphs (b–c) to contradict the unilateral obligation to treat the sick and wounded based solely on urgent medical need.

Each citation describes an aspect of military medical practice, whether civilian, enemy, or compatriot care, that cracks the monolithic concept of impartiality. A more detailed discussion unfolds in subsequent chapters. Here, we see how the exigencies of armed conflict alter a firm principle of peacetime medical ethics. One relevant factor is available assets. When resources are scarce, military planners devote what is necessary to maintain their war effort. Another factor turns on the unequal rights of different patient classes to receive medical care. In apparent violation of the principle of impartiality, similarly ill or wounded compatriots, enemies, and local nationals will receive very different care during armed conflict (Chapter 1). Finally, consider how associative duties impose a special obligation on compatriots that further turns military medicine away from strict impartiality.

Associative Duties of Care

Associative duties reflect the moral significance of a small, tightly knit, and interdependent family or community and demand preferential care for those who are close (Mason 1997; Miller 2005; Simmons 1996). Few doubt that friends, family, and compatriots owe duties of aid and assistance to one another that they do not owe to strangers. At one level, conditional commitments of mutual aid—"You watch my back and I'll watch yours"—ground associative duties. But we also expect friends and comrades-in-arms to watch our back because they are our friends, not because they are returning or banking a favor. In this vein, associative duties evoke an "ethics of care" that speaks to an emotive rather than contractual bond that calls for "personal concern, loyalty, interest, passion and responsiveness to the uniqueness of loved ones, to their specific needs, interests [and] history" (Held 2006: 95). Associative duties reflect intense existential interdependence. "How *we* fare at a fundamental level," observes Saba Bazargan-Forward (2019: 2364), "depends on how *they* fare." Relationships among friends and family can confer a firm sense of well-being, self-esteem, and personal identity and engender a special moral duty to safeguard their lives and interests.

Military units also constitute a moral community that generates special obligations of care akin to those among family or friends. By their training and shared experiences of war, comrades-in-arms often bond into a "primary group" (Kirke 2010; Siebold 2007; Wong et al. 2003) that generates associative duties in military organizations. Primary groups are not merely a collection of well-coordinated, self-interested individuals, but a cohesive band woven together by "mutual affection, interdependence, trust, loyalty . . . peer bonding and teamwork" (Siebold 1999: 15; also King 2013: 24–39). The resulting sense of belonging engenders self-sacrifice and commitment that afford service personnel emotional and physical security, a sense of purpose, and the social capital necessary for resilience.

True, this may be changing. Preliminary evidence, for example, suggests that male-dominated primary group bonds are weakening as women assume a growing role in the military (Miller 2017) and as respect for professional skills motivate interpersonal cooperation as much as deep friendship does (King 2016). None of these developments, however, deny the benefits of associative duties nor the importance of developing personal bonds and obligations. That some groups, such as women, do not find a place in male-dominated primary groups does not count against the value of such groups. Instead, it reinforces demands for the inclusion of women so they may enjoy the same benefits of the moral community.

Although military necessity justifies preferential treatment for those who return to duty, associative duties may override necessity. Faced with lightly injured host-nation allies and severely incapacitated compatriots who cannot return to duty, military necessity directs our attention to the former. At the same time, associative duties dictate priority care for the latter (Chapter 5). Associative duties are often overwhelming, but they are not definitive. Casual reflection suggests that associative duties cannot justify preferential treatment for compatriots when others are in exceptionally dire straits. This line is not always easy to draw. Nonetheless, associative duties, military-medical necessity, broad beneficence, and limited resources temper the principle of impartiality during contemporary armed conflict. Doing so also impinges upon the commitment to medical neutrality.

Medical Neutrality and Immunity

The duty to remain neutral is bound up with impartiality. Impartiality is a medical precept that requires caregivers to ignore everything but urgent medical need. Neutrality is a political notion. By demanding indifference to a belligerent's identity and to the justice (or injustice) of his cause, neutrality places any medical worker above the fray. By remaining neutral and impartial, medical (and clerical) personnel enjoy a special status that confers immunity and protects them and their facilities from direct attack (ICRC 1949a: Art. 19, 24). Two distinct claims might justify medical immunity.

1. Military medical personnel have no truck with war. They threaten no one and carry no arms. Medical units do not make an "effective contribution to military action," nor does their "total or partial destruction, capture or neutralization . . . offer a definite military advantage" (ICRC 2016: §1794).
2. Medical immunity is a necessary condition of combatants' right to health care. Without protection from attack, medical staff and facilities cannot meet their obligation to provide warfighters with proper care and maintain unit readiness. As a result, sovereign nations agree to protect their military medical personnel out of mutual self-interest.

The first claim is twofold. First, medicine is inherently neutral because it pursues impartial humanitarian care. Second, army medical personnel pose no military threat because they are willing to treat friends and enemies alike. In this view, military surgeons and their staff do not serve war but peace (Messelken 2018). Indeed, mid-18th-century civilian nurses who tended the wounded across Europe under the aegis of the nascent ICRC did just that. Today, humanitarian NGOs retain the same protections. However, NGO staff members enjoy immunity because they are civilian noncombatants, not because they are nurses and doctors. In these cases, medical service confers no special protection; noncombatant innocence alone anchors immunity from attack.

Medical members of military organizations, however, are not innocent. Instead, military surgeons threaten their adversaries as they fulfill their medical mission to return their compatriots to duty. Nor does the medical staff manage the sick and wounded irrespective of combat status or national affiliation. On the contrary, doctors or nurses may first tend their own, defer care of local civilians, and ignore hostile enemy forces. Military medical personnel do not pose a direct lethal threat, but their services, like any support service, are essential to maintain military capabilities. Military medicine is not inherently neutral or nonthreatening. Therefore, there is no reason to offer physicians the equivalent of noncombatant immunity any more than any other support service.

If immunity does not draw from the innocence of medical providers, it may draw from the rights soldiers enjoy to receive the health care necessary to fulfill their military mission. To meet this claim, military organizations must protect their medical personnel and facilities from attack. They are too valuable to risk. Belligerents may, therefore, agree to extend immunity to their respective medical corps on the condition they remain neutral. "Neutral" says nothing about abjuring a preference for one's own as it did when Red Cross nurses populated the battlefield. Instead, it merely prohibits medical personnel from taking up offensive arms.

To preserve immunity and reinforce medical neutrality, international law vigorously condemns any attack on, or belligerent use of, medical personnel or facilities (ICRC 1949a: Art. 19–22). Either is a war crime (ICRC 2020: Rule 28). The norm is functional. It does not speak to any violation of noncombatant rights as much as it incentivizes respect for a mutually beneficial convention. Medical immunity, like clerical immunity, stems from reciprocity and contract, that is, explicit or tacit agreements among belligerents to preserve valuable and highly trained personnel. There is nothing in the nature of medical or clerical service to substantiate a prima facie case for immunity. As such, medical immunity and the duty of neutrality persevere only as long as mutual interest does. In a conventional war between nation-states, the prospect of mutually destroying one another's medical facilities usually affords sufficient motivation to respect immunity. In asymmetric war, however, guerrilla forces seldom command the means to threaten their enemy's medical facilities significantly.

In asymmetric war, violations of medical neutrality often proliferate as insurgents exploit immunity to stage attacks from hospitals or use ambulances to transport personnel and materiel (Israel MFA 2009; Gross 2006: 187–193). In response, state armies counterattack, often without discrimination (Brown 2015; WHO 2016). The law condemns both but without significant disincentives, the motivation to respect the law wanes. Insurgents are willing to risk harm to innocents when they abuse medical neutrality, while state armies face little risk by attacking medical facilities that they claim violate the law.

If asymmetric war undermines medical neutrality among adversaries, it does not release belligerents from their obligations toward civilians (Barilan and Zuckerman 2013). When the United States staged a fake hepatitis B vaccination campaign to collect DNA to capture Osama bin Laden in 2011, for example, medical workers knowingly violated medical neutrality. In response, officials argued that the United States needed to use "all the tools at its disposal to find bin Laden" (Terry 2013: 37). As it stands, the claim is unconvincing. Although military-medical necessity describes the medical means to attain legitimate military objectives, the "tools at their disposal" must be proportionate and attentive to fundamental human rights. By most accounts, they were not. During the fake campaign, many local nationals did not receive the full course of vaccinations. In its aftermath, local citizens proved reluctant to accept polio vaccinations for their children, while attacks on vaccination workers increased significantly (Kennedy 2017). This violation of neutrality is egregious. The fake campaigns brought no harm to military personnel but did violate patient rights and practitioner duties by unnecessarily jeopardizing patients' health and the safety of aid workers.

Narrowly construed, medical immunity and neutrality facilitate care for compatriot warfighters and allow aid workers to promote public health. Sweeping immunity and any duty to maintain absolute neutrality, however, obscure the constraints of warfare. Accounting for associative duties and military-medical necessity restores equilibrium and helps resolve charges of dual loyalty that sometimes plague military medicine.

Dual Loyalty

Offering an ethic for military medicine, Thomas Beam and Edmund Howe (2003: 853) propose:

> that a military physician is primarily a physician and in most instances makes decisions on this basis rather than as a military officer. Although this statement appears to emphasize the differences between medicine and the military, the instances of there being a significant conflict are very rare.

Beam and Howe endorse the two-hatted, one-head depiction of military physicians struggling with incompatible roles: doctor and soldier. They soften the blow by suggesting that conflicts are rare. Perhaps, but why should there be any conflict at all or any hint of betrayal should one serve one role rather than the other?

Suggesting conflicting practitioner duties, dual loyalty is the bugbear of military medical ethics. The International Dual Loyalty Working Group defines dual loyalty as "a role conflict between professional duties to a patient and obligations, express or implied, real or perceived, and to the interests of a third party such as an employer, an insurer, the state or . . . military command" (London et al. 2006: 382). More specifically, dual loyalty reflects a tension between professional judgments and obeying orders, between healing and harming and, ultimately, between preserving human rights and violating them to serve state interests (London et al. 2006: 383–385; also PHR 2002).

Dual Loyalty and the Practice of Military Medicine

To speak of dual loyalty is to misconstrue the practice of military medicine as two competing vocations—medicine and military service—when it is, in fact, a singular social practice. Following Alasdair MacIntyre (1981), a social practice comprises its aim, that is, the goods it hopes to provide, the rules governing its activity, and the virtues or standards of excellence necessary to participate in the practice and realize its goals (also van Burken and de Vries 2012). Table 2.2 summarizes these attributes across the practice of medicine, military service, and military medicine.

Table 2.2. The Goals, Rules, and Virtues of Medicine, Military Service, and Military Medicine

	Goal	Rules Regulating the Practice	Virtues
Medicine	Health Care	Impartial Care Do No Harm Narrow Beneficence Medical Urgency	Compassion Discernment Trustworthiness Integrity Conscientiousness
Military Service	Self or Other Defense	Military Necessity Proportionality Discrimination	Fidelity Trustworthiness Chivalry Courage Honor
Military Medicine	Health Care to Enable Self or Other Defense	Military-Medical Necessity Associative Duties Broad Beneficence	Discernment Trustworthiness Compassion Courage

Medicine and military service differ. Medicine's primary goal is to maintain or restore physiological and psychological health, while the purpose of military service is to preserve or restore national sovereignty (*self*-defense) or human security (*other*-defense). In terms of justice, medicine fulfills a human claim right for health care while military service addresses claim rights for security. The rules regulating each practice are also different. Medicine imposes a duty of impartial care and narrow beneficence guided by urgent medical need. Despite the incidence of therapeutic harm, its guiding maxim is "do no harm." Military service begins with controlled, lethal violence. Regulation is crucial to protect combatants from gratuitous harm and civilians from disproportionate harm. Military necessity, not clinical-medical necessity or urgent need, offers the ends-means calculus for operational decisions that serve the collective good of broad beneficence.

Finally, consider the virtues or excellences necessary for each practice. Beauchamp and Childress (2009) describe five "focal" medical virtues. Compassion (sympathy, generosity, and kindness), discernment, and trustworthiness are other-directed and pertain to practitioners' relationship with their patients. In contrast, the virtues of integrity and conscientiousness are self-directed. Other-regarding military virtues embrace fidelity, trustworthiness, and chivalry (protecting the innocent). The first two extend to comrades-in-arms, the latter, chivalry, to civilians or enemy prisoners. Self-directed military virtues include courage and honor (Olsthoorn 2011: 32–43; Mehlman and Corley 2014).

Military-medicine is a unique practice. Its goal is to maintain and restore the physiological and psychological health of a fighting force that prosecutes a defensive or humanitarian war. Force conservation is not a byproduct of military medicine but a good internal to its practice. Unlike civilian medicine, the rules governing military medicine turn on military-medical necessity, mission requirements, associative duties to compatriots, and broad beneficence. These rules and norms enable practitioners to maintain a battle-ready force effectively.

Looking at the virtues of military medicine, Table 2.2 appears to amalgamate those of medicine and military service and, indeed, might include all nine attributes. Closer inspection reveals that the substance of each virtue changes significantly. Consider four examples. In civilian medicine, discernment calls on insight and understanding "to make fitting judgments and reach decisions without being unduly influenced by *extraneous considerations, fears, personal attachments*, and the like" (Beauchamp and Childress 2009: 40, emphasis added). In military medicine, discernment may require physicians to infringe on a patient's right to privacy, informed refusal, or medical treatment to sustain operational capabilities. In doing so, discernment subordinates urgent medical needs to *extraneous considerations*, such as military necessity, and to the *personal attachments* or associative duties. As a result, deliberations surrounding eligibility for military medical care, for example, can be exceptionally trying (Chapter 5).

Trustworthiness crosses most social practices, although the objects of trust-building expand in military medicine to include patients *and* comrades-in-arms. Conflicts may arise if patients and comrades-in-arms do not understand the reach of discernment (and, for example, complain if left untreated for a less wounded soldier who can return to duty). Integrity, too, is familiar to any social practice but may be wrongly impugned, again, if observers do not appreciate the demands of discernment that require setting aside medical urgency as conditions demand or adopting a narrow interpretation of neutrality. Likewise, compassion is a virtue central to medical practice but is tempered by military medicine's commitment to mission success. One does not renounce compassion when tending to a lightly wounded compatriot before a more severely wounded compatriot who cannot return to duty. But one does subordinate medical urgency, a decision that reframes one's interpretation of compassion. Finally, consider courage. Physicians and fighters each exemplify courage. Each requires the mettle to make life and death decisions at personal risk whether from infectious disease or hostile fire. Military medicine embraces both risks, sometimes simultaneously.

Dual Loyalty Reconsidered

Dual loyalty is an inappropriately castigating term to describe the dilemma of striving for legitimate but conflicting moral goals. Dilemmas are prevalent in medical ethics because fundamental rights and duties often conflict. Few ethical systems are so hierarchically ordered that one can easily rank rights and obligations. The perennial conflict between life and liberty animates the euthanasia debate, while recurrent opposition to mandatory measles vaccines or sheltering at home force public health officials to navigate between individual rights and collective well-being. No one ever calls this "dual loyalty." Yet, the charge is frequent in military medical ethics because military physicians swear two professional oaths: one to Hippocrates and one to defend their country against all enemies. How does defending the Constitution of the United States (or her majesty, the Queen, as the case may be) collide with the modern Hippocratic oath's duty to "apply, for the benefit of the sick, all measures that are required, and . . . remain a member of society, with special obligations to all my fellow human beings" (McMaster University 2019).

Much depends on interpretation and what it means to be a "member of society." A cosmopolitan reading might require one to choose between military service to protect the political community and medicine to protect the health of all human beings. A narrower reading speaks more closely to the aims of military medicine, namely, to protect the "health of my fellow human beings" so they can defend the society of which one is a member. This reading ranks individual and collective good lexically but subordinates the former to the latter in wartime. Military-medical necessity, therefore, justifies the medical means required to save lives or improve their quality in pursuit of national self-defense or humanitarian intervention. In this way, broad beneficence and military-medical necessity coalesce into a single obligation for military medical practitioners that avoids confusion about dual loyalties. Broad beneficence and military-medical necessity offer grounds to address questions about triage, medical diplomacy, medical rules of eligibility, and detainee care from a unified perspective subject to effectiveness and rights-protecting proportionality. Military-medical necessity does not eliminate moral deliberation. Hard questions about balancing rights and utility remain. These are not dual loyalties but the stuff of ethical dilemmas more generally. Unilaterally asserting that military healthcare professionals must always and impartially prioritize urgent medical need does little to ease military medicine's moral difficulties.

To return then to Hippocrates. Conflicting obligations did not confound him as he refused the Persian king's request to treat his plague-infected troops (Chapter 1). Instead, Hippocrates misunderstood the full import of military medical ethics. His decision to deny the Persian army is misguided, not because one should always and unconditionally care for one's enemies, but because the Persian army no longer threatened Greece. Had Hippocrates faced Xerxes bearing down to subjugate Greece, any Persian appeal for aid would have been presumptuous. An enemy's right to demand medical attention is reserved for those who no longer pose a threat. Alternatively, Greece might be at war on other fronts. With resources scarce to the breaking point, foreign aid is not feasible. But Xerxes is dead, and Sparta has yet to invade Athens. Hippocrates's animus is only a vestige of a previous war. He faces no moral dilemma, dual loyalty, or pangs of conscience. He only lacks the moral courage to aid his former enemies, a common aversion when wars end.

Patient Rights and Practitioner Duties

If patient rights drive practitioner duties, they must share a common moral framework. Patient rights begin as claim rights for health care. War redefines these to restrict the rights of informed consent, refusal, and privacy while expanding the rights of others to receive priority treatment when they substantially contribute to military operations or when they benefit from special, associative duties in austere environments. The principles of broad beneficence and military-medical necessity in just wars of national defense or humanitarian intervention afford the appropriate moral framework for patient rights during armed conflict.

Utilizing the same framework to understand practitioner duties questions prevailing notions of impartiality, neutrality, and dual loyalty. Impartiality works well *within* moral and political communities, but absent a cosmopolitan world order, it does not easily extend across them. Associative duties create special obligations toward compatriots. When assets are limited, as they inevitably are during war, patient rights break down by national identity rather than medical urgency. More generally, national sovereignty, security, and mission success co-opt neutrality. But they also strengthen each side's motivation to confer special protection or immunity on medical personnel and facilities. Neutrality and immunity, therefore, should not be confused. As early as 1906, L. Renault, a member of the French delegation to Conférence de révision réunie à Genève, which updated the rules of medical neutrality, wrote:

> to say that doctors are neutral would suggest that they are indifferent with respect to the conflict that sets the fate of their country at stake; they are, in actual fact, enemies, albeit enemies with a special task, and protection and special immunities must be accorded them precisely to enable them to perform that task. (Kalshoven 2007: 1002)

Understanding that this special task is inexorably linked to one's country's fate helps resolve the incongruity between patient rights and practitioner duties, and eases charges of dual loyalty. It further informs this book's subsequent chapters, as military medical practitioners confront the moral and logistical challenges of tending the sick and wounded during 21st-century armed conflict.

3

Moral Reasoning in Military
Medical Ethics

The turn from principles to practice is dynamic. The previous chapters outlined a theory of military medical ethics and patient rights drawn from two major norms of political philosophy: sovereignty and human rights. These two norms, together with such justificatory principles of war as necessity, distinction, and proportionality shape military medical ethics. Military medicine provides health care to serve the collective ends of just war (broad beneficence) by effective, proportionate, and necessary means (military-medical necessity) and appropriate attention to associative duties. With these principles tentatively in place, the next question is, "How do they work in practice?"

Models of Moral Reasoning

Answering this question is essential to seeing how an integrated view of military medical ethics differs from models that bifurcate military and medical necessity. Beam and Howe (2003: 855) offer a flowchart model (see Figure 3.1) to reason through medical decisions that may carry significant risk to service personnel.

Military necessity is paramount. "Military physicians must give absolute priority to military needs . . . when society's interests would be significantly sacrificed as a result of not doing so" (p. 853; Boxes A and B). Absent existential threats, however, the medical officer asks after two local effects: a treatment's contribution to the military mission (Box C), and the risks of medical treatment (Box D). When the risk of medical treatment is significant, then the soldier's autonomous wishes always prevail (Box E). When the risk is low, the mission's needs prevail unless the medical intervention has no particular military purpose (Box B).

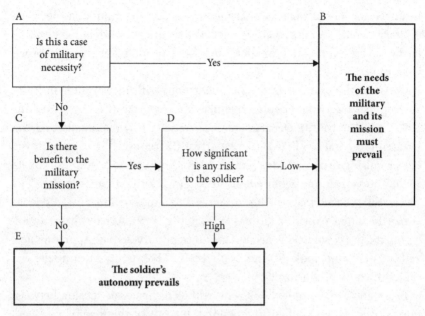

Figure 3.1. Military medical ethics decision making.

This model is problematic for several reasons. First, by focusing solely on threats that compromise a nation's survival, the model construes military necessity too narrowly. While a country facing genocide might permissibly subject its troops to limitless risk, another facing loss of territory (e.g., the Falklands/Malvinas) must, on this model, act with greater restraint. A broader, more useful conception of military necessity is precisely the one this model overlooks, namely, the means required to benefit a military mission. As such, a medical intervention that does not benefit a military mission, that is, is not militarily necessary, falls to the soldier's autonomy. This claim is not controversial. On the other hand, the risky medical intervention that benefits a mission is what generates the intricate and provocative dilemmas of military medical ethics. Some missions, other than those allaying existential threats, also might justify high risks.

To evaluate costs and benefits, therefore, it is insufficient to ask whether a soldier faces *high* risk from a therapeutic intervention. Instead, *relative* costs and benefits are determinative. A critical mission will permit greater risk than one less consequential. High risk alone is insufficient to establish disproportionate harm if the military benefits are significant. Finally, the

Beam-Howe model suggests that medical needs are shunted aside when military needs prevail, when, in fact, they work in tandem. Integration is the virtue of military-medical necessity, proportionality, and broad beneficence.

Consider the example of treating US troops with investigational drugs. Fearing that Iraq would deploy chemical or biological weapons during the 1990 Gulf War, the US Department of Defense (DoD) requested Food and Drug Administration (FDA) waivers to treat US troops with two unapproved but promising drugs: pyridostigmine bromide (PB) and botulinum toxoid (BT). To override the requirement to obtain informed consent, the DoD successfully argued that permitting soldiers to refuse treatment would jeopardize the military mission (Annas 1998; Rettig 1999). As a result, treatment was mandatory; soldiers refusing faced disciplinary action. Approximately 250,000 personnel took PB, and 8,000 received BT vaccines during the war (Fulco, Liverman, and Sox 2000).

Beam and Howe's model does not help us navigate the tension between mission success and patient rights. First, the fate of the Republic was not at stake. Even if the war was lost because numerous troops succumbed to nerve gas, defeat in the Gulf did not threaten America's survival. Turning to the second question, "Was the vaccine of benefit to the military mission?" Assuming it worked as expected, US troops would gain protection against a virulent biological agent. But what of proportionality? Do the risks of treatment outweigh its military benefits? Putting aside the purported benefits, what constitutes *significant* risk? Given that soldiers risk their lives all the time, medical risk should track military risk. If a military commander may permissibly order a mission that poses a 50% risk of death (e.g., Rush 2001: 280–282), the medical risk can be no less in similar circumstances. Suppose a military physician must default to autonomy when a soldier faces significant medical risk. In that case, the commanding officer must do likewise and pull soldiers from a mission when military risk is similarly high. Alternatively, if military commanders are willing to risk high casualties to achieve their objective, why does it matter if the losses come from enemy fire or prophylactic measures to protect troops? There is no compelling reason that medical risk counts any more than military risk. Finally, the model provides no answer to the question, "Who decides?" Some decisions are the purview of medical officers; others are the purview of military officers. Deliberative forums range from individuals to committees to public decision-making bodies.

An Integrated Model of Moral Reasoning

A comprehensive and integrated model of moral decision-making resists a flow chart because it is not linear. Instead, one can think about three distinct tasks to articulate and resolve moral dilemmas of military medicine:

1. Define the Military and Medical Mission
2. Articulate the Ethical Questions
3. Weigh the Pertinent Moral Factors

At first glance, these tasks may seem like discrete, consecutive stages. Sometimes they are, but very often decision-makers will double back to re-define the military or medical mission if either proves unnecessary or dis-proportionately costly. Returning to mandatory inoculation during the Gulf War, the following sections work through each task before highlighting the pivotal role of private deliberation and public discourse.

Define the Military and Medical Mission

The military mission guides the medical mission. The first Gulf War was an international effort to curb Iraqi aggression in Kuwait. Under Chapter VII of the UN Charter, the United Nations approved military action to contain a threat to international peace and security. No Coalition nation's survival was at risk. Nevertheless, each country had an interest to thwart aggression and defend Kuwaiti sovereignty. This was the military mission. Among the conditions necessary for military success was a force capable of prevailing in a chemical/biological war (CBW). To meet the CBW threat, the military medical mission called on the medical corps to deliver the vaccines and pro-phylactic agents necessary to maintain its force capabilities.

Articulate the Moral Questions

Two moral questions dominated the debate: "Is it permissible to use an in-vestigational drug?" and "Is it permissible to treat service personnel without informed consent?" These questions cannot be answered in parallel, only serially. First, there must be sufficient grounds to use an unapproved drug independent of informed consent. Second, there must then be adequate grounds to override informed consent.

Weigh the Pertinent Moral Factors

Resolving military and medical moral dilemmas requires careful assessments of effectiveness, necessity, cost and benefits (utility), and proportionality. Consider each in the context of mandatory BT and PB vaccines.

1. *Effectiveness*: Are BT and PB effective? "Effective" has two dimensions. Will BT and PB protect a single soldier from harm? Second, will BT and PB maintain unit readiness? A drug or vaccine that poses an n% risk that a single soldier will suffer severe side effects or long-term disability may not necessarily impair force capabilities if the military deploys sufficient troops. Whether the risk is unacceptably high depends on the value of the military mission.

2. *Necessity (1)*: Is the vaccine medically and militarily necessary? Are there military or medical alternatives to maintain the fighting force? Therapeutic options may include other drugs or protective clothing to prevent infection. Military means to diminish the threat may strike at the source and include air attacks on chemical and biological facilities or credible threats of retaliation that undermine the will to deploy chemical weapons.

Answering "no" to effectiveness and necessity (1) may lead policymakers to redefine the medical mission. Answering "yes" affords reasonable grounds to consider administering BT and PB. Is informed consent necessary?

3. *Necessity (2)*: Is it feasible to attain informed consent from service members? Feasible may mean: Do deployment conditions offer sufficient time for service personnel to mull things over? The DoD thought not and convinced the FDA to issue a waiver of informed consent. In other words, there was no alternative policy to accomplish the mission while securing informed consent. Were there, decision-makers would then weigh the costs and benefits of each.

4. *Costs, Benefits, and Proportionality*: Costs and benefits evaluate broad (collective) and narrow (individual) beneficence. Does the benefit of

treating soldiers with investigational drugs outweigh the costs of a policy that requires consent? There are medical, military, and moral costs and benefits to assess. The immediate medical benefits compare the protection from disease gained by the entire military population (if treatment is mandatory) to the immunity afforded only to those who consent (if treatment is consensual). The countervailing medical costs are short- and long-term mortality, morbidity, and the attendant cost of care. The military benefits compare how each policy contributes to mission success while accounting for the attrition of soldiers who refuse consent and must leave the military. The moral benefits of foregoing consent confirm the military's responsibility to protect all its soldiers, while the costs highlight the affront to dignity from imposing treatments without full consent or full disclosure of risk.

Proportionality, Costs, and Benefits: A Closer Look

To assess proportionality accurately, decision-makers must carefully evaluate costs and benefits. Calculations of expected utility weigh magnitude and probability. Magnitude reflects the absolute cost or benefit of action. On some scale, say 1 (minimal) to 10 (weighty) one can assess the value of outcomes: the ability of troops to withstand CBW, the military benefits of a particular mission, the worst-case medical effects of a vaccine, or moral affronts to dignity. Comparing two military operations, for example, one operation may bring significant benefits while another offers only minimal gain. Assessing magnitude requires metrics. Some measures, such as lives saved/lost or projected morbidity, lend themselves to quantification. In contrast, deterrent capability, morale, or respect for autonomy and dignity are far harder to measure and compare.

Probability also matters. During the Gulf War, the chemical, biological threat never materialized, and ultimately, vaccinations were never needed. Introducing probability alters the cost-benefit calculation. Were the chances of CB warfare great and the attendant costs of vaccination low, then the potential harms to service personnel are justifiable. But were the likelihood of war low and the attendant risks and costs of vaccination to individual soldiers high, then the same harms may be disproportionate and without justification. Utility focuses on the interest of all the relevant parties. In this case, the rights and interests of compatriot warfighters and their nations are at issue.

In subsequent chapters, the rights and interests of host-nations and their citizens are at stake and central to calculations of utility.

Finally, justice and fairness matter. Avoiding undue burdens generally requires a firm, universal baseline so that no one suffers excessive harm. Patient rights ensure a minimal baseline of health care that broad beneficence, associative duties, or military medical necessity cannot undermine. When considering mandatory vaccination, fundamental rights of self-determination and respect for dignity prohibit physically coercive measures. No one would vaccinate a soldier by force but may think of imposing onerous costs for opting out, such as imprisonment. Is incarceration, for example, disproportionate? Answering this question affirmatively demands a significant benefit, and lack of less costly alternatives before mandatory vaccination backed by the threat of jail can outweigh the substantial harm of detention.

Costs, Benefits, and the Lesser Evil

While many utility calculations compare costs and benefits, some must choose among the many ills of war. Military operations will kill, injure, impoverish, and debase civilians and soldiers who have done nothing to deserve their fate. In some cases, it is necessary to choose one evil to avoid a greater evil and do good. Circumstances may excuse but never justify evil deeds. The lesser evil defense is not a feature of mandatory vaccination but pervades many decisions concerning civilians and detainees (Chapters 6, 7). Consider the Allied bombing of Hiroshima, part of a pattern of saturation bombing in World War II to break civilian morale. Today, we commonly view injury to civilians through the lens of collateral harm that justifies civilian deaths as the unavoidable but proportionate side effect of a necessary military operation. This was not true of Hiroshima. Instead, Hiroshima's civilian population was the target. Civilian deaths were not a side effect, but the operation's primary goal. Americans chose to kill civilians directly to avoid a long war and numerous American casualties, a greater evil from the US perspective.

The lesser-evil defense demands two strict tests. First, the lesser evil must prevent the greater evil with high probability. Second, the lesser evil is a necessary and last resort, so that there is no less evil or harmful action that can mitigate or prevent the greater evil. The nuclear bombing of Hiroshima and Nagasaki are extreme cases that fail to meet each test. If direct attacks on civilians are ever permitted, it might only be when the attacking nation faces an existential threat. This is Michael Walzer's doctrine of supreme emergency (1977: 251–268). The United States would incur significant casualties to invade Japan, but not loss of its political community. At the same time, alternative means of forcing surrender went untested. Nor did the Allies ever moderate their demands of absolute surrender to end the war.

Greater and lesser evils abound in war. When appropriate, the lesser-evil defense only offers an *excuse* because intentionally harming another, even to achieve a greater good, retains shards of evil. As subsequent chapters argue, excused harm may mitigate the perpetrators' punishment but requires compensation for the victim whose rights are infringed.

Proportionality, Costs, and Benefits: A Second Case

Commenting on military mental health care, Johnson, Grasso, and Maslowski (2010) write: When ethical–legal conflicts arise, it is always important to ask, "What will be in my client's best interest and how can I avoid causing him or her harm?" These questions are not always appropriate. The right questions are, "What will be in the *mission's* best interest," and then, "how can I avoid causing my client disproportionate harm?" This is to reframe the problem in terms of broad beneficence and military-medical necessity.

Consider, briefly, a second case:

> You are the GDMO (General Duties Medical Officer) detached to a Forward Operating Base (FOB). One of your soldiers was close to an explosion. Although he was not physically injured, he complains of deafness and tinnitus in both ears. He is the unit's only Unmanned Aerial Vehicle (UAV) pilot. He is seen at a field hospital where he had an audiogram which shows his hearing is below deployable standard and indicates his return to the UK. The CO (Commanding Officer) of the FOB needs the soldier to stay at the FOB as he is "so essential and losing him may cost lives". He may still have to go out on patrol. The CO is adamant about this, and is getting very angry at the prospect of losing him. As a GDMO you recommend his [evacuation] back to UK. (Coetzee, Simpson and Sharpley 2010: 207)

The authors present this hypothetical case as "unit need vs. individual need." This already starts on the wrong foot. The proper question turns on military-medical necessity: Is medical evacuation or retention of higher value to the mission? To answer requires one first to define the mission.

There are two missions: the narrow mission to maintain the FOB force and the broader mission to maintain the entire deployed military force. Without specific regard for "individual need," the physician can invoke the broader mission and evacuate the injured soldier to receive medical attention and so return to duty another day. To consider the FOB force, necessity asks whether retaining the soldier is the least costly option to maintain FOB readiness. Are there other options? The vignette does not say. Are the costs of retaining or evacuating the wounded soldier disproportionate? How much will the unit benefit or suffer if he stays? These are the material costs and benefits of retention or evacuation. Will the retained soldier suffer if he remains? Does he face undue medical risk? These are the medical costs. Finally, what of the soldier's wishes? Should he consent or even demand to stay, does evacuation undermine respect for autonomy and self-determination? These are the moral costs of retention.

The authors acknowledge that "the final outcome of a medical problem may be difficult to predict." "In the end," therefore, "the quality of information is the only thing that distinguishes a calculated risk from a gamble" (p. 207). To push their point further, I note that information about the *medical* problem is necessary but insufficient without quality data about the military and moral issues. It is also essential to understand that civilian medical ethics does not usually allow physicians to take calculated risks unless for the patient's good. In contrast, military medical ethics permits, in fact, enjoins calculated medical risks for a mission's good. This is not to play off two disparate goods: the individual's and the mission's, but to place military medicine in the service of war. Military medical ethics offers an integrated decision-making process that avoids unnecessary and confusing dualism.

This case and the previous highlight two types of decision-making. One is top-down. Wrestling with mandatory vaccinations, military and government officials, that is, high-level bureaucrats, formulate policy. As the debate unwinds, academics, jurists, ethicists, and other interested parties join in. Evacuating a single wounded soldier (Case 2) is not a policy decision but its street-level implementation. This deliberative process involves at least three individuals and, perhaps, their subordinates or peers: the medical officer, the military officer, and the wounded soldier. In each case, the process is inclusive, dynamic, and deliberative. Inclusive, vigorous deliberation is the hallmark of legitimate moral decision-making so that the question "Who decides and how?" is fundamental when nations go to war and practice military medicine.

The Deliberation Process: Who Decides and How?

There are many actors in military medicine: patients, medical practitioners, unit commanders, military organizations, nongovernmental organizations (NGOs), the departments (or ministries) of defense, and commanders-in-chief. The media, academics, public intellectuals, and ultimately, the body politic all weigh in. Military medicine begins with war. Justifying war is not only a private exercise but also one of public deliberation and discourse. Early in the Iraq war, the role of medical personnel in the interrogation of detainees garnered considerable debate (Chapter 6). Less heated but no less critical discussions coalesced around veteran care and postwar reconstruction following withdrawal from conflict areas. In each case, private individuals and public forums struggled to reconcile the norms and practices of medicine and war.

Private Moral Deliberation

Confronted with a moral challenge, individuals first may turn to the principles at hand. Sometimes, these provide ready guidance. Sometimes they do not. To steer through conflicting norms, one may seek reflective equilibrium. Reflective equilibrium is an introspective reasoning process "reached after a person has weighed various proposed conceptions [of justice] and he has either revised his judgments to accord with one of them or held fast to his initial convictions" (Rawls 1971: 48). Moral agents constantly compare their moral judgments that arise in particular situations with the principles they hold dear. When the two conflict, each may give way to the other to allow the moral agent to reach a state of equilibrium that reinforces one's sense of justice. While Rawls (1971: 50) hopes that the principles of justice as fairness "give a better match with our considered moral judgments on reflection" than alternative theories of justice, the process is dynamic and fluid. Individuals seek the best fit.

Incorporated into modern bioethics, Beauchamp and Childress (2009: 382) advise practitioners to derive "guides of action" from their norms of right and wrong and then test these in real life. If they "yield incoherent results . . . we must go back and readjust the guides further." To use their example, the principle "always put the patient first" may yield incoherent results in practice when conducting research or when triaging battlefield casualties. Reaching a coherent decision requires alternative principles that modify what is discordant. In these cases, concern for the collective benefits of research and of national self-defense temper the priority of patient interests.

Although Rawls, Beauchamp, and Childress paint an isolated picture of moral deliberation, the same process animates groups. Public moral discourse is reflective equilibrium writ large and complicated by the messiness of people trying to reason with one another and reach agreement. Like its rarified cousin reflective equilibrium, moral discourse toggles between norms and practice but in a way that speaks to the competitive and cooperative urges of human association. Public discourse is well suited to the contentious nature of war and military medical ethics.

Public Moral Discourse

Public, moral discourse is a dynamic political and consultative process among free and equal individuals *and* their communities. Its vehicles include ethics committee deliberation, interest group competition, town hall meetings, judicial activism, and the legislative process.

At its best, democratic deliberation legitimizes institutional or political policy by putting it through the mill of public discourse. Joshua Cohen (1998: 224) summarizes its conditions:

> Given that citizens have equal standing and are understood as free, and given the fact of reasonable pluralism, we have an especially strong showing of legitimacy when the exercise of state power is supported by considerations acknowledged as reasons by the different views endorsed by reasonable citizens, who are understood as equals. (also Gutmann and Thompson 2009: 1–63)

Unpacked, the conditions of public discourse and deliberation include:

1. *Maximum participation*. Free and equal standing underscore the conditions of participation: equality of access and opportunity, freedom of expression, tolerance for diverse opinions, open-mindedness, rationality, and mutual respect (Habermas 1990: 200). Participation exposes individuals to well-reasoned arguments so they may evaluate their preferences and enlarge their outlook (Cooke 2006: 60).

2. *Well-reasoned arguments*. Moral discourse is argumentative. Each participant is free to challenge another. Well-reasoned arguments reflect an avowed interest in the public good and present claims that are sincere,

factual, and undistorted by manipulation, falsehoods, censorship, or coercion (Habermas 1979: 53; Risse 2000). Well-reasoned arguments are rational, that is, parsimonious, consistent, and suggest actions "that take effective means to ends" (Rawls 1971: 25). Well-reasoned claims utilize universalizable forms of moral argumentation that cut across divergent worldviews. These include deontological arguments about duties and fundamental human rights, and utilitarian arguments that invoke costs, benefits, and greater or lesser evils regarding liberty, security, sovereignty, and public order.

3. *Reasonable pluralism.* Public discourse does not require nor strive for consensus to reach legitimate outcomes. On the contrary, "the deliberative model," writes Habermas (2006: 414–416), "expects the political public sphere to ensure the formation of a plurality of considered public opinions." To do so, moral discourse works through many layers that include the courts, legislature, administrative agencies, NGOs, mass media, lobbyists, advocates, experts, moral entrepreneurs, and intellectuals who respect the rules of participation and well-reasoned argumentation.

4. *The centrality of community.* Moral discourse is strongly communitarian. "Morality," writes Habermas (1990: 200), "cannot protect the rights of the individual without also protecting the well-being of the community to which he belongs." The two are intertwined so that private moral discourse is unintelligible without the community-constructed norms and rules that guide it. Community—local, national, or international—is the forum for moral discourse and deliberation. In military medical ethics, this includes the military, medical, and political community as well as suggestions for an independent ethics unit to evaluate individual and collective interests (Benatar and Upshur 2008).

5. *Responsive public policy.* Citizens debate policy, not just ideas. The outcomes of the debate should influence national and international policymakers. As the discussion evolves, there is every expectation that public policy should respond accordingly. For this reason, public discourse demands democratic institutions.

Meeting these conditions, deliberative democracy does not always generate the best or most justified outcome. But nor are the results inconsiderate of justice. Instead, by adhering to background conditions that respect liberty and security, and to operating conditions that ensure free and equal access, respect diverse opinions, and generate reasoned arguments, resulting policy decisions gain a firm measure of legitimacy. On this model, dissenters do not revolt but remain within the deliberative paradigm to respect its outcomes as they work the same mechanism to reform public policy. At various times, outcomes may be ineffective, intemperate, and worse than the alternatives. Still, one hopes that the mechanism is self-correcting over time in a well-functioning national and international system.

The debate surrounding mandatory inoculation met many of the crucial conditions of public discourse. Mostly transparent and accessible, discourse stretched across the DoD, the FDA, the judiciary, veterans' groups, drug manufacturers, and the legal, bioethics, and medical community. Lacking definitive data, researchers investigated the long-term effects of vaccinations and treatment protocols as they assessed claims for compensation (Nass 2002). Collectively, participants to the debate built reasonable moral arguments that weighed costs, benefits, and proportionality and remained attentive to shared convictions that inoculation served the troops' welfare and the public interest. Ultimately, Congress enacted the Project BioShield Act of 2004 to allow the FDA to permit the DoD to use investigational drugs during a "declared emergency" (Parasidis 2012). The transparent and discursive attention of private citizens and interest groups, public servants, and the appropriate branches of government legitimizes subsequent policy. In contrast, deliberation accompanied by factional participation, incomplete or falsified data, and selfish rather than public-spirited reasoning is defective and cannot legitimate the policies it endorses.

Moral Reasoning in Military Medical Ethics

Many layers and dimensions of ethical deliberation exist in military medicine. The principles of broad beneficence and military-medical necessity capture the integration of the medical into the military mission. Choosing the appropriate means to ensure mission success depends on assessments of effectiveness, military-medical necessity, and proportionality to yield the optimal balance of medical, military, and moral costs and benefits. In this context, fundamental patient rights constrain actions but do so in ways that differ from civilian medical ethics. Sometimes, patient rights limit practice by regulating military medical research more tightly than civilian medical research (Chapter 8), and sometimes less so by permitting mandatory inoculation. The principles of military medical ethics, patient rights, and practitioner duties are crucial ingredients of judgment but insufficient without a large stage for private and public deliberation.

Not all military-medical challenges enjoy broad public debate. The controversy surrounding mandatory vaccines was exceptionally well attended but did not reach the general public. In contrast, the controversy surrounding interrogation enjoyed vigorous public deliberation until marred by deliberate misinformation (Chapter 6). Other issues were less public but no less energetic as practitioners, policymakers, and the occasional ethicist wrestled with medical diplomacy, medical rules of eligibility, and the fraught relationship between military units and humanitarian NGOs. On the other hand, postwar policy suffers from neglect rather than any surfeit of attention. Lack of interest calls attention to our neglected moral duties, which plague us all the more when the fighting winds down, the urgency subsides, and moral fatigue paralyzes responsive deliberation.

The subsequent chapters take up these and other subjects. More precisely, the following discussions reason through the principles of military medical ethics to justify, repudiate, or revise fundamental aspects of military medical practice and set the stage for future conduct. Part II opens with an overview of military medicine in the Iraqi and Afghan theaters following 9/11 before addressing the unique dilemmas and challenges of providing health care to combatants, detainees, and civilians.

PART II

ON THE BATTLEFIELD:
CARING FOR THE
WOUNDED OF WAR

4

Military Medicine in Contemporary Armed Conflict

Iraq and Afghanistan Revisited

For the longest time, medicine could do little more than bind superficial wounds, splint broken bones, and amputate mangled limbs. Helpless against infection and contagion, military surgeons could only watch as disease, sepsis, and gangrene carried off far more soldiers than enemy shells. Rarely did anyone expend the resources to evacuate the injured until after the fighting ended. Technological development and emerging Enlightenment ideals about citizen-soldiers changed all this. By the 19th century, the Napoleonic Wars (1803–1815) and the American Civil War (1861–1865) saw attempts to organize military medicine to evacuate and care for troops. By the Franco-Prussian War (1870–1871) and Russo-Japanese War (1904–1905), successful vaccines, antiseptics, and wound debridement elevated the role of military surgeons. By the First World War, military medicine could claim the dubious achievement of reducing death by infection and disease to the level of combat fatalities. Things continued apace. By World War II and beyond, the advent of antibiotics, innovative surgical and resuscitation technologies, and timely evacuation during battle further reduced military casualties, and returned many wounded to the line.

As the names of these conflicts suggest, American, European, and Asian nations mostly fought conventional state-on-state wars through the mid-20th century. The postwar period, however, brought a surge in colonial and guerrilla warfare in Africa, the Mideast, and Southeast Asia as peoples fought for independence. These wars were morally, materially, and legally asymmetric. Seizing the moral high ground of national self-determination, guerrillas were, nonetheless, poorly equipped and without standing in international law. As international conventions recognized the rights of national liberation movements, guerrilla war moved out of the shadows. "New" vicious wars of ethnic conflict, civil war, and regime change disrupted international peace and stability. Places as far-flung as Lebanon (1982–1983), the former Yugoslavia (1991–2001), and Somalia (1992–1995) drew in the Western powers to battle insurgents, terrorists, and rogue states.

Following 9/11, international forces entered Afghanistan and Iraq. With this, the small, asymmetric wars of the late 20th century morphed into large, asymmetric wars of the early 21st century. If the small wars struggled to contain hotspots, the large wars aspired to alter the world order, depose rogue regimes, and install constitutional democracies. To that end, international forces put big budgets and big guns into play. Significant numbers of boots hit the ground. Nevertheless, the conflicts remained attritional, long drawn-out affairs whose success remains undetermined. In many ways, however, the wars in Iraq and Afghanistan portend future conflicts. Some will be proxy wars and some will comprise hybrid affairs that blend kinetic and nonkinetic force in an array of local and regional venues. Some will pit states against insurgents; others will depose errant regimes. Proactive warfare will not disappear but will, at best, be more judicious. In this way, the wars in Iraq and Afghanistan bridge the wars of the 20th and 21st centuries, as exemplars of far less than total war, but far more than armed policing. Iraq and Afghanistan exemplify the challenges of armed conflict on many levels: tactics, strategy, resource allocation, public opinion, and foreign policy.

Military medicine seeps into many of the same issues, while its ethics gleans lessons for future consideration. Among the first concerns of any nation going to war is battlefield care to maintain combat readiness, return the injured to duty, and save lives. Maintaining combat readiness is a function of routine and acute medical care. Returning service personnel to duty and saving lives rests on emergency, life-saving treatment on the battlefield, and swift evacuation to the appropriate military medical facilities. As the wars in Iraq and Afghanistan demonstrate, the logistic and moral challenges of providing superlative care in an austere environment to a large and diverse patient base are enormous.

War and Medicine in Iraq and Afghanistan

The nearly two decades of fighting in Iraq and Afghanistan were among the longest and most expensive Western military operations since World War II. Among the largest contingents of multinational forces, nearly three million American soldiers and 300,000 British soldiers served in Iraq and

Afghanistan (UK MoD 2015; Watson Institute 2015) where they suffered 6,951 and 633 dead, and approximately 53,000 and 13,000 wounded, respectively (Farmer 2014; UK MoD 2019a, 2019b; Guardian 2019). This number excludes more than 7,500 US contractors who lost their lives (Crawford 2018). The American injured included at least 1,045 amputees, 320,000 cases of traumatic brain injury (TBI), and 300,000 incidents of post-traumatic stress (PTSD), depression (Krueger, Wenke, and Ficke 2012; Tanielian and Jaycox 2008: xxi), and moral injury (Frame 2015). Despite these casualties, warfighters enjoyed better medicine, better evacuation, and better protection than in all previous wars. But the call to treat military personnel was only half the challenge. It was soon apparent that host-nation allies and civilians would make growing demands on multinational healthcare facilities, which they were neither funded nor prepared to meet effectively.

As a prelude to the ethical dilemmas that animate this book, the following sections survey medical care during wars in Iraq and Afghanistan. At issue are three distinct phases of wartime care that describe the invasion, transition, and reconstruction periods. Neither war was a seamless progression—quite the contrary. Buoyed by early and what seemed to be decisive victories in Afghanistan and then Iraq, multinational forces found themselves unprepared for a resilient and renascent insurgency that would quickly belie "mission accomplished." Although the Taliban would not reorganize until 2006, a potent combination of deposed Baathist fighters and radical foreign jihadis put multinational forces on the defensive within a year of arriving in Iraq. With the local healthcare network in shambles, Coalition authorities soon faced growing and urgent demands from the local civilians, police, and army personnel.

A War Chronology: From Invasion to Reconstruction

To map medical management, it is useful to divide Coalition presence in Iraq and Afghanistan into three periods: invasion, transition, and reconstruction. Throughout each period, politics and medical care changed dramatically. Political changes mark the ebb and flow of the insurgency and efforts to develop local governing capacity. Operationally, the invasion, transition, and reconstruction phases mirror the counterinsurgency stages of "Shape, Secure, Hold and Develop" or, to adopt David Petraeus's medical metaphors: "Stop the Bleeding," "Inpatient Care—Recovery," and

"Outpatient Care—Movement to Self-Sufficiency" (FM3-24 2006: §5-3). In response to the exigencies of war, medical care answered to the demands of a rapidly changing patient population, novel wound types, fluctuating assets, and the presence of new actors.

Pinpointing precise dates for each stage is difficult because local politics was a fluid, unstable, and protracted affair. Nevertheless, each period affords a useful analytic device to chart the development of military medicine in the wars and the dynamic relationship between medical management and po-litical/military events in each country. In Afghanistan, the invasion and ini-tial occupation period extended from the original assault in October 2001 to oust the Taliban government and capture bin Laden until the establishment of an interim government in June 2002. The duration of the invasion period is fluid. It may easily extend to 2004 when the Council of Elders ratified a new constitution in January or when Hamid Karzai was elected president in October 2004. In Iraq, the invasion period began when multinational forces invaded in March 2003 and stretched until the United States transferred sovereignty to the interim government in June 2004 or, later, with national elections and a constitutional referendum in 2005. At this point, Iraq and Afghanistan became "host" nations as fledgling nationhood transformed the nature of the forces in Iraq from invader and occupier to a force invited to offer military assistance (Benard et al. 2011: 52–53; also Bassiouni 2010). During this one- to two-year period, the local government in each country was up but not entirely running. Multinational forces provided much of the medical care local nationals required.

In the invasion stage, military medicine tends the wounded. Although one might expect the greatest need during the initial invasion, such was not the case in Iraq and Afghanistan. On the contrary, rapid victories in the early fighting did not overly stress Coalition medical resources. Once the insur-gency erupted, however, first in Iraq in late 2003 and Afghanistan in 2006, defeating insurgents and establishing control over a newfound territory and population assumed overriding importance. Here, front-line care and rapid evacuation drove military medicine and powered the race for resources to serve the urgent needs of multinational soldiers, detainees, host-nation allies, and civilians.

The following period was one of transition and nascent development. Politically, the local government gained a foothold, held elections, and un-dertook to govern. In Iraq, the transition period ran four to five years, from the first steps toward local government until the Status of Forces Agreement (SOFA) and the Security Framework Agreement (SFA), which called for the withdrawal of combat forces from Iraq by June 30, 2008. The transition period in Afghanistan was longer, running eight to ten years until the United States and Afghanistan signed a Strategic Partnership Agreement (SPA) in May 2012.

The transition stage consolidates invasion-stage gains and is particularly intense. With a rebound of insurgent activity, the pressure increased for multinational forces to develop the rudimentary institutions of human security, including schools, police, courts, financial institutions, and health care. Attention to human security imposes a medical and political function on military medicine. Medically, multinational facilities ramp up to treat military casualties and offer limited care to the local population. Politically, military medicine supports counterinsurgency operations with stability operations, medical diplomacy, and medical humanitarianism to bolster support for the local government and undermine support for guerrillas. Sometimes characterized as "winning hearts and minds," medical humanitarianism utilizes health care to resuscitate civil society and legitimize the new government by providing high profile but not always sustainable medical care.

In the reconstruction or "outpatient" phase of the war, medical humanitarianism turns from transition-phase pacification to state-building. At this stage, international forces struggle to establish a self-sufficient and stable government consistent with the rules of good governance. Following the transition period, each Coalition nation reduced its military presence while undertaking reconstruction, a process that continues to this day and remains heavily dependent on US funding (Chapter 11). Healthwise, Coalition authorities collaborated with the local government to deliver primary health care and hospital services to ensure maternal, pediatric, and public health; control infectious disease; and provide mental health, disability care, and essential medicines (Senlis Council 2007). Beyond improving health, medical reconstruction strives to enhance state-building by empowering local communities and conferring legitimacy upon the state. These aims are no less political, or controversial, than medical stability operations. Ultimately, intervening military forces hope to cede control to the local government so they may leave the nation in an orderly fashion and in somewhat better shape than they found it. Neither is a foregone conclusion.

Military Medicine on a Changing Battlefield:
Military and Civilian Players

Five providers offered various levels of care and undertook an array of medical missions in Iraq and Afghanistan. Each also served a very diverse patient population. At the beginning of each war, multinational forces operated medical facilities designed and funded to deliver on-the-ground treatment for US and Coalition troops, as well as detainees. However, they soon found it necessary to expand their services to treat members of the Iraqi and Afghan security forces who fought alongside multinational forces and to treat local civilians who suffered severe illnesses and war-related injuries. As such, four distinct classes of patients emerged to vie for medical resources: multinational service personnel, detainees, host-nation allies, and local civilians. In contrast to civilian medicine where a single class of patients all enjoy the same right to health care, military medicine in Iraq and Afghanistan catered to different categories of patients, each of whom enjoyed the disparate medical rights and privileges described in Chapter 1.

Several providers managed these patient groups.

US and Coalition Facilities
Multinational military forces built an impressive medical infrastructure in-theater and out to offer battlefield care for service personnel and, when feasible, host-nation allies and local nationals. To regulate access and preserve limited resources, Coalition facilities established restrictive medical rules of eligibility (MRoE). These would pose a unique and overwhelming challenge for military medical ethics (Chapters 5–7). Active throughout the war, multinational facilities were the primary providers of health care in the invasion period, slowly winding down as troop levels decreased.

Medical Civic Action Programs and Provisional Reconstruction Teams
Medical Civic Action Programs (MEDCAPS) were modest medical units that afforded limited care to the local population. Medical interventions included vaccination campaigns, dental care, and acute care that could be provided on the spot with limited facilities and did not require extensive or long-term treatment. Provincial Reconstruction Teams (PRTs) were small, dedicated civilian/military units charged with laying the foundations for local services. Funded by their respective Coalition governments, PRTs engaged with local nationals and nongovernmental organizations (NGOs) to

build and staff schools, roads, water projects, and medical clinics and to train local civilians in these fields. PRTs were most active in the transition period and later were phased out as NGOs and the local government took over the management of medical care.

The US Agency for International Development
The US Agency for International Development (USAID) is an independent US government agency. Working closely with local government officials and NGOs, USAID funded civilian projects in health, education, agriculture, private sector development, and governance. Supporting PRT activities and large-scale projects, USAID was a major player in the short- and long-term reconstruction of Iraq and Afghanistan and active throughout the entire period.

Nongovernmental Organizations and International Organizations
Nongovernmental organizations (NGOs) and international organizations (IOs), such as the World Health Organization (WHO) and the International Committee of the Red Cross (ICRC) provide funding, staff, and expertise to enable local governments to develop healthcare and hospital services. Domestic, foreign, religious, and nonsectarian NGOs were active throughout the wars but gained a significant foothold in the transition period once better security enabled them to operate safely. As one of many providers during this period, these NGOs often clashed with MEDCAPs and PRTs whom they accused of infringing on their "humanitarian space" and endangering patients. Together with the local government and USAID, NGOs took on a significant role during reconstruction expecting to decrease their support as local healthcare infrastructures and budgets stabilized.

Local Government
Ultimately, the reconstruction of their decimated and ill-functioning medical infrastructures fell to the local governments. In Iraq, sanctions and the flight of trained medical personnel devastated what had been a relatively efficient healthcare system (Jaff et al. 2019; Library of Congress 2006, 2008). Before the imposition of sanctions following Iraq's 1990 invasion of Kuwait, most Iraqis enjoyed access to health care (SIGIR 2013: 110). In the years following, funding collapsed and "health indicators fell to levels comparable to some of the least developed countries" (Iraq MoH 2004: 5; also Jones et al. 2006: 228–238). In contrast, Afghanistan never enjoyed an efficient or

modern healthcare system. Its health indicators are among the worst in the world (Jones et al. 2006: 189–196). Following armed intervention, Coalition military facilities were the only source of medical attention. In time, NGO-run hospitals supported by USAID took on the burden of medical care as the local government slowly implemented a basic healthcare package.

Military Medicine in the Invasion Period

In a period marked by swift military victory and the collapse of essential in-frastructure, occupying multinational forces faced growing pressure from the local population to deliver health care. Initially, the war went well. Casualties were low. In Afghanistan, US forces suffered 161 killed and 423 wounded from 2001 to 2004. In Iraq, 138 soldiers died and 542 were injured by the time President Bush declared mission accomplished (icasualties 2019). Light casualties, coupled with an overabundance of resources allocated for the chemical and biological war that never was, led Douglas Galuszka (2006: 60) to conclude the "combat health support system was not stressed enough to show if it was truly capable of performing up to the Army's expectations." This assessment was premature; American and Coalition medical facilities soon faced overwhelming stress as the insurgency intensified.

The Insurgency Grows

In the early months of each war, US and other multinational forces fought and won a conventional war against government forces. These victories were, however, short-lived. In Iraq, de-Baathification decommissioned about 400,000 members of the military, leaving large numbers of Sunni soldiers and officers unemployed and disgruntled (Gordon and Trainor 2006: 475–507; Global Security 2019). Many of these would later organize, finance, and lead the insurgency (Ricks 2006: 190–192). At the same time, foreign jihadis, soon to be called al Qaeda in Iraq, flocked to Iraq to take on Western forces. Their contributions were initially minor, but with the support of former Baathists, they soon coalesced into a capable insurgent force by late 2003 (Bacevich 2016: 5072).

Similarly, in Afghanistan, the Taliban regrouped in the South. Fueled by an opium economy, an open border with Pakistan, local discontent, rising nationalism, and growing animosity toward the foreign invaders, they would gain significant support from local warlords (Barfield 2010: 30–31). By 2006, Taliban forces tripled the number of armed attacks they launched previously. Improvised explosive devices (IEDs) were the weapon of choice, and IED causalities skyrocketed from 113 in 2005 to 415 in 2007 to over 1,800 in 2009 (Cordesman, Allison, and Lemieux 2010.)

The Improvised Explosive Device Threat

Early IEDs were roadside bombs, car bombs, or suicide bombers that targeted soldiers on foot or in armored and unarmored vehicles. If most of the early injuries in Iraq resulted from small arms fire (Kelly et al. 2008), IED attacks soon claimed the highest percentage of victims. In Afghanistan, IED attacks accounted for 30% of multinational forces killed in combat in 2002; 50% in 2004; and 65% in 2008–2010 (Livingston and O'Hanlon 2011). Similarly, in Iraq, IED attacks rose from zero in June 2003 to 59 in November/ December to 332 in 2004. By 2007, nearly three quarters of all combat deaths in Iraq resulted from IEDs (Cordesman, Loi, and Kocharlakota 2010; Goldberg 2010).

IED attacks on foot patrols cause blast and thermal injury, blunt trauma, and penetrating fragment wounds. Attacks on vehicles cause burns, penetrating wounds, traumatic brain injury, or near-drowning if vehicles roll over into roadside sewage canals (Hennessy 2016: 1920–1929). Technology developed apace. As Coalition nations improved personal and vehicle armor, insurgents developed increasingly powerful IEDs and explosively formed projectiles (EFPs) to achieve significant armor-piercing capabilities. Coalition casualty rates were high but would drop from 22% to 6% once Coalition forces deployed Mine-Resistant, Ambush-Protected Vehicles (MRAP) to replace the more vulnerable High Mobility Multipurpose Wheeled Vehicle (HUMVEE) at the cost of $43.5 billion (Feickert 2010).

Despite improvements in body and vehicle armor, IED attacks cause unprecedented injuries. Occupants of targeted vehicles often suffer severe, multiple injuries, including open wounds, wounds to the extremities, fractures of the heel, pelvis, and spine, and traumatic brain injury (TBI) (Bricknell, Jones and Hatzfeld 2011; Eastridge et al. 2012b). Although brain injuries are a frequent cause of death in armed conflict, they are increasingly survivable owing to helmets, body armor, and protected vehicles. Karen Hennessy (2016: 1148) describes how TBI, the signature injury of the wars, "occurs when a blow or jolt to the head or a penetrating head injury disrupts brain function and damages brain tissue." Symptoms include memory loss, dizziness, sleep-lessness, cognitive impairment, and mood changes. Approximately 22% of wounded soldiers and 11% to 23% of all deployed soldiers from Iraq and Afghanistan suffered some measure of TBI (Risdall and Menon 2011; also Pazdan et al. 2019). The US Department of Defense (DoD 2018) estimates that over 383,000 service personnel suffered TBI from 2000 to 2018, of which 82% were mild, 12% moderate, and 1% severe or penetrating; the balance of the injuries were unclassified.

In addition to TBI, multiple-body-site injuries were the norm. In one British hospital, the mean injury rate ranged from 2.6 affected body regions among survivors to 4.7 body regions among nonsurvivors in 2006 (Brevard, Champion, and Katz 2012: 53). Multiple battlefield injuries and catastrophic wounds were significantly different from what most medical personnel had seen in their civilian practice. The severity of battlefield injuries led to sig-nificant consumption of resources that would compel Coalition medical forces to develop medical rules of eligibility to ration available bed space and reserve substantial resources for the expected military casualties of the fighting.

Battlefield Medical Care for Warfighters

During the invasion period, multinational forces established medical facil-ities to serve Coalition forces. Five medical *echelons*, or *levels* (in US termi-nology) or *roles* (in UK terminology) managed health care. Each echelon represents an increasingly sophisticated treatment facility that forms an evacuation chain to move the wounded up the chain until they receive ap-propriate care. Echelons I–III are located in-theater, while Echelons IV and V are in Europe and the United States (Lane et al. 2017; Schoenfeld 2012).

Echelon I: Battalion Aid Station
A front-line aid station staffed by a combat medic and/or physician to control hemorrhaging and evacuate to a Level II, Forward Surgical Team (FST) or Level III, Combat Support Hospital (CSH) within one hour of injury.

Echelon II: Forward Surgical Team (FST)
Following evacuation from the field or aid station (Echelon I), a 20-person Forward Surgical Team attends the wounded. FSTs employ orthopedic surgeons, general surgeons, medics, and nurses. A typical FST has two operating tables and a blood bank to allow 30 operations without resupply. Most FSTs have portable ultrasound monitors rather than X-ray machines. Serving three to five kilometers behind the front lines, Echelon II facilities provide damage control resuscitation and surgery until casualties are returned to duty or evacuated to a higher level of care (Rush et al. 2005).

Echelon III: Combat Support Hospitals (CSH)
Combat support hospitals and ancillary recovery facilities in-theater in Kuwait and Qatar afforded the highest level of battlefield medical care. The medical staff provides orthopedic, ocular, thoracic, oral, and maxillofacial surgery, intensive care, and psychiatric treatment. All have X-ray imaging equipment, and some have CT scanners. Although equipped to handle as many as 250 beds, operational capacity was usually much less. At the height of the fighting in Iraq, for example, three Army Combat Support Hospitals and one Air Force Theater Hospital provided five to ten trauma bays, two to five operating rooms, and 10 to 20 ICU beds each. Together they offered services for 141,000 US service personnel in 2005, while 274 operational hospital beds served 150,000 deployed troops in Iraq between 2006 and 2008 (Beekley, Bohman, and Schindler 2012; Belasco 2009; Richardson 2008). The USNS *Comfort,* a 1,000-bed hospital ship that included 80 ICU beds, and additional facilities operating from neighboring Kuwait, supported Operation Iraqi Freedom until June 2003 (Nessen 2005; Paine et al. 2005).

In Afghanistan, five Echelon III facilities operated in Kabul (30 beds), Kandahar (35 beds), Bagram (50 beds), Camp Bastion (25–50 beds), and Mazar-e-Sharif (36 beds) during the height of the fighting in 2010–2011 (Brondex et al. 2014; Lee et al. 2015; Schulz et al. 2012; Vassallo 2015, Doscher 2007). Led by France, the United States, the United Kingdom, and Germany, these hospitals served International Security Assistance Force (ISAF) soldiers and Afghan civilians and security forces. The configuration of the Kabul unit with seven ICU beds, 30 hospital beds, and an outpatient clinic was typical (Brondex et al. 2014). During this period, the ISAF forces numbered 132,000 service personnel (NATO 2011).

Echelon IV: Landstuhl Regional Medical Center (LRMC)
Facilities in Landstuhl, Germany, provided advanced trauma and intensive care for US service personnel that was unavailable in-theater. Medical services included general surgery, orthopedics, pulmonology, critical care, infectious disease, gastroenterology, burn care, and TBI screening and treatment. Most patient visits were short-term. Of the 61,000 patients evacuated to LRMC, 21% returned to duty, and 85% transferred to the United States in less than 96 hours. The dominant injuries were burns, amputations, penetrating wounds, and open and closed head injuries. About 20% of the patients sustained battle-related injuries. Other injuries resulted from disease and accidents, including many sports-related accidents (Hennessy 2016).

Echelon V: The Continental United States and Europe
Following Landstuhl, Walter Reed Army Medical Center, San Antonio Military Medical Center (formerly Brooke Army Medical Center), and the National Naval Medical Center at Bethesda provided continuing treatment for US casualties. In the United Kingdom, The Royal Centre for Defence Medicine (RCDM) at the Queen Elizabeth Hospital Birmingham (QEHB) managed British casualties. Other Coalition nationals received continuing care in their respective countries.

For the most part, these facilities offered excellent care for multinational troops injured in Iraq and Afghanistan. Survival rates improved over time with advances in armor and emergency medicine. Improved body and vehicle armor prevented many fatal injuries and decreased the percentage of soldiers killed in action to the lowest in military medical history. The rate of soldiers killed in action (KIA), that is, direct combat deaths dropped from 21% in Vietnam to 7.1% in Iraq and Afghanistan while the "case fatality rate," that is, the percentage of fatalities among all wounded, dropped from 23% to 9.3%, respectively (Berwick, Downey, and Cornett 2016: 47–48).

Emerging Technologies

Battlefield medicine owes much of its success to rapidly developed technologies without which the tiered infrastructure for delivering care would have been far less effective. Some innovations were decidedly low technology. Improved extremity tourniquets saved an estimated 1,000–2,000 lives between 2005 and 2011 (Berwick, Downey, and Cornett 2016: 40; Kragh et al.

2009). Other innovations reflected advances in hemostatic (blood clotting) agents, hypothermia care, burn management, noninvasive monitoring technologies, and fluid resuscitation (transfusions and blood products). Once stabilized, the wounded benefited from prompt air and ground evacuation to the definitive echelon of care. If it took a month or more for a soldier injured in Vietnam to reach the United States for treatment, severe American casualties reached Germany or the United States within 36 hours of injury (Beekley, Bohman, and Schindler 2012). New and old tools allowed many patients with previously nonsurvivable injuries to live (Bridges and Biever 2010; Perkins and Beekley 2012).

Civilian Medical Care in the Invasion Period

Estimates of civilian deaths ranged from 100,000 to 200,000 in Iraq and 40,000 in Afghanistan (Tapp et al. 2008; Crawford 2018). That number, if not more, suffered war-related injuries (Watson Institute 2019). Owing to the wretched state of health care in Iraq and Afghanistan, civilian medical care in the invasion period suffered considerably. Following sanctions against Iraq after the first Gulf War, widespread shortages of essential commodities increased infant mortality and severely impacted maternal and child care (SIGIR 2013: 110). As the situation deteriorated, medical workers fled Iraq, leaving the country severely shorthanded. American occupation in 2003 brought the dismissal of 20,000 military medical personnel and the closure of 31 military hospitals, further crippling the healthcare system (Bowersox and Al-Ainachi 2006). To provide rudimentary treatment, multinational forces mobilized Medical Civic Action Programs (MEDCAPs) to offer basic clinical care while drawing up plans to rebuild shattered facilities.

Administered by a small military staff and funded by Coalition units, MEDCAPs utilized temporary clinics or mobile medical vehicles to provide direct but short-term treatments. First launched during the Vietnam war, MEDCAPs had been established in conflict zones worldwide with varying degrees of success (Gross 2006: 202–208). MEDCAPs administered vaccinations, conducted health screening, and offered therapy for malnutrition, joint pain, cold symptoms (Lougee 2007; Shafran 2007). At first, individual military units ran MEDCAPs as independent medical operations (Avery and Boetig 2010: 70–71). Later, many came under the purview of Provincial Reconstruction Teams (PRT) (Malsby 2008: 94). MEDCAPs, like PRTs, were often part of concerted public diplomacy to use medicine to win the hearts and minds of the local population. MEDCAPs and their sister PRTs pursued two, sometimes disparate, aims: medical support to upgrade local health care, and medical stability operations to mobilize domestic backing for Coalition forces and the national government. Neither was easy to achieve, and the tension between the two created difficult ethical dilemmas for military and medical practitioners in the field (Chapter 10).

Apart from MEDCAP operations staffed directly by military personnel, US authorities and USAID formulated ambitious plans to deliver primary care and wellness services to 25% of the entire population and 50% of mothers and children (SIGIR 2013:110). These plans were slow to take root. Cumulative healthcare aid would eventually reach close to $1 billion in Iraq (SIGIR 2013: 110) and $1.5 billion from USAID in Afghanistan (SIGAR 2017). But development was sluggish. Contracts awarded in 2004 for $360 million to build primary healthcare centers and $103 million for the Basrah Children's Hospital in Iraq, for example, were only completed four to six years later (SIGIR 2013: 111). As these projects stalled and MEDCAP facilities could only offer minimal care, combat support hospitals had to take up the slack and manage civilian patients. The task would prove daunting and lead authorities to formulate restrictive medical rules of eligibility. These rules, the subject of Chapters 5 through 7, granted preferential treatment to multinational forces but permitted combat support hospitals and forward surgical units to treat local civilians whose wounds were the direct result of Coalition action (i.e., collateral casualties). As such, the medical rules of eligibility severely limited access of local nationals. Iraqi and Afghan civilians could not receive medical attention at military facilities for injuries resulting from accidents, disease, or insurgent fire. In such cases, civilians could only seek care at local hospitals and clinics. Spending on health care increased slowly in Iraq and more slowly in Afghanistan. Per capita health expenditures grew from $16 and $28 in Afghanistan and Iraq during the invasion period to $67 and $210, respectively, in 2017 (WHO 2020). Compare $170 to $341 in nearby Jordan from 2002 to 2017.

Host-nation soldiers fared only slightly better. Among Iraqi and Afghan allies, over 100,000 soldiers and police officers died in the fighting (Crawford 2018). The injured probably numbered at least that many, but there are no reliable figures. Wounded in battle, local security forces could receive initial stabilizing care in a Coalition facility but had to turn to indigenous facilities for follow-up treatment. When local hospitals could not handle the influx, multinational facilities picked up the slack. Initially small, the number of Iraqi security personnel aiding multinational forces soon grew to 60,000–80,000 soldiers (Pollack 2006). By 2006, Iraqi soldiers occupied more than 80% of hospital bed days in US military medical facilities (Bowersox and Al-Ainachi 2006: 1769). But when fighting surged in 2007–2008, the burden of caring for multinational forces increased. By mid-2008, US military personnel accounted for more than 40% of admissions to US military medical facilities, while Iraqis accounted for less than 38% (Richardson 2008). With security precarious, available bed space in military facilities fluctuated considerably during the invasion and into the transition phases.

Medical Care in the Transition Period

> According to existing US military logistic doctrine, no provision exists for US forces to become decisively or exclusively engaged in providing essential services to the populace. However, this doctrinal position does not prohibit units from applying skills and expertise to help assess HN [host-nation] essential services needs. Along with these assessments, logistic and other units may be used to meet immediate needs, where possible and in the commander's interest. These units can also assist in the handoff of essential service functions to appropriate US agencies, HN [host-nation] agencies, and other civilian organizations. (FM 3-24 2006: §8–35)

As the invasion period wound down, multinational facilities maintained their multi-tiered system while continuing to treat Coalition casualties. Differential rules of eligibility led Coalition medical staff to shuttle host-nation nationals to strapped local facilities, causing considerable resentment among host-nation allies. Taking note, counterinsurgency policies shifted civilian care away from combat support hospitals to MEDCAP, PRT, and NGO-supported institutions. High on their projects list were clinics in remote areas, support to restore hospital services, medical training, and preventive medicine (FM 3-24 2006: §8–41). Nevertheless, the army field manual is telling. Counterinsurgency doctrine makes no provision for providing essential services apart from the commander's, that is, military interests.

Recognizing the need to partner with local authorities, multinational forces augmented existing MEDCAPS with PRTs to help raise small-scale projects, including clinics, schools, roads, and water projects (GAO 2008). In contrast to MEDCAPs, PRTs were joint military-civilian ventures staffed by military medical personnel and NGO personnel, defended by multinational forces, and funded by the US Department of Defense (DoD), Department of State, and USAID. In Iraq, four PRTs were established at the end of 2005 and peaked at 25 by 2008. Only one remained in 2011 (SIGIR 2013: 44). In Afghanistan, 26 PRTs (12 US-led and 14 others led by Coalition allies) operated between 2006 and 2012 (GAO 2008: 1) dropping to 13 by 2013 and phased out by mid-2014 (Mitchell 2015). Staff numbers were relatively small, ranging from 80 in American PRTs (5% civilian) and 100 in British facilities (30% civilian) to 400 in German PRTs (5% civilian) (GAO 2008: 4,7). The total numbers were not large. In Afghanistan, for example, 1,021 military personnel and 49 civilians staffed the 12 US PRTs in 2008.

Like MEDCAPs, PRTs have distinct welfare and political agendas. To enhance welfare, they fund and build sanitation and water facilities, utilities, schools, and courthouses in addition to medical clinics and training institutions. These projects benefit the local population directly and enhance their health and economic well-being. Politically, they endeavor to improve the provincial government's credibility to deliver public services. In this way, better medical care, among other welfare projects, could strengthen support for and trust in the national government and wean local civilians from insurgents (Israel 2010; Sargent 2008). When successful, PRTs are an important counterinsurgency tool. But they were never tasked to revamp the entire local healthcare system. Reconstruction would come later as the DoD would bow out, and PRTs would slowly unwind. As the military medical mission phased out, NGOs would cooperate with the local government to rebuild hospitals and clinics with funds provided by the US government and other donor nations.

Military Medicine and Reconstruction

Postwar reconstruction emphasizes the obligation to rebuild a nation ravaged by war. When armed military intervention brings regime change, the ensuing political vacuum exacerbates the plight of the local population. Stepping in, intervening forces and donor nations must tend to the chaos. It is not enough to restore the status quo ante bellum. Nations must go further. Rebuilding, therefore, moves along a continuum. At one end, are plainly stated goals: The purpose of healthcare reconstruction is to enhance health by improving infant mortality, life expectancy, and resistance to infectious disease. In partnership with the local government, NGOs conduct immunization campaigns, train healthcare workers, provide essential drugs, build hospitals and clinics, and improve access. There is no political subtext. At the other end of the spectrum, however, are more ambitious political aims that utilize medicine for governance, state-building, and democratization.

Each faces formidable obstacles. Despite significant funding by donor nations and international organizations, government health care in Iraq and Afghanistan could only deliver 15%–20% of what the inhabitants needed. Private facilities, doctors, and pharmacies provided the rest at a high out-of-pocket cost to patients. Nevertheless, progress was steady in Iraq until a surging ISIS brought the healthcare system to the brink of collapse. Afghanistan moved more slowly and remains heavily dependent on international aid that will steadily diminish.

If the simple goal of improving health outcomes proved challenging, achieving the larger, more complex goals of enhancing governance seem almost beyond reach. Conceptual and material challenges confront state-building. Conceptually, healthcare reconstruction can help establish and strengthen political legitimacy. Assuming an open, collaborative process that engages donors, local communities, stakeholders, and public officials, and which culminates in a fair and equitable healthcare system, medical reconstruction can nurture trust and civic responsibility. It is a very tall order that remains elusive. In theory, community participation does not always translate into state legitimacy. Practically, no donor state or organization can commit the funds necessary to create anything resembling a first-world medical program. Shorn of funds, a solid middle-class tradition of civic responsibility, solidarity, and sufficient human capital, Iraq and Afghanistan are not the same candidates for successful nation-building as postwar Japan and Germany.

Aside the obligation to repair war-torn nations, postwar reconstruction cannot ignore the same duty to reintegrate veterans into civil society. Veteran care is the neglected, flip side of a nation's obligation to rebuild. Of the nearly three million soldiers deployed to Iraq and Afghanistan, one million have filed claims with the US Veterans Health Administration (VHA). To serve veteran patients from Iraq, Afghanistan, and previous conflicts, the VHA maintains dedicated outpatient clinics and medical centers (Chapter 12). In the United Kingdom, the National Health Service (NHS) treats discharged warfighters while national healthcare institutions in Canada, France, Germany, and Australia afford similar services. As estimates of veteran healthcare costs reach hundreds of billions of dollars, each nation finds itself falling short. When nations go to war, they try to estimate their costs. Usually, they are wrong, but they are very wrong when they ignore the price of rebuilding at home and abroad.

Medical Care in the Conflict Zone: Key Points

This overview of military medical management in Iraq and Afghanistan affords the backdrop for a plethora of novel and challenging ethical dilemmas. Initially, multinational forces fought a conventional war that saw overwhelming firepower to shock and awe opponents into submission. Those victories were short-lived and soon usurped by a counterinsurgency that pitted multinational troops against guerillas who sought cover in the civilian population and utilized rear-guard tactics to harass and demoralize the US, British, and other NATO armies. As IEDs became the weapon of choice, the imperative to develop a practical medical doctrine assumed overriding importance. At the same time and typical of insurgencies, the civilian population suffered greatly while each side tried to win them over. Multinational forces mainly utilized positive incentives, including medical care. Insurgents did not shy away from terrorism, extortion, kidnapping, and murder (Gross 2015: 153–212).

War brought intense pressure on military medical infrastructures. Organized for warrior care, US forces experienced a surfeit of resources during the early invasion stage of the war. However, as the fighting dragged on, Coalition forces commanded insufficient assets to treat their own *and* tend local civilians, host-nation allies, and detainees. Whether Coalition governments should or could have mobilized sufficient personnel and materiel for these purposes is one question the subsequent chapters hope to answer. But the legal and ethical principles for providing medical care in a counterinsurgency such as that in Iraq and Afghanistan remain murky. International humanitarian law and medical ethics dictate neutrality and impartiality, but battlefield practice made room for different standards for treating compatriots, enemies, local civilians, and host-nation allies. Changing mission requirements and limited resources, coupled with legal and moral ambivalence about how to best use them, raised the normative questions that occupy the subsequent chapters: Are disparate standards of care for various patient classes defensible? What is the proper balance of medical care for humanitarian purposes and force protection? What level of medical attention do detainees deserve when host-nation *allies* command but pitiable resources? How might medical research enhance warfighters to prevail in counterinsurgency warfare? When does rebuilding a war-torn country end, and what obligations remain to veterans long after all is forgotten?

Answers to such questions are not solely the purview of medical ethics. Instead, they require a political context that asks about the justice of war, how soldiers fight, and the state's duty to rebuild shattered societies and warfighters. As the United States and its Coalition allies unwind military operations in Iraq and Afghanistan after nearly 20 years, many far-reaching strategic, tactical and logistical, legal, and ethical questions confront us. We ask ourselves whether this war was the best way to protect American and Western interests, or is the world better off and safer than before 9/11? We want to know if the war was prosecuted efficiently and whether mistakes were recognized and rectified. And, we want to see if we did our best to care for the men and women sent to fight in a distant, brutal, and inhospitable corner of the world.

5

Combat Casualty Care

As the primary provider of medical care in Iraq and Afghanistan during the invasion period, Coalition medical personnel faced large numbers of host-nation military and civilian casualties as well as Coalition wounded. With only limited resources to attend to local nationals, multinational facilities established medical rules of eligibility (or medical rules of engagement) to regulate the flow of local nationals seeking medical attention. Systematic regulations to govern the management of other than compatriot wounded are unique to 21st-century asymmetric war. More confounding, perhaps, is how emerging practice violates norms of impartiality by institutionalizing preferential treatment for multinational forces. The medical rules of eligibility are not exceptions to the principles of medical ethics but the rule. Justifying these new rules leans heavily on military-medical necessity and associative duties toward compatriots.

The Medical Rules of Eligibility

Under the medical rules of eligibility, local civilians facing an imminent threat to "life, limb, and eyesight" only qualify for treatment if:

Rule 1: Bed space is available at a combat support hospital that is not needed to treat multinational forces, *and*
Rule 2: Their injuries are the direct result of Coalition action (UK MoD 2014: §2.6–2.8; FM 4-02 2013: §1–43).

In practice, there is little ambiguity about the rules of medical eligibility. "Delivery of neurosurgical care is clearly defined by medical rules of engagement," write Paul Klimo and his colleagues (2010: 108), for example. "The *obvious top priority* is to care for all US and Coalition troops with battlefield injuries. Care is also rendered to Afghan National Security Forces, contractors, and local nationals, including children and enemy combatants who are injured as a result of combat operations (emphasis added)."

In each formulation, the medical rules of eligibility defy the principle of impartial medical care so dominant in bioethics. Rule 1 introduces disparate classes of patients and stipulates preferential treatment for multinational forces. Under Rule 1, Coalition forces have absolute priority regardless of the severity of their injuries when presenting for in-theater care at forward surgical units or combat support hospitals and exclusive access to out-of-theater care in their home country. In-theater medical care is short-term. Its purpose is to return the lightly and moderately wounded to duty and evacuate critically wounded multinational soldiers to facilities abroad. In-theater care was neither designed nor funded to afford extended care to the local population or provide more than emergency treatment to host-nation warfighters.

When local nationals present for treatment, eligibility depends on the type of injury, the source of injury, and the patient's identity. Identity is definitive. There are no restrictions on the care of multinational forces. For all others, medical attention is contingent upon an imminent threat to life, limb, or eyesight. Host-nation allies, that is, Iraqi or Afghan security forces fighting alongside multinational troops, receive initial emergency treatment in a Coalition military facility. Once treated, they either return to duty or transfer to the local healthcare system for continued care. Host-nation allied soldiers are not eligible for treatment at Echelon IV or Echelon V facilities. On the other hand, captured insurgents enjoy the high standard of care the Geneva Conventions require (Chapter 6). Civilians fare the worst. They are only eligible for emergency care at Coalition facilities when facing a threat to life, limb, and eyesight (Rule 1) *and* when they suffer injuries as the direct result of Coalition military action (Rule 2). Otherwise, civilians must seek treatment at indigenous facilities. By granting victims of collateral harm an exclusive right to medical care and compensation, Rule 2 pushes far beyond anything ever seen on the modern battlefield. Its ramifications for military medicine during asymmetric war are the subject of Chapter 7. The present chapter focuses on the right to preferential treatment the medical rules of eligibility afford to compatriot warfighters.

Preferential treatment for compatriot warfighters stands in sharp contrast to the conventional principles of civilian medical ethics that prohibit discrimination based on anything but urgent medical need. Whether and how these rules are justified and whether there are better rules to distribute health care is a question that affects battlefield medicine, veteran care, and postwar reconstruction. Traditionally, rules of triage govern the distribution of medical assets. As the following section elaborates, these rules turn on military-medical necessity that permits patients' combat roles, not medical need, to define the order of treatment. But necessity only tells half the story. To explain why compatriots merit better care than host-nation allies when both share the same combat role, one must turn to associative duties. These distinctive duties permit the medical rules of eligibility to carve out a special place for compatriots and establish the cogency of new rules. The following section returns to the norm of medical impartiality I first discussed in Chapter 2. The subsequent sections explain why preferential treatment for compatriot warfighters is not morally objectionable despite the language of international humanitarian law.

The Duty of Impartial Care

International law emphasizes the duty to administer impartial care based solely on a patient's medical needs. The 1949 Geneva Conventions set the stage, instructing belligerents to provide treatment, "without any adverse distinction founded on sex, race, nationality, religion or any other similar criteria," further emphasizing that ". . . Only urgent medical reasons will authorize priority in the order of treatment to be administered" (ICRC 1949a: Article 12). The commentary to Article 12 of the Geneva Convention I (ICRC 2016: Article 12, §2a) drives the point home: *Each belligerent must treat his fallen adversaries as he would the wounded of his own army.* Written in the aftermath of World War II, this rule only embraces members of the armed forces, irregular forces, and some civilian military employees. It did not extend to local civilians or to allies whose care was ordinarily the responsibility of their respective governments. To clear up any misunderstandings, Additional Protocol 1 (1977) puts everyone on equal footing:

> Wounded and sick mean persons, whether military or civilian, who, because of trauma, disease or other physical or mental disorder or disability, are in need of medical assistance or care . . . shall receive, to the fullest extent practicable and with the least possible delay, the medical care and attention required by their conditions. There shall be no distinction among them on any grounds other than medical ones. (ICRC 1977a: Articles 8, 10; ICRC 2016: Article 12, §1325)

The Practice of Impartial Care

This strict interpretation currently infuses the duty of impartial medical care during armed conflict. But if the Geneva Conventions stiffened the principle of impartiality, practice soon loosened it. By 2016, the revised commentary to Article 12 woke up to the reality of asymmetric warfare:

> One difficult question that arises is whether the prohibition of "adverse distinction" prohibits preferential treatment for one's own personnel in situations where enemy personnel receive an acceptable standard of medical care. Reportedly, during the armed conflicts in Iraq and Afghanistan, wounded US soldiers were stabilized and shipped to Germany or the United States as quickly as possible for further treatment, but "Iraqi prisoners and civilians, on the other hand, receive[d] all their care in Iraq." (ICRC 2016: §1396)

To rescue Coalition practice from a clear violation of international humanitarian law, the commentators explain how "it could also be argued that as long as Iraqi soldiers in the power of the United States received the same standard of medical care as US soldiers who were being cared for in Iraq, there is no *adverse* distinction in the sense of paragraph 2 (§1396)."

The argument fails in theory and practice. In theory, there is no convincing reason to think that shipping US soldiers to Germany or the United States and leaving Iraqis to the limited medical attention combat support hospitals can deliver is not a meaningful adverse distinction. In practice, as the subsequent discussion demonstrates, it was not always possible to afford compatriots and host-nation allies or prisoners the same standard of in-theater care. Local health care was far from Coalition standards and could not always provide proper follow-up treatment. As a result, host-nation wounded did not always receive the same sophisticated surgeries that military doctors offered multinational soldiers.

The medical rules of eligibility deviate from the principle of impartiality, and military physicians know it. Medical rules of eligibility "may conflict with medical ethics" notes one handbook for army medical officers (Fish 2014: 42). "The differential treatment of casualties based on nationality does seriously distance the military physicians' responses from those of the civilian humanitarian physician," concludes Stuart Gordon (2014: 425) following interviews with 74 British military medical personnel. The medical rules of eligibility do not attend to patients impartially or without distinction. By focusing on a patient's identity, the rules are discriminatory. But the duty to ensure nondiscriminatory treatment leaves intervening nations only two options. Either military planners must allocate sufficient resources to manage *every* patient at a level commensurate with Western medicine or reserve their scarce resources solely for patients facing imminent threats to life, limb, or eyesight regardless of their national identity. Demanding enormous expenditures that might easily impair a war effort makes the first option unfeasible. Leaving some compatriot soldiers needlessly dead, blind, or crippled makes the second option unpalatable. How might we navigate this dilemma and vindicate preferential treatment for compatriots?

Justifying the Medical Rules of Eligibility

It is tempting to appeal to necessity to substantiate preferential treatment for compatriots. Clinical-medical necessity registers the therapeutic care required to save life and limb, and permits differential care for similar wounds when external factors affect the success of treatment. Military-medical necessity positions medical management in the context of a just war and makes room for preferential consideration when it aids the war effort. Neither can fully justify the medical rules of eligibility, however, without invoking associative duties.

Preferential Treatment for Compatriots:
Clinical-Medical Necessity

Determinations of medical need require medical practitioners to treat similar cases similarly. In some instances, however, clinical-medical necessity may dictate otherwise. A typical example is organ transplantation. Successful transplants depend upon postoperative compliance with rigid therapeutic regimes. Factors militating against compliance, such as drug use or alcoholism, afford good reasons to treat similar transplant cases differently and prioritize certain classes of patients whose behavior or history suggests a better prospect of recovery. Otherwise, a valuable organ goes to waste.

In Iraq and Afghanistan, care for local nationals, whether soldiers or civilians, also depends upon follow-up health care in local facilities. When the facilities cannot deliver appropriate care, there may be grounds for denying or restricting *initial* treatment and offering host-nation allies a different standard of care than comparably wounded Coalition soldiers receive. Consider the following cases:

- . . .doctors were told not to intubate any of the Afghans with burns exceeding 50%. Without a burns unit, those patients would be doomed. The Coalition patients, on the other hand, could be repatriated to their home countries to obtain high-quality burn care. Such divergent treatment is hard to bear and highlights the need to develop local healthcare infrastructures, but what are the immediate alternatives? (Sokol 2011; also Rush, Martin, and Cocanour 2017).

- An Iraqi interpreter presented at a combat support hospital with a shattered elbow. As a local national, there was no follow-up care available that would have permitted surgeons to successfully rebuild the elbow or replace his forearm with an advanced prosthetic device as they would a Coalition soldier. Instead, surgeons performed an elbow arthrodesis that fused his elbow at 90 degrees immobilizing his arm but leaving him the use of his hand (Nessen, Lounsbury, and Hetz 2008: 251–252).

- When eye repair is possible, but the ultimate prognosis for vision or globe survival is slim to nonexistent, repair should be attempted whenever technically feasible . . . This guidance is appropriate in cases where the availability of proper follow-up and ophthalmic surgery can be reasonably assured, such as is the case for service members being evacuated to higher levels of care (Level IV and V facilities). However, if a patient in the same clinical situation may not be able to obtain proper follow-up care (e.g., host-national in a country with no reliable healthcare system), primary enucleation [removal of the entire eye] may be more advisable for the patient's long-term welfare (Cho and Savitsky 2012: 323–324).

- Based on similar observations in head-injured children and adults during our rotation, host-nation casualties with devastating head injuries received palliative care in circumstances in which some Coalition casualties did not. The most recent Joint Theater Trauma System (JTTS) guidelines for the care of patients with severe head trauma have aligned with this management paradigm (Martin et al. 2010: 254; also McCafferty et al. 2018: 3).

In each of these cases, local allies receive differential and inferior medical care for the same injuries that warrant comprehensive treatment for Coalition soldiers. The reality of local health care affords a compelling reason to treat similar injuries differently. One option, of course, is to improve local care. As subsequent discussions demonstrate, however, ethics only demands a basic healthcare package commensurate with local resources, not the level of care available in Western countries (Chapter 12). No basic package has room for the follow-up services necessary to facilitate the advanced trauma care these cases describe. A second option is to exclude local nationals from sophisticated therapies based on clinical-medical necessity.

Clinical-medical necessity conditions medical care on the type of wound or illness, not on the patient's identity. If injuries are equally treatable and do not, for example, require intense follow-up care, then local nationals should receive treatment on par with multinational forces. So, while burns and limb injuries might not enjoy equal treatment, other surgical interventions that do not require sophisticated follow-up should be treated without regard for the patient's identity. However, the medical rules of eligibility are not sensitive to wound types when resources are scarce. Regardless of wound type, host-nation patients move to the end of the queue. Clinical-medical necessity, therefore, does not animate the medical rules of eligibility. Might the principles of military-medical necessity justify their logic more convincingly?

Preferential Treatment for Compatriots: Military-Medical Necessity

Recall how military-medical necessity justifies the least costly medical means a military force requires to effectively pursue just war. Considering medical care for warfighters, Edmund Howe (2003a: 316) suggests that military-medical necessity offers grounds for preferential treatment when it (1) preserves fighting strength by returning the maximum number of soldiers to duty, (2) maintains morale, and (3) fulfills obligations to provide compatriots with the best possible care. Each claim, however, is incomplete. First, military-medical necessity might defend "reverse triage" but does not justify the medical rules of eligibility that reach beyond the demands of triage. Second, there is no compelling evidence that preferential treatment, or lack thereof, affects morale. Third, the moral obligation to treat compatriots before strangers or enemies draws on associative duties rather than necessity.

Preferential Treatment and Force Conservation

Although the Geneva Conventions and the Additional Protocols empha-size the imperative to tend the wounded based solely on medical urgency without distinction, they offer no firm practical guidelines. "Medical need" and "urgent medical reasons" remain undefined. In civilian medicine, urgent medical need often refers to life-saving care. Conventional hospital triage relies on sufficient resources so that all those requiring medical attention will eventually receive it. Patients suffering from imminent life-threatening inju-ries receive care first. At the same time, an abundance of necessary resources assures that those less severely injured or sick will receive care before their condition deteriorates irreversibly. Everyone receives adequate medical at-tention using rules that maximize the number of lives saved.

Disaster or mass casualty triage, on the other hand, sets different constraints when medical assets are scarce and insufficient to attend all ad-equately. Resource scarcity requires policymakers and caregivers to choose eligible patients carefully to maximize lives saved (Horne and Vassallo 2015; Lerner et al. 2011). In what is sometimes called "reverse triage," armies will, under extraordinary conditions, return the moderately injured to duty first, rather than first attending to those with life-threatening injuries (Gross 2006: 137–154). Similarly, mass casualty triage regimes often allow wounded first responders to jump the queue so they can guarantee law and order and attend to the other sick or injured. The logic is utilitarian: salvaging or re-turning as many soldiers as possible to duty will save more lives than trying to save the critically wounded who, if they survive, cannot return to duty and contribute to the war effort. The distributive principles of social utility (maintaining law and order) or military-medical necessity (conserving a fighting force) replace the principle of urgent medical need. Although re-verse triage is rare (DoD 2015: 39–41), the reasoning is sound if there is in-sufficient time, personnel, or equipment to treat all the injured according to need *and* if favoring the less critically injured saves more lives.

Although military-medical necessity can prioritize treatment for combatants who can return to duty, it cannot justify preferential treatment for severely injured compatriots. On the contrary, military-medical neces-sity demands that *all* wounded soldiers, whether compatriots or host-nation allies, compete equally for medical attention based on their chances of reassuming their combat roles. If neither can return to duty, then military-medical necessity demands that each relinquish his claim to scarce medical resources. In practice, however, only local nationals must step aside.

Wayne Kondro (2007: 131), for example, describes the case of a severely wounded Afghan soldier who was allowed to die "because treating him would drain the blood bank":

> We can either continue on for hours and hours and see what we can get to, or if you guys don't think this is going to be successful, let's not use all of our resources because there are a lot of conflicts going in the area. And so a decision was made to stop at that point. . . . [But] this guy, he was a healthy young guy. If he landed in our OR [operating room] here [i.e. stateside], we would go at him all day and all night and do everything and get him to the ICU [intensive care unit]. He may well then die of complications a few days after but still, you're not going to make that conscious decision in the operating room.

Were this patient a Coalition soldier rather than a local ally, doctors and nurses would probably "go at him all day and all night." For local patients, on the other hand, "there was inexorable pressure to just 'stabilize and move [patients] along,' because beds had to be kept open in the event Coalition soldiers from Western nations needed treatment, knowing that Afghani patients were being transferred to a hospital in Kandahar that does not have the ability to mechanically ventilate to keep the patients alive and that their chances of survival were decidedly slim" (Kondro 2007: 131; also Cereste 2011).

Combat medical facilities kept beds open for multinational forces without regard for the severity of their injuries or the likelihood that they could return to duty. Military-medical necessity, therefore, does not explain why the policy of preferential treatment is morally permissible. But concern for soldiers' morale might.

Preferential Treatment and Morale

"It is essential to the morale and combat effectiveness of our Soldiers and their units," declares US Army field manual FM4-02 (2013: §2–7), "that Soldiers recognize and believe they will receive the best and most effective medical care possible should they be wounded or injured." Medical support, suggest NATO policymakers, "reinforces morale through the knowledge that personnel will receive the same standard of care irrespective of their location in theatre" (NATO 2015: 10–12). And, if in-theater resources are insufficient to provide every patient with the highest standard of care, then preferential out-of-theater treatment for compatriots is necessary to preserve morale and conserve the force capabilities. By this reasoning, the medical rules of eligibility fortify morale and help ensure mission success. How sound is this conclusion?

Morale denotes "the enthusiasm and persistence with which a member of a group engages in the prescribed activities of that group" (Manning 1994: 4). Military morale is a positive frame of mind necessary to undertake a dangerous or difficult task. A variety of factors affect military morale. Body armor, up-to-date weaponry, swift evacuation, and health care reduce the risk of death and severe injury. Commanders in Vietnam attributed morale to "creature comforts such as recreational facilities, rest and recuperation, open channels of complaint and information and, the rotation systems" (Kellet 1982: 247). Additionally, military psychologists emphasize the role of organizational factors: group cohesion and a shared sense of purpose, competent leadership, proper training, a responsive organization, and a steady flow of pertinent information (Farley and Veitch 2003).

Surveys in Iraq and Afghanistan paint a picture of dwindling morale since the war's inception. In the fall of 2003, 66% of army soldiers reported medium or high morale, but that figure dropped to 47% by 2010 (Cohen 2015b; Josar 2003). Reviewing the trend in 2015, Raphael Cohen (2015a) concludes that declining morale "stems from the dissonance between the commitment to, and pride in, the mission in Iraq and Afghanistan and the knowledge that these sacrifices have not yielded the desired results." "This mismatch," reasons Cohen, "may also explain why so many soldiers question the army's direction and doubt their senior leadership."

Organizational factors—poor leadership, unattainable military goals, and lack of mission success—underlie discontent far more than the level of medical care. This is not to say that there were no complaints about health care, from going into battle with inadequate medical supplies to the long waits for care in stateside military healthcare facilities (Tilghman 2014). Responding to the lack of adequate mental health care in 2009, the US army decided "to combat the falling morale and lack of mental health professionals in the field" by doubling the number of mental health providers (Mount 2009). In general, however, the troops in the field did not lack medical care nor face the prospect of abandonment that historically decimated morale among soldiers. Lack of medical care inevitably affects morale, but its effects are difficult to isolate. Instead, inadequate care in a modern army reflects the breakdown of the military organization more generally. An army that cannot manage its

wounded is also unable to deliver replacement troops, war equipment, trans-
portation, or even food as needed. It is an army on the verge of defeat, and
morale suffers accordingly.

The Vietnam War underscores the complex factors that affect morale.
Armed with strong leadership and a firm sense of mission, North Vietnam
could maintain high morale with a minimum of medical services as long
as troops were assured of evacuation from the battlefield and fair access to
whatever meager treatment North Vietnamese doctors could offer (Gross
2006: 79–80). This is precisely the lesson we glean from South Vietnam.
Morale was abysmal, and desertion was a constant drain. And while Robert
Brigham (2006: 71–73) cites substandard medical care, additional factors including lack of food, low pay, inadequate housing, corrupt officers, and arbitrary conscription laws contributed to demoralization. Meager food, pay,
health care, and housing also afflicted the North, but unlike their enemies,
South Vietnamese soldiers suffered a crisis of confidence in their military
and political leadership. A similar crisis of morale bedevils Afghan Security
Forces where high casualties, poor pay and living conditions, corrupt leadership, intimidation by insurgents, and lack of medical care fuel desertion
(Cordesman 2017; Jalali 2016). Morale may be essential for military success,
but medical care is neither necessary nor sufficient to maintain the requisite
fighting spirit. The futility of war, rather than poor medical management, de-
moralized multinational and local troops in Vietnam, Iraq, and Afghanistan.

Despite the diffuse effects of medical care more generally, *differential*
treatment may impair morale directly. Facing a host-nation soldier with
catastrophic injuries, participants in a British workshop chose to evacuate
the soldier rather than terminate treatment and let him die "because of the
negative effect of morale for partnered ANA of perceiving different levels of
care being provided based on nationality" (O'Reilly 2011: 409; also Brigham
2006: 69–72). In contrast, undifferentiated, impartial care may impair
Coalition morale if the same Afghan soldier receives medical attention at a
Coalition soldier's expense. Which argument is more persuasive?

There are two dimensions to each claim: the underlying moral principle
and the practical effects of differential treatment. The Afghan soldier dreads
just what the previous case studies describe: premature termination of treatment and discharge to a substandard healthcare system that affords little
hope of recovery. Similarly, Coalition soldiers fear they will be denied life- or
limb-saving care if local nationals occupy the beds they need. Without sufficient resources for all, there is no way to alleviate these fears entirely. In an

austere environment, one can only try to formulate morally defensible principles of resource distribution. Military-medical necessity does some of the heavy lifting when it affords grounds to offer priority care to those who can return to duty. But this principle does not decide among those who cannot return to duty, or between a lightly wounded Coalition soldier and a more seriously injured host-nation ally.

Morale does not provide the requisite principle because it cuts in two directions. If preferential treatment weakens morale among those who receive fewer medical resources, it strengthens morale among those who receive more. To break this stalemate, one might invoke special obligations toward compatriots.

Preferential Treatment for Compatriots: Gratitude and Associative Duties

Warfighters benefit from two special obligations that afford a prima facie justification of preferential treatment. The first reflects the debt civilians owe those fighting on their behalf. The second calls on associative duties and the special obligation of care due to compatriots. Considering the first, Howe (2003a: 316–317) describes how "treating soldiers, POWs, and civilians equally could undermine the present implicit promise made to all soldiers to give them the best medical care possible." This sentiment is a common one and draws on the intuition that those risking their lives for their nation deserve unmatched care. I return to this claim in detail when I consider veteran care (Chapter 12) and only suggest here that the argument is problematic for two reasons. First, it introduces desert into claims for medical resources, a factor foreign to civilian medical ethics, and without any apparent justification in military medical ethics. Second, risk-based claims, if compelling, extend to all those warfighters defending one's country and offer no grounds to exclude allies. If risking one's life generates a unique right to receive medical care, then allies fighting side by side should enjoy it equally. In contrast, associative duties encompass exclusive rights and responsibilities specific to compatriots.

Associative Duties, Special Obligations, and the Ethics of Care

Although discomfited by the way medical rules of eligibility upend their commitment to impartial care, military medical personnel often sense a special obligation to tend compatriots. Consider the following case:

One US soldier and one Iraqi Army [allied] soldier present with a gunshot wound to the chest. Both have low oxygen saturations. There is only enough lidocaine for local anesthesia for one patient, and only one chest tube tray. One will get a chest tube with local anesthesia, and the other will get needle decompression and be monitored by the flight medic.[1]

In this case, medics assess a field injury before evacuation to a second or third level echelon facility. The choice they make does not determine who lives but who gets a better standard of care (the chest tube). Working through the dilemma in a workshop at the Walter Reed National Military Medical Center in 2009, the moderators (including the author) asked participants, all military medical service personnel, "Who gets the chest tube and local anesthesia and why?" The decision was nearly unanimous: The American gets the better treatment. Why? Because "He's our brother" (Gross 2013).

The principle of military-medical necessity is unhelpful in this case. Each soldier's contribution to the war effort is presumably equal. Clinical-medical necessity would generally carry the day based on which patient is the most severely ill, is expected to best benefit from medical attention, or has access to better follow-up care. With the Iraqi soldier facing continuing care in a poorly equipped local facility, one might reasonably invoke clinical-medical necessity to justify better treatment for the Coalition soldier. But this was not the response. Instead, participants disregarded necessity entirely to invoke the special obligation one owes comrades-in-arms. These are associative duties and lie at the heart of the first rule of medical eligibility.

"Associative" duties, outlined in Chapter 2, reflect the special obligation of care individuals owe family, friends, and compatriots. As do family and friends, compatriots often will aid one another without expectation of payment in kind, often at high personal cost, and while knowing that the same aid might benefit a stranger more. Like other special relationships that generate associative duties, the bond among soldiers affords a defining element of personal identity and contributes to individual and collective survival. At many levels, military units comprise a moral community that generates "particularistic" or special obligations to its members that do not extend to everyone (Etzioni 2002: 577). Failure to fulfill this obligation and fully support comrades bonded by friendship ties and camaraderie may precipitate profoundly intense trauma and guilt (Grossman 2014: 89). For a military medic, doctor, or nurse, fulfilling this obligation of support often requires preferential treatment for compatriots.

Nevertheless, it seems that extending compatriotism and associative duties to other members of a multinational force is tenuous. Americans might owe a unique duty of care to other Americans, but do they owe the same obligation to other Coalition soldiers? Two reasons explain why compatriotism pushes beyond narrow parochialism in humanitarian war. First, multinational forces delineate a moral community or association bonded by a shared sense of humanitarian mission that engenders associative duties of its own. More powerfully, Coalition members agree to help one another fulfill their associative duties toward compatriots as a condition for participating in humanitarian war. No single nation can meet its responsibilities to fellow citizens without assistance from its partners.[2]

By creating a unique class of privileges, associative duties run afoul of justice when foreigners or anyone outside the association are in greater need but receive poorer care. With this in mind and assuming that soldiers fear substandard care should they fall captive, Paul Gilbert (2013) expects warfighters to reject associative duties and demand a general rule of impartial care. Perhaps some do, but the chances of Coalition soldiers falling captive in Iraq and Afghanistan were exceptionally low. And whether soldiers can relinquish their associative duties, any more than a parent can, is a perplexing question seemingly at odds with human experience. Associative duties generate overwhelming claims for preferential treatment that draw inexorably from "our specific historical and social identities, as they develop and evolve over time, [and] continue to call forth claims . . . which are not reduced to silence by general considerations of need," observes Samuel Scheffler (2002: 64). Parochial human identities, considerations of need, and justice make inherently incommensurable demands and, therefore, yield competing, compelling, and irreconcilable prescriptions for thought and action.

Nevertheless, one may take steps to reduce the tension between justice and the duties of association by paying attention to the facts on the ground. When resources are abundant, associative duties hold no sway because there are sufficient time, personnel, and medical provisions to treat according to urgent medical need. However, when resources are scarce and medical needs radically disparate so that strangers are critically wounded and compatriots only lightly injured, then the duty to ensure "moral minimums" of care prevails (Held 2006: 71; Miller 2005). At this juncture, associative duties bump up against the fundamental right to health care that any soldier or civilian enjoys. Moral minimums take precedence and require military medical personnel to attend to a severely injured local national before a superficially wounded compatriot unless the imperative to return the latter to duty dictates otherwise. Ensuring minimal care, moreover, may also obligate intervening forces to maintain sufficient medical resources for local allies or civilians (Chapter 7) throughout their operations. As resources grow to meet the need, conflicts between associative duties and human rights claims attenuate.

Scarcity, however, plagues battlefield medicine. Here, associative duties play out. When medical needs are equal, as characterized the Iraqi and American soldiers with gunshot wounds, associative duties function as a tiebreaker. "He's our brother" affords extra moral weight that tips favored treatment toward one's compatriot. Tiebreaking exemplifies the weak role of associative duties that the medical rules of eligibility implicitly acknowledge. They do not override medical needs but offer an additional moral criterion to decide between two equally needy cases.

But what if resources are scarce and the extent of injuries only moderately unequal? May associative duties permit military medical personnel to tend compatriots first when others require more urgent attention? Intuitively, the answer is yes. A father need not, and indeed should not, falter even if saving his drowning child means that two others whom he can save perish instead. Medical rules of eligibility reflect this intuition by allowing military medical caregivers to treat compatriots while letting higher numbers of non-compatriots go untreated when resources are scarce. This rule can only apply, however, when injuries are *moderately* disparate. When injuries are radically unequal, moral minimums trump associative duties.

Wounds are difficult to evaluate precisely, particularly at the point of injury. Still, moderately unequal injuries among the wounded may translate into a preference for saving fewer compatriot lives rather than a higher number of non-compatriot lives, or restoring injured compatriots to reasonable functioning (by saving their limbs or eyesight) instead of saving the life of a non-compatriot (Gross 2013). In these cases, associative duties can play a substantial role and override relative medical need when compatriots face life- and limb-threatening danger. The argument is not instrumental; compatriots do not merit preferential treatment because they, rather than local troops, can return to duty. Instead, associative duties reach beyond utility to commitments that draw on and maintain the emotive bonds and unique relationships that vouchsafe membership in a moral community. As an essential element of what it means to be human, associative relationships and commitments are intrinsically good and worthy of protection in their own right. This aspect of associative duty is the subtler, noninstrumental meaning of "He's our brother" that justifies medical rules of eligibility that give preference to compatriots when utility might dictate otherwise.

But if associative duties are of overriding importance, why don't they apply to peacetime medical management? Workshop participants understood that it would be inappropriate to give preferential treatment to their biological brother if, for example, there were many deserving patients and only one bed left in the ICU. Associative duties should not function as a tiebreaker in this case; a lottery is morally preferable. Avoiding conflicts of interest is one way to explain the difference between the two cases. In a civilian hospital, chaos and conflicting claims would ensue if each caregiver gave preference to his or her sibling. In the military setting, however, there is a consensus: all compatriots are brothers and sisters to whom practitioners owe a special obligation of care. This view mirrors associative rules in many national healthcare systems that attend to indigent compatriots but not destitute foreigners. Full eligibility turns on national identity; foreigners must either pay for services or return home for all but emergency care.

When resources are limited, hard moral dilemmas bedevil military medicine. Even when funded by a country as wealthy as the United States, scarcity plagues wartime medical care. Under these circumstances, providers often are torn among legal norms, military-medical necessity, clinical-medical necessity, and associative duties. These are not easy dilemmas to navigate, but in cases such as those described, medics, nurses, and doctors should feel no moral compunction about providing priority care to compatriots. Associative duties augment necessity and explain when and why it is permissible to tend a more severely injured compatriot before less severely injured host-nation soldiers. Nevertheless, associative duties cannot run roughshod over fundamental moral norms or permit abject neglect. But do associative duties permit bumping active host-nation patients when compatriots present for medical care? The short answer is no.

Regulating Triage and Bumping Patients

Consider a commanding officer who orders a surgeon to interrupt the surgery of a local national to treat incoming Coalition casualties or to vacate ICU beds occupied by host-nation patients to hospitalize Coalition wounded with multiple injuries (Easby, Inwald & McNicholas 2015: 464). In contrast to choosing among untreated patients, a strong moral intuition prohibits interrupting surgery to tend another unless the first patient can be safely set aside for the time required to manage the incoming casualty. This obligation is not peculiar to medicine. Imagine a lifeguard who rescues a drowning swimmer only to have another flail his arms as he approaches the shore. Had both presented simultaneously, his choice might rest on the probability of success and associative duties. Once he undertakes to rescue one swimmer, however, he cannot abandon him to his death for another.

In these cases, the rescuer answers the injured or drowning person's call for help. Once she does, she agrees to fulfill the obligation of rescue. The rescuer's agreement reinforces the rescuee's claim right to aid. One can only imagine extreme circumstances that might allow the rescuer to abandon one rescuee for another, say to save another lifeguard who can then help save many more. But abandoning one's acknowledged obligation to aid another in this case depends on the certain knowledge that the rescuer can save the second rescuee so that he is fit to save others. Rarely is this the case. The attending surgeon is situated similarly. Apart from a justified concern that withdrawing treatment is akin to murder, the surgeon enters into a privileged relationship once he begins treating any wounded person. This new relationship carries substantial obligations of care of its own that a medical practitioner cannot readily abandon unless medical treatment is futile.

When care is futile hospital staff may reasonably limit available treatment. Consider the following case:

> A severely wounded soldier arrives by helicopter at your Combat Support Hospital or Forward Surgical Team. Half of his abdominal wall is missing with exposed viscera and active bleeding. He arrests on arrival and you get him back. In the operating room, you start on his abdomen while anesthesia continues to resuscitate with blood products . . . Seven "urgent surgical" patients are inbound, and your anesthesiologist tells you he just hung the tenth unit of blood, which is half of your total blood supply (Rush, Martin, and Cocanour 2017: 750).

The authors ask: Do you continue and exhaust your unit's blood supply on this patient with a low probability of survival? Do you stop and make this patient "expectant," allowing him to die so that you can attend to other injured patients?

There are two decisions here, first to stop treatment and second to tend others. The decision to stop treatment is a medical decision subject to an assessment of futility irrespective of available resources. If the probability of survival is low, then ceasing care is permissible and worlds apart from abandoning a patient who will most likely survive surgery. The second decision is whom to tend among the seven incoming. Under the current rules of eligibility, multinational forces enjoy priority care while host-nation allies will receive emergency care subject to available resources. The goal is to evacuate the Coalition casualties out-of-theater and discharge host-nation allies to local hospitals. Lack of requisite follow-up care may affect initial treatment decisions for allies. Subject to moral minimums, however, the decision may be different. When all seven incoming wounded suffer comparable injuries, associative duties function as a tiebreaker if resources are scarce. Were they suffering widely disparate injuries, however, the moral minimum of care dictates prior treatment for the most severely wounded.

Medical Care for Compatriots and Allies: A Sustainable Rule of Eligibility

"When the military hospital system is full," writes Martin Bricknell (2014: 459), former Surgeon General of the British Armed Forces, "local security force casualties and captured persons would still be eligible for emergency care. Once treated [local security forces] transfer to a local hospital or discharge while insurgent forces transfer to a detainee facility." These regulations are the crux of medical eligibility for warfighters.

Carefully splitting hairs, one might argue, as the Geneva Conventions commentators do, that no warfighter, whether Coalition or host-nation ally, receives differential emergency care at a military medical facility. Narrowly true, perhaps, this narrative ignores how host-nation wounded will not necessarily receive anything more than emergency treatment or will not receive the *same* emergency care due to lack of suitable facilities for follow-up treatment after discharge. As a result, the medical rules of eligibility repudiate the long-standing norm of impartial medical care on the battlefield.

The changing circumstances of asymmetric war, particularly humanitarian war, alter the norms of military medical ethics. In conventional war, state military organizations typically attend to their own. Modern histories of military medicine detail the health care that state armies in World War I and World War II provided their troops (Gabriel 2013: 193–244) but offer few details about if and how they tended local allies. When war turns from self-defense to intervention, host-nation allies often shoulder a consider-able portion of the fighting without adequate health care. In South Vietnam, for example, 1,000 doctors served the entire nation during the war, and of these, 700 serviced the South Vietnamese Army (Brigham 2006: 70–73). South Vietnamese troops frequently complained of inadequate resources to evacuate the wounded, shortages of medical staff, lack of supplies, and inad-equate care at local hospitals. Indeed, more than 10,000 wounded and dis-abled soldiers returned to their villages rather than accept medical care at "overcrowded and poorly supplied" healthcare facilities (Brigham 2006: 72).

Three decades later, medical rules of eligibility in Iraq and Afghanistan introduced measures to address the needs of host-nation allies but did not overcome the antagonism accompanying differential treatment protocols. Explaining how "the Afghan people are painfully aware that the international military and NATO bases benefit from sophisticated medical services," and warning that "the anger that this generates further endangers the lives of the military troops who are doing their best to bring peace to Afghanistan," the SENLIS Council (2007: v) captures the downside of medical eligibility rules. Short of an enormous infusion of resources to provide host-nation allies with the same high level of care that multinational forces receive, there is no way to fully assuage Afghan or Iraqi anger.

One way to narrow the medical-care gap between intervening and local forces is to step back from equal health care for all and equalize military outcomes instead. If the overriding goal of combat casualty care is to main-tain fighting strength, and host-nation forces are as proficient as Coalition forces, then each should receive the care necessary to return moderately and lightly wounded troops to duty. Among US forces in Iraq, for example, 55% returned to duty within 72 hours (Goldberg 2010: 221). Due to poor record-keeping and relatively high rates of desertion in some areas, it is dif-ficult to calculate the return-to-duty (RTD) rate for Afghan and Iraqi secu-rity forces. Nevertheless, utility demands that military medical policy ensure sufficient resources to equalize RTD rates by providing more than emer-gency care to wounded local allies. Absent broader directives for host-nation allies, the requisite care might mirror the "resuscitative care, limited hospi-talization for stabilization and short-term medical treatment, with an em-phasis on return to duty . . . " that contractors accompanying military forces enjoy (Hodges 2010: 54). Under this revised rule of eligibility, host-nation allies will receive broader in-theater care than they currently enjoy, but not out-of-theater evacuation unless additional resources are forthcoming. As a result, the revised rule cannot entirely equalize RTD rates because multinational forces will benefit from care in Germany or their home nations. Among some 60,000 US forces treated in Landstuhl, Germany, for example, more than 20% returned to duty (Hennessey 2016: 1051). Local forces will not enjoy this advantage. For this reason, the revised rule, too, violates the principle of impartiality.

A rule of medical eligibility that guarantees broader in-theater casualty care to equalize return-to-duty rates helps to narrow the care gap among all service personnel while respecting the contribution of local allies. But the gap is not bridged entirely. Nations requesting intervention to oust a rapacious regime strike a bargain with international forces. In return for military assistance and the prospect of a better life, the host-nation is willing to suffer the devastating effects of war, including inadequate medical attention. Nevertheless, the ensuing bargain calls for military and economic assistance to train personnel and build the infrastructures necessary for the host-nation to defend itself alone and secure a decent life for its people. Under these circumstances, the host-nation may reasonably request the health care, equipment, and training necessary to fight well and preserve its respect and dignity. The cost is high, but the duty of humanitarian intervention does not require a state to bankrupt itself to appreciably improve the lives of another people (Chapter 11). Nor is the rescuer obligated to forego its associative duties to its fighters. An information campaign to explain the rights and duties of intervening forces and host-nation peoples is undoubtedly a helpful adjunct to the medical rules of eligibility.

Neither measure, whether an expanded rule of medical eligibility or an accompanying information campaign, directly addresses medical care for detainees or civilians. Detainees prod our moral intuitions when enemy forces receive significantly better health care than allied forces. This is one subject of the following chapter. In contrast, civilians have no claim to medical care under a rule that equalizes return-to-duty rates. Instead, civilians appeal to another rule, unprecedented in warfare, that recognizes liability for collateral casualties and offers its victims medical attention and monetary compensation. Civilian health care during armed conflict is the subject of Chapter 7.

6

Detainees and Prisoners of War

When host-nation troops fight alongside those intervening on their behalf, the rules governing medical care for detainees are morally puzzling. The medical rules of eligibility offer Coalition forces and detainees access to superlative medical facilities but only provide short-term emergency treatment to host-nation allies. After that, host-nation allies return to the local health-care system to manage as best they can, while detainees stay on in multinational medical facilities. In the previous chapter, I explained how associative obligations and military-medical necessity justify preferential treatment for compatriots. In this chapter, I consider the ethical challenges of a system that prioritizes detainees over allies, but, at the same time, ignores or limits other healthcare rights.

In the wake of abuses at Abu Ghraib (Fay and Jones 2004), many may question any assertion of decent, let alone preferential, care for detainees in Coalition-run prisons. But following significant command and policy changes in late 2004, conditions steadily improved (Benard et al. 2011: 49–82), and the ICRC conducted regular inspections (e.g., ICRC 2006; 2007b; 2009a). The following section describes detainee care and asks how medical care on par with compatriots is morally justified. The answer is that it is not. There are no grounds to offer detainees better care than host-nation allies. If anything, it seems that allied warfighters deserve *better* treatment than captured enemy insurgents. The subsequent sections move from medical care for detainees to interrogation, torture, and force feeding. I will not review the interrogation debate in any great detail. Instead, I will ask about complicity and suggest that the public debate, particularly in the United States, met many, but not all, the conditions of moral discourse and democratic deliberation that mitigate charges of war crimes. Force feeding often is described as an adjunct of torture. Closer analysis, however, reveals a complex issue that tempers unconditional respect for patient autonomy with security concerns when detainees employ nonviolent resistance to press political claims during armed conflict.

Medical Care for Detainees

To qualify for medical care, wounded and sick enemy combatants must "refrain from any act of hostility." Sensing confusion, the commentary to the First Geneva Convention continues: "Thus, contrary to the ordinary meanings of the terms 'wounded' and 'sick', persons who continue to engage in hostilities do not qualify as wounded or sick under humanitarian law, no matter how severe their medical condition may be" (ICRC 2016: Article 12, §1345).

Explaining a detainee's right to health care, the commentary emphasizes a fundamental difference between civilian and military medical ethics. Although a "severe medical condition" is ordinarily sufficient to trigger a person's right to medical attention, a wounded enemy soldier must "refrain from any act of hostility" to gain access to care (ICRC 2016: Article 12, §1345). No state is obligated to tend an enemy whose further inability to fight is not ensured. Once disarmed and detained, enemy personnel join the pool of all eligible wounded—compatriots and local nationals alike—whom the medical staff must treat based on urgent medical need alone. The 1952 commentary attending the First Geneva Convention emphasizes how "each belligerent must treat his fallen adversaries as he would the wounded of his own army" (ICRC 1952: Article 12, §2a).

Article 12 and its related provisions set the legal standards for detainee care. Following revelations of detainee abuse in Abu Ghraib, Iraq, in 2003 and 2004, the Army Inspector General found "significant shortfalls in training and force structure for field sanitation, preventive medicine and medical treatment requirements for detainees" (Schlesinger et al. 2004: 57). Later regulations for detainee care mirrored Article 12:

> Healthcare personnel charged with the medical care of detainees have a duty to protect detainees' physical and behavioral health and provide appropriate treatment for disease. To the extent practicable, treatment of detainees should be guided by professional judgments and standards similar to those applied to personnel of the US Armed Forces. (DoD 2006: §4.1.2; also FM4-02.46 (2007): §1–29)

British regulations for treating captured persons also stipulate medical standards "equivalent to those applied to members of the UK Armed Forces" (Simpson, Wilson, and Tuck 2014: 4).

As the medical rules of eligibility developed, there was little ambiguity about the medical attention that detainees were entitled to receive. In practice, and despite American doubts about the applicability of the Geneva Conventions to detainees, American and Coalition medical facilities endeavored to offer detainees in-theater care on par with that of multinational forces. Consistent with revised regulations for detainee care, the US government deployed combat support hospitals to Abu Ghraib and southern Iraq to tend military personnel and detainees in mid-2005 (Lee 2012; Sheaffer 2007). In general, detainee medical care sought the same level of in-theater medical attention Coalition troops received. Detainees, however, did not qualify for out-of-theater evacuation to Europe or the United States (Chalela 2017; Murray et al. 2005; Patton 2009; Tuck 2005). And although ICRC prison visit reports are confidential, a leaked summary of its January 2008 inspection of Camp Bucca, Iraq, a facility housing 20,000 detainees (AFPS 2008), describes "no allegations of abuse, misbehavior or mistreatment against any US personnel" (Sasahara 2008).[1] If multinational troops received five-star care, detainees enjoyed the right to four-star care. Host-nation allies and civilians, on the other hand, had to contend with poorly staffed and maintained indigenous medical facilities offering them three-star care at best.

Why do detainees merit greater medical attention than host-nation allies? If the right to health care turns on means necessary to maintain a dignified life as previous chapters contend, then they do not. This right does not vary with the patient's identity. But this is only to say that each deserves the same primary care. Medical ethics does not necessarily prohibit differential treatment beyond the baseline of moral minimums. And, in contrast to the 1952 Geneva Convention commentary, the 2016 commentary offered conditional support for differential treatment:

> The gist of [Article 12] is not to prevent one's own soldiers from receiving the best possible medical care, but to ensure that enemy soldiers receive the kind of care required by their medical condition and that the standard of care that enemy soldiers receive is not lowered in order to make personnel and other resources available for the treatment of one's own forces. (ICRC 2016: Article 12, §1396)

Coming too late to affect detainee care in Iraq and Afghanistan, the 2016 guidelines pose a new challenge for future wars. Rather than demand equal treatment for detainees, the commentary sets a floor that implies some minimal standard of care. One challenge is to flesh out these requirements. This standard should comprise the medical resources required to maintain a dignified life and is no different from the basic package of healthcare services (BPHS) local governments must implement during reconstruction (Chapter 11). The second challenge is for intervening forces and donor nations to allocate the resources necessary to maintain this level of care for any local national, whether allied warfighter, civilian, or detainee. Each task is daunting; but once achieved, there is no moral justification for treating one's fallen adversaries as one's own. Instead, the rule is to treat one's fallen adversaries as one treats any local national.

Reciprocity, however, might afford another reason for equal standards of care among belligerents and their prisoners. The underlying norm is self-interest, not unilateral humanitarian duties. On this view, enemies offer one another comparable care with the expectation that one's wounded will enjoy adequate medical attention if captured. Whether reciprocity holds in asymmetric warfare is an open question. First, guerrilla armies usually have inadequate medical resources to tend their soldiers, let alone enemy prisoners. More telling, only a handful of American soldiers, for example, fell captive to insurgents in Iraq and Afghanistan. Therefore, it is unlikely that reciprocity drives Coalition concern for captured insurgents. Instead, Coalition facilities care for their prisoners because this is their legal obligation. In the early years of each war, detainees remained in Coalition-run detention centers where they received a relatively high standard of medical attention. Only after the consummation of status-of-forces and similar agreements with newly constituted governments in Iraq (2008) and Afghanistan (2012) did detainees transfer to locally managed prison facilities where they received a standard of care commensurate with indigenous health care (SOFA 2008, Article 22; Holman 2008; MOU 2012). In the interim, however, detainees enjoyed a higher level of healthcare than host-nation allies.

The moral justification for providing or funding a superior level of health care for detainees is elusive. Reciprocity is irrelevant. Detainees have no superior right to medical care and, therefore, the three categories of host-nationals—civilians, soldiers, and detainees—warrant the same standard of medical attention. Achieving this aim requires occupying powers to transfer detainees to the local healthcare system just as they do host-nation wounded, and to work assiduously to rebuild local healthcare institutions to deliver the healthcare services essential to maintaining a dignified life.

Medical Personnel and Interrogation

Despite policies to provide detainees with a relatively high level of health care, interrogation and detainee abuse captured many observers' attention. The debate over enhanced interrogation ravished military medical ethics during wars in Iraq and Afghanistan following charges that medical personnel participated in CIA interrogation sessions (Lifton 2004; Miles 2004). Looking back at the CIA interrogation program, it is useful to start at the end of the debate following calls to prosecute medical professionals for war crimes or censure them for violations of medical ethics (McColl, Bhui, and Jones 2012; Miles 2020; Miles, Alencar, and Crock 2010; O'Connor 2009). Throughout the wars and after, however, successive US administrations shielded interrogators from prosecution claiming their orders to participate were not manifestly unlawful. Establishing manifest unlawfulness turns on an appeal to public conceptions of justice that emanate from moral discourse and democratic deliberation.

This chapter does not adjudicate the ethics of interrogation. After outlining how medical personnel supported interrogation, the discussion focuses instead on civic discourse: Did the public debate affirm the manifest injustice of interrogation and, thereby, afford grounds for refusing superior orders? The short answer is "no," but there are important qualifications about the lack of credible information.

Medical Support for Enhanced Interrogation

Enhanced interrogation describes aggressive techniques that include hooding, stress positions/wall-standing, loud music, sleep and sensory deprivation, threats and humiliation, and waterboarding. Between 2002 and 2007, the CIA's detention and interrogation program utilized these techniques to interrogate 39 detainees (SSCI 2014). The CIA's Office of Medical Services (OMS) first detailed the role of medical personnel in a heavily redacted report in 2004, later released in 2009, and in a 2007 report publicly released in 2018 (CIA 2004; 2007). Many details did not emerge until 2014 with the publication of the 2012 *Report of the Senate Select Committee on Intelligence of the CIA's Detention and Interrogation Program* (hereinafter SSCI). This report confirmed many earlier accounts about the role military psychologists, physicians, and physician assistants played during enhanced interrogation. (e.g., Bloche and Marks 2005; Bloche 2011; ICRC 2007a; Miles 2006; Pope 2011). Psychologists questioned detainees or advised interrogation officers about effective techniques (SSCI 2014: xix–xx; 72; 107). Physicians and physician assistants monitored and treated detainees for the effects of waterboarding, stress positions, wall-standing, or sleep deprivation (SSCI 2014 42; 70; 84–87; 132, 415–416, 419).

The authority of medical personnel to halt or modify interrogations is unclear. Although the Senate report describes how authorities discontinued enhanced interrogation because medical officers voiced concern about "unacceptable medical or psychological risks" (SSCI 2014: 148), the Committee largely rejected CIA claims that "an interrogation session would be stopped if, in the judgment of the interrogators or medical personnel, medical attention was required" (SSCI 2014: 113; 420; 490). The reaction of medical officers to interrogation varied from support to reproach. Some acknowledged the utility of waterboarding to control detainees or "vet information on an as-need basis," while others noted the ineffectiveness of waterboarding and other enhanced interrogation techniques. Medical assessments were similarly disparate. Some medical personnel criticized the CIA for exceeding guidelines for the number of permissible waterboarding sessions, while others offered suggestions to "avoid water intoxication and dilution of electrolytes" by using saline in future sessions (SSCI 2014: xxiii; 84–89).

Echoing the ICRC (2007a), the US field manual *Medical Support to Detainee Operations* permits healthcare personnel and psychologists to "provide advice concerning interrogations of detainees when the interrogations are fully in consonance with applicable law," and do not entail physical, emotional, or sexual abuse (FM 4-02.46 2007: §1-42; 57). Whether CIA interrogations met these conditions was the question that fed the American government's response and the broader debate about the legitimacy of enhanced interrogation.

Enhanced Interrogation: The American Response

Evaluating accusations of war crimes for complying with superior orders requires answers to two questions. First, could military medical personnel have acted differently? Second, did medical workers recognize that CIA interrogation techniques were manifestly unlawful or immoral? Juxtaposing the common understanding that "ignorance of the law is no excuse" with "legal reassurances that illegal practices are, in fact, legal," Clare Finkelstein and Stephen Xenakis (2020: 501–503) describe how "uniformed personnel are in a difficult position." On the one hand, senior officials approved interrogation procedures and issued orders accordingly. On the other, service personnel refusing superior orders face disciplinary action. High-level approval speaks to ignorance; the threat of court-martial speaks to coercion. Either may mitigate charges of war crimes (Dinstein 1985: 236–238). Coercion, however, is secondary to ignorance. One needs to understand that an order is unlawful before considering the consequences of disobedience.

Recognizing the exculpatory power of ignorance, the 2005 Detainee Treatment Act (Sec. 1004 and 42 USC §2000dd-1) specifies how "it shall be a defense that such [interrogation] officer or other agent did not know that the practices were unlawful and a person of ordinary sense and understanding would not know the practices were unlawful. Good faith reliance on the advice of counsel should be an important factor, among others, to consider in assessing whether a person of ordinary sense or understanding would have known the practices to be unlawful." President Obama reaffirmed US policy in 2009 when he pronounced that those carrying out their duties would not be subject to prosecution (Obama 2009).

Adopting this formulation, the US administration offers a blanket, a priori defense to any interrogator or medical facilitator who complied with superior orders. Referring to the US Department of Justice (2002) memorandum authorizing enhanced interrogation, "advice of counsel" is, however, too thin an authority to command sweeping exculpatory power. More compelling, instead, is to evaluate the entire public debate and ask: Did the ensuing discussion offer reasoned arguments for a person of ordinary sense and understanding to comply with US interrogation policy, despite (or because of) evidence that the CIA lied about interrogation techniques from its inception? The test of manifest unlawfulness is not so much to parse isolated legal documents but to think carefully about how persons of ordinary sense and understanding would reason through and understand enhanced interrogation together with the other members of their political community. This process is the essence of democratic deliberation.

Enhanced Interrogation: Democratic Deliberation and the Public Debate

The conditions of democratic deliberation speak to the structure of discourse, not its outcome. Ensuring free and equal access, respecting diverse opinions, and invoking reasoned claims, fellow citizens deliberate principles of justice, norms of conduct, and public policy (Chapter 3). As they do, "the exercise of state power" to use Joshua Cohen's (1998: 185) phrase, gains political legitimacy. Legitimacy does not mean that all the outcomes of public discourse meet consistently high standards of justice. Instead, the claim is weaker: collective judgments following appropriate deliberation are sufficiently just to offer reasonable grounds for complying with superior orders. Evaluating the controversy surrounding interrogation and torture on these terms is complex. Invoking the civic discourse does not afford recourse to ignorance as much as it affirms the knowledge that American interrogation policy was sufficiently legitimized to forestall charges of complicity or war crimes.

The contours of current debate settled after the American Psychological Association permitted military psychologists to "adhere to the requirements of law, regulations and other governing legal authority" should they equivocate when required to take part in interrogations (APA 2002: §1.02). Construing "regulations" as superior orders, the APA was reproached for offering its members the same "Nuremberg defense" exercised by Nazi war criminals (Hoffman et al. 2015: 55). Objections to the superior-order defense and, with it, calls to military medical personnel to refuse orders to aid interrogators and prosecute those who do not, appeal to manifest unlawfulness. Because enhanced interrogation disregards universal laws against torture and indefensibly violates human dignity, its unlawfulness and injustice are self-evident. Cogent as these arguments are, however, they represent only one side to a public exchange that addressed these very questions.

Determining whether enhanced interrogation violates legal and moral proscriptions of torture or is conducive to "normal, lawful interrogation," as the ICRC permits (2007: 23), drove democratic deliberation. The discourse was robust across the political spectrum as it engaged the government, judiciary, military, media, and academy. Proponents and opponents alike offered reasoned legal or moral arguments for medical personnel to refuse or agree to participate in interrogation sessions. Nevertheless, later revelations that the CIA destroyed videotapes of waterboarding and misled the US government about the effectiveness of enhanced interrogation jeopardized the legitimizing function of democratic deliberation. With CIA subterfuge undermining the epistemic conditions necessary for moral discourse, opponents and defenders could only speculate about the efficacy of enhanced interrogation as they formulated policy options.

Echoing Sanford Levinson's (2003) early review, several arguments dominated the debate from the beginning.

1. Torture Is Impermissible

Defined by the Convention against Torture (CAT 1984: §1) as an act inflicting severe physical or mental pain or suffering to obtain information, inflict punishment, or effect intimidation or coercion, torture violates fundamental human rights. No one questions this assertion. Instead, the debate revolves around two other claims: enhanced interrogation is not torture, and torture is a permissible lesser evil.

2. Enhanced Interrogation Techniques Are Not Torture

Claims that enhanced interrogation is not torture go back at least as far as the 1972 Parker (UK) (Brownlie 1972) and 1987 Landau (Israel) commissions, and the 1978 rulings of the European Court of Human Rights. There, the court, and later governments in Israel and the United States, agreed that five interrogation techniques—hooding, wall-standing and stress positions, sleep deprivation, food deprivation, and exposure to loud music (or temperature extremes) "did not occasion suffering of the particular intensity and cruelty implied by the word torture" (Ireland v The UK 1978: §167). And although the European Court and Israeli Supreme Court ruled that these techniques amounted to ill-treatment, there was considerable discussion about whether and how they violated international laws prohibiting torture (e.g., Israel Law Review 1989). Attempts to clarify severe suffering in terms of intensity and duration only set the stage for some to distinguish between the permanent disabilities and harm occasioned by mutilation, beating, and electric shock, and the transient effects of enhanced interrogation or "torture lite" (Ignatieff 2004: 136–144; Miller 2005). This debate touches on the distinction between *interrogational torture* to obtain information, defensible perhaps in extreme cases, and unconditionally proscribed *terrorist torture* to intimidate the local population and stifle political dissent by inflicting severe bodily harm (Posner 2006: 83). To opponents of enhanced interrogation, these distinctions ignore the severe sequelae of interrogational torture and its use to punish or disable detainees in addition to, or instead of, eliciting information.

3. Torture Is the Lesser Evil

The lesser evil is a utilitarian argument: If enhanced interrogation can save lives, then its affront to dignity is less evil than letting many innocent people die (Allhoff 2012; Casebeer 2005). The lesser evil is a moral defense that appeals to exceptional circumstances to excuse torture and enhanced interrogation. Weighing the magnitude and probability of foreseeable harm (such as a ticking bomb), the lesser-evil argument compares the value of public order, the security of *many* civilians, and the integrity of the political community, with the usually nonlethal but substantial harm the torture victim suffers. The argument reaches into Michael Walzer's claim that an existential threat or supreme emergency might allow a nation to save the lives of many compatriots (or its very way of life) by targeting innocent enemy noncombatants (1977: 251–269). Both arguments require the same provisos: (1) an emergency that threatens catastrophic harm that alternative, less destructive means cannot avert, and (2) a significant probability that the lesser evil will prevent the greater (Chapter 3). The lesser-evil argument enjoyed broad appeal among many writers who "seem to agree that under some extreme conditions ('extreme' being a subjective determination), torture could be excused, justified, and even necessary" (Blum 2010: 42).

Several responses meet the lesser-evil argument.

3.1. The prohibition on torture, ill-treatment, or enhanced interrogation is absolute.

After once asking an Israeli human rights lawyer whether enhanced techniques were effective, he replied, "we don't know, and we don't care." They are unconditionally wrong, "an absolute and unforgivable evil" (Melzer 2020: ix). Absolute arguments mirror CAT and are usually deontological. They invoke a basic justice argument that does not permit violating human dignity under any circumstances (Waldron 2005). In response, proponents of the lesser evil argue that an absolute prohibition falters when fundamental rights—life, liberty, dignity, and security—conflict. Resolving contention among competing universal norms requires a ranking that will, in some cases, subordinate one to the other.

3.2. The slippery slope

Failing to convincingly distinguish between the harsh interrogations that democracies may practice and the brutal torture that repressive regimes may not, opens the road to equate the two. Domestically, attempts to limit enhanced interrogation to intelligence agencies may fail and allow torture to seep into law enforcement during peacetime (Luban 2005). Internationally, if democracies can invoke the lesser evil to torture terrorists, why can't other regimes torture their political opponents? In either case, utilitarians may slide toward two lesser evils they are probably loath to accept: (1) inflicting brutal torture when enhanced methods prove futile or (2) torturing bystanders who may have incidental knowledge of terrorism (e.g., the cook) or who may induce a subject to speak (e.g., the suspect's child).

3.3. Torture is not the lesser evil

This, too, is a utilitarian argument: the short- and long-term evil of torture (e.g., a cancer on democracy) never trumps the short-term benefits employing torture to defuse a ticking bomb. The benefits of torture are, moreover, contingent upon a rare constellation of events: sufficient knowledge about where the bomb is located, when it will explode and how to defuse it, adequate time to act on actionable intelligence, and reliable data that enhanced interrogation will elicit truthful answers (Brecher 2007; Ginbar 2008; Statman 1997). The ticking bomb scenario misconstrues intelligence gathering from a gradual accumulation of necessary and sufficient information to a one-time, decisive "big bang" event.

These arguments are not exhaustive, nor will I attempt to decide among them. Instead, they demonstrate how a public debate invoked reasoned moral arguments in multiple arenas and drew on universalizable deontological and utilitarian principles in the process.

Arenas of Debate

Public discourse and policy evolved dynamically, each shaping the other throughout the war years. But the process was not linear. Stakeholders did not first debate and then implement policy in an orderly fashion. Instead, the interrogation program evolved in secret, and only media disclosure in April 2004 sparked the public debate. The ensuing controversy highlights the crucial role of investigative journalism and independent NGOs in the deliberative process. By May 2004, members of the Senate Intelligence Committee met with the CIA and executive branch "to focus on detainee issues" (SSCI 2014: 134). The result was to suspend but then to reinstate enhanced interrogation techniques without waterboarding two months later. By then, 33 of the 39 detainees ultimately subjected to enhanced techniques had been interrogated (SSCI 2014: 458–461).

While sensitive to the public debate, Congressional support for extending greater latitude to the CIA relied on Office of Legal Counsel (OLC) memoranda from May 30, 2005, and July 20, 2007, "determining that the techniques were legal in part because they produced 'specific, actionable intelligence' and substantial quantities of otherwise unavailable intelligence" that saved lives (Del Rosso 2015: 130–158; SSCI 2014: 174–175). Responsive policy drove the debate forward. Moving to the legislature in the wake of intense public interest, the Senate voted overwhelmingly, 90–9, to approve the Detainee Treatment Act in October 2005. This bill restricted all military interrogations to those techniques authorized by the Army and prohibited physical, emotional, and sexual abuse. The Act, however, did not explicitly ban the CIA from conducting enhanced interrogation. After the Supreme Court affirmed the United States' obligation to protect captured members of al Qaeda under the Geneva Conventions (Hamdan v. Rumsfeld 2006), Senator Kennedy introduced an amendment to the Military Commissions Act (2006) to deem waterboarding, sexual humiliation, physical pain, and other enhanced interrogation techniques a punishable offense under international humanitarian law (Congressional Record 2006). The amendment failed. Similarly, Congressional attempts to extend the 2005 restrictions on Army interrogations to the CIA could not override a presidential veto in 2008.

The vicissitudes of the public debate resonated in the academic literature. Two early, influential anthologies by Sanford Levinson (2004) and Karen Greenberg (2006) published essays by prominent academics on both sides of the torture debate. By 2018 Scott Anderson and Martha Nussbaum published *Confronting Torture*, rehearsing some earlier arguments and providing a critical overview. Yet, "while none of the chapters here can be said to be favorable toward the use of torture," explain the editors, "they are all sensitive to the . . . difficulties in thinking about torture" (2018: 5). This sensitivity defined most of the almost 15-year debate and set the stage for reasoned and deliberative arguments that split public opinion evenly into the Trump administration (Gronke et al. 2010; Tyson 2017; Wike 2016.)

As it evolved, the debate focused on past and future policy. Looking back at the debate helps to understand the stance required of a "reasonable person" or "reasonable soldier." Manifest unlawfulness characterizes orders that a person of ordinary sense and understanding knows to "obviously involve the commission of a criminal act" (Green 1985: 282; also Chapter 1). Before the public debate, medical personnel in interrogation facilities did not have the fruits of public deliberation to rely upon. But if the crucial question is, "How do persons of ordinary sense and understanding evaluate the events around them?" the subsequent debate demonstrated what a reasonable answer to this question might look like. There were, to be sure, several answers, some testing the limits of law and ethics more than others. Nevertheless, the plurality of considered public opinions serves a retroactive validating function that undercuts the manifest unlawfulness necessary to demand unequivocal opposition to regulations that permit enhanced interrogation. Information constraints, however, may sorely test this conclusion.

Information Constraints in the Torture Debate

Throughout most of the debate, proponents and opponents crafted their arguments in the absence of definitive information about the effectiveness of enhanced interrogation. Uncertainty, however, is a fixed feature of moral discourse. Although information is the keystone of deliberative democracy, proponents acknowledge that it is frequently incomplete. Bargaining parties often withhold information but incomplete or unobtainable data do not impair the legitimizing function of democratic deliberation unless the authorities alter or fabricate pertinent information to mislead and subvert civic discourse.

Although the CIA confirmed the effectiveness of enhanced interrogation, the Senate Committee Report analyzed the "eight most frequently cited examples of 'thwarted' plots and captured terrorists" and found the CIA's representation to be "inaccurate and unsupported by CIA records" (SSCI 2014: 225). The Report reverberated widely because reliable data about effectiveness are the lynchpin of the torture debate. There is no call to distinguish enhanced interrogation from torture if the former has no utility. The necessity defense is no defense at all if the enhanced interrogation techniques never work. Without the presumption that the lesser evil could prevent a greater evil, the former has no purchase. And although deontological opponents of torture do not require empirical data, many made claims about the ineffectiveness of enhanced interrogation that we now realize might have been verified. Of course, it may be that the Senate report is incomplete. Or, it may be that CIA officials believed enhanced interrogation worked, and, perhaps, it sometimes did. The CIA adamantly contested some of the Committee's findings (SSCI 2014: 648–649). Regardless, inaccurate and misleading information would have affected every significant aspect of the torture debate. One result was to reassess legislative support for enhanced interrogation as new facts emerged.

Armed with the Senate Select Committee's repudiation of the CIA, the Senate voted 78–21 to reaffirm President Obama's 2009 ban on enhanced interrogation across all services in 2015. Reasons for assent varied and not all agreed that enhanced interrogation was ineffective. Some thought it was no longer necessary, while others opposed the amendment, reluctant to "deny future commanders in chief and intelligence officials important tools for protecting the American people and the US homeland" (Lewis 2015). The decade-long debate was often partisan but also significantly dialogical. The nine Senators voting against the 2005 Detainee Detention Act were Republicans who, presumably, did not want to limit the Army's interrogation techniques any more than the CIA's. In 2008, only a presidential veto defeated bipartisan support to prohibit the CIA from employing enhanced interrogation. And although committee approval of the SSCI Report split 9–6 on mostly partisan lines, three fourths of the Senate subsequently voted to ban enhanced interrogation in 2015.

Medical Involvement in Enhanced Interrogation

Where does the preceding discussion leave military medical personnel stationed in interrogation facilities? Congressional and executive decisions reverberated in the medical community. In 2006, the American Medical Association adopted strict guidelines prohibiting physicians from participating in or monitoring interrogations (AMA 2006). By 2010, the American Psychological Association dropped its advice to practitioners to adhere to the law or other "governing legal authority," and now instructed them not to "justify or defend violating human rights" (APA 2010). Reiterating the themes of the broader political debate, the medical community addressed dual loyalty, the lesser evil of enhanced interrogation, and the duty to care for detainees despite the undesired outcome of aiding interrogators (Allhoff 2008; Annas 2005; Goodman and Roseman 2009; Howe et al. 2009; Lepora and Millum 2011). This discourse, like the broader one that occupied the public at large, first carved out a place for enhanced interrogation and later closed it. Each stage moved the bar of manifest unlawfulness.

Still, there are nagging epistemic questions. It seems gratuitous to excuse anyone because they didn't know. There is a difference, however, between information that is hiding in plain sight but ignored and information manipulated to stay out of plain sight. Permeated with disinformation, moral discourse can only offer the semblance of legitimacy. The result is to afford a person of ordinary sense and understanding reasonable grounds to accept the outcome of collective deliberation, and then to change course when better information is forthcoming. In the meantime, interrogations that exceed the parameters set by public discourse remain indefensible. These constraints prohibit unnecessary suffering, terroristic torture, greater evils, and disproportionate harms. Outside the pale of moral discourse and, therefore, manifestly unlawful, these cases and those responsible are the appropriate subjects of judicial proceedings. Among them are those who designed the CIA interrogation program with full knowledge of the false and misleading data they disseminated.

The deliberative process also demonstrated how the utilitarian arguments overpowered all others. There was little support for a "we don't know, and we don't care" posture that did not include some speculation about the effectiveness of enhanced interrogation. Empirical data drives this debate but was either absent or false. In this regard, the Senate Committee Report is critical but not determinative. It awaits additional data, and those emerging (e.g., O'Mara 2015) will impinge on present and future deliberation. Current debates ask about the humanity of such permissible interrogation techniques as solitary confinement or sensory deprivation (Finkelstein and Xenakis 2020). Another looks to the efficacy of rapport-building interrogation techniques developed by the US government's High-Value Detainee Interrogation Group (HIG) Research Program since 2010 (Meissner et al. 2017; Stein 2018). Future debates may look much different if pharmacological agents, neuroimaging, or neuro-stimulating technologies replace waterboarding. These techniques may violate dignity painlessly but, perhaps, no less egregiously than earlier methods (Blitz 2017: 45–58; Wolpe, Foster, and Langleben 2005; Langleben and Moriarty 2013). Proponents of enhanced interrogation may feel vindicated as they hope to detach the new techniques from the ambit of torture and ill-treatment entirely, move away from the slippery slope, and obviate any need for lesser-evil arguments. Opponents may waver unless they can force a new dialog about violations of dignity and cognitive liberty in an age of galloping neuroscience. As previously, democratic discourse leaves room for a plurality of reasoned arguments to inform policy.

Finally, one should look askance at the speed with which the successive US administrations exonerated interrogators and medical facilitators based on little more than the "advice of counsel." Although robust democratic deliberation offers a much more comprehensive context than legal memos to evaluate interrogation and torture, neither endorses any defense a priori. Rather, the fruits of public discourse only provide food for that defense. If *defense* has any purchase whatsoever, then it comes after an indictment and during a trial, not before. Medical personnel participated in many ways. Some facilitated enhanced interrogation, while others forged death certificates or abused detainees (Miles 2020: 111–121). And although a person of ordinary sense and understanding can call on the opinion of counsel and the ensuing public debate as he constructs his defense, his success in court will vary with the character and severity of his actions. No single defense fits every charge. Moreover, assessing the cogency of any defense of superior order is the purview of the judiciary and not the executive or legislative branches of government.

Enhanced Interrogation: From War Crimes to Censure

In contrast to calls to indict medical workers for war crimes, demands to censure medical workers for participating in enhanced interrogation turn on violations of medical ethics, not criminal activity. Enhanced interrogation, nonclinical body cavity searches, and medically unnecessary procedures elicit charges of violating the ethical principles of beneficence and "do no harm" that no appeal to public order or military necessity can overcome (Berger, Rubinstein, and DeCamp 2018).

Berger, Rubinstein, and DeCamp pursue two claims. Recalling the legal debate, one argument repudiates the lesser evil defense because enhanced interrogation is equivalent to torture, and torture knows no defense of necessity. This argument was an integral part of the broader debate and raises similar counterarguments. The second argument is about burdening patients with superfluous and harmful medical procedures. Charges that specific procedures, such as rectal infusion, violate medical ethics merit close investigation. No public discussion of rectal infusion (or rehydration) in connection with interrogation appears in the literature until the SSCI Report disclosed the practice in 2014 as a method of delivering nutrients rectally to end hunger strikes by detainees (pp. 100, 488). The Senate report criticizes rectal infusion as either medically unnecessary or as a form of behavior control to discourage hunger striking. Surely, physicians deserve censure for inflicting a useless and painful invasive procedure. A larger question, however, turns on the ethics of medical intervention and force feeding to end hunger striking.

Force Feeding Hunger Strikers

When detainees refuse to eat, prison officials may decide to feed them by force. In Guantanamo Bay, Cuba, the United States adopted an aggressive approach, strapping inmates to a chair and inserting a nasogastric tube to deliver nutrients following hunger strikes of as little as 72 hours (JTF 2013a: 8). Elsewhere, in Israel, for example, officials often wait weeks until prisoners lose consciousness before a physician or nurse delivers nutrients intravenously (parenteral nutrition) or through a feeding tube (enteral nutrition).

The following sections address the ethics of force feeding in light of the political challenges that hunger strikes pose. Hunger striking is an integral part of a social or political struggle. Domestic criminal inmates, for example, may strike for better prison conditions. Foreign or enemy inmates often integrate hunger striking as part of a nonviolent campaign to gain concessions from their adversary. In Iraq, Afghanistan, Turkey, and Israel, these campaigns supplement armed resistance. As such, force feeding and hunger striking are the purview of military medical ethics as much as of medical ethics alone. Nevertheless, medical ethics and the pronouncements of the World Medical Association (WMA) and the International Committee of the Red Cross (ICRC) are the starting point. From there, the discussion moves to address the central issues of force feeding: patient autonomy and dignity, public order, and the politics of hunger striking.

Force Feeding: Legal and Professional Guidelines

The World Medical Association prohibits force feeding unequivocally:

> All kinds of interventions for enteral or parenteral feeding against the will of the mentally competent hunger striker are to be considered as forced feeding. Forced feeding is never ethically acceptable. Even if intended to

benefit, feeding accompanied by threats, coercion, force or use of physical restraints is a form of inhuman and degrading treatment. (WMA 2017b: §23)

Similarly, "The ICRC is opposed to forced feeding or forced treatment; it is essential that the detainees' choices be respected and their human dignity preserved" (ICRC 2013).

The prohibition invokes respect for a competent patient's autonomy to refuse nutrition. As such, "physicians may rarely and exceptionally" force feed a striking patient only when (1) the patient has been coerced to refuse food or (2) force feeding is necessary to preserve a person's life when the patient is no longer conscious *and* "left no unpressured advance instructions" to continue to refuse food or fluids (WMA 2017b: §20–21).

The central questions for medical ethics, therefore, turn on autonomy and beneficence. First, are hunger strikers truly autonomous if prison inmates or detainees face enormous pressure to join hunger strikes? Second, is dying always the best outcome? The WMA (2017b: §20) believes, "It is ethical to allow a determined hunger striker to die with dignity rather than submit that person to repeated interventions against his or her will" (also Crosby, Apovian, and Grodin 2007; Irmak 2015). In rebuttal, a moderate vitalist claim that values the sanctity of life will look at this argument askance. After considering these two questions, I turn to military medical ethics. Here the issue is very different: Does the state have the right to end a hunger strike that threatens a nation's political interests, particularly during armed conflict?

Force Feeding, Coercion, and Autonomy

When inmates in California undertook a sustained hunger strike in 2013, state authorities petitioned the court to permit force feeding. Consistent with the WMA, the court allowed prison authorities to feed hunger strikers if a hunger striker were at risk of near-term death or significant bodily injury and either (1) failed to execute a valid Do Not Resuscitate (DNR) order or (2) was coerced to refuse nutrition (Plata v Brown 2013). Knowing that they would be fed and not allowed to die, prisoners called off their strike without gaining any substantial concessions.

Emphasizing respect for autonomy, the California court ruling permits medical staffers to force feed inmates if they are coerced to hunger strike.

Having in mind imprisoned gang members taking orders from their leaders, one could make the same argument about captured insurgents. Prison inmates, particularly political detainees, face significant pressure to join hunger strikes as peers, leaders, or military superiors compel, threaten, or order detainees to refuse food. Depression and dejection may further contribute to their proclivity to strike (Garasic 2015; Glick 1997). If these conditions undermine autonomy, then detainee instructions to refuse food are invalid, and the authorities might permissibly force feed striking political inmates to save their lives.

Coercion reflects social pressure to strike and refuse nutrition. Despite suspicions that inmates receive orders to strike there is no prima facie reason to think that taking orders constitutes coercion. Although some might construe autonomous decision-making as radically individualistic—the lone patient weighing available information impartially and making a decision free from any interference—consent is a social construct, the product of one's shared political, social, and moral environment. Personal decision-making is always responsive to norms of fidelity, social cooperation and peer pressure, religious or civic duties, mutual responsibility, and personal well-being. Although some are skeptical about attributing robust consent to those who accept payment for services (e.g., organ donors) or who fear sanctions or punishment (e.g., taxpayers or hunger strikers), these conclusions are too severe. A person's motives are often mixed, and a hunger striker who complies with orders to strike may be acting from collective responsibility, political or religious duties, and fear of sanctions. None of this impairs autonomous decision-making but is, indeed, part and parcel of the consensual process.

Some individuals, moreover, exercise "second-order autonomy" when they freely entrust their decisions to others. This choice, too, is a form of consent and particularly salient when hunger strikers (particularly those who belong to a military organization) entrust their leaders with the task of pursuing their collective good and negotiating with the state. There is no reason to think that the decision to participate in a hunger strike is not free unless accompanied by *overt* coercion, that is, by the threat of physical or severe psychological harm. Absent such evidence, inmates' refusals to accept any food or medical treatment remain valid irrespective of any orders they may have received from above. The bar of impaired decision-making, therefore, sits very high, particularly when detainees are members of a military organization that uses punishment to maintain discipline. Seldom, then, is autonomy defective. As such, one must look for another reason to force feed hunger strikers. If medicine's duty to preserve life is paramount, then infringing upon autonomy and self-determination to force feed humanely might be permissible.

Force Feeding, Vitalism, and the Duty to Protect Life

Vitalism is a unilateral imperative to save a life, a secularized form of the sanctity of life, that some believe trumps autonomy. In response to the Israel Medical Association's (IMA) condemnation of force feeding, some health-care professionals pushed back in a public petition:

> We, the undersigned believe that in extreme circumstances, when all persuasive efforts have failed and when there is a clear and present danger to the prisoner's life if the fasting continues, the ethical value of preservation of human life and the professional responsibilities of the physicians to save human life takes precedence over the infringement of the individual's autonomy. (Rinat 2015)

There is no sure formula to balance vitalism against respect for autonomy except to note that in practice, physicians often opt for creative ways to save their patients' lives. During a 2013 hunger strike in Israel, physicians injected hunger strikers with Vitamin B without their consent and revived them sufficiently so detainees could make an informed decision about continued care (Even 2013). And, indeed, some decided to end their strike. But unless prisoners leave explicit instructions to accept vitamin injections, this, too, is force feeding. Although this kind of workaround may relieve moral distress, it does not necessarily serve the patient's best interest. Waiting until a patient loses consciousness to revive him risks serious illness (Reyes, Annas, and Allen 2013). If physicians take vitalism seriously, then their medical associations should permit infringements of autonomy to make it easier for caregivers to treat their patients before starvation causes extreme suffering and irreversible harm.

Vitalism also underlies medical ethics in prisons, where states have a custodial duty to protect those entrusted to their care by the courts. During armed conflict, Common Article 3 of the Geneva Convention obligates states to "protect the physical well-being of persons deprived of their liberty . . . by providing them with the requisite medical assistance" (Özgül

v. Turkey 2007). In civilian prisons, "correctional authorities should protect prisoners from physical injury, corporal punishment, sexual assault, extortion, harassment, and personal abuse, among other harms" (ABA 2010: §23-5.1). Prison authorities face severe criticism if they cannot prevent inmates' deaths.

Despite some cogency, neither defective autonomy nor vitalism affords sweeping grounds to permit force feeding. Defective autonomy is seldom convincing. Expanding stark individualism to consider the social-military context of decision-making makes room for sufficient autonomy to competently refuse food. Vitalism may reasonably override autonomy. But bioethics offers no supreme principle for choosing between saving lives and respecting self-determination. Patient self-determination gains its force when a patient decides to end a life one deems of little value. In contrast, the healthy hunger striker faces no such prospect. Young, vigorous strikers leave physicians to struggle with two fundamental duties: preserve life or respect autonomy. Their choice will fall as they weigh the merits of one or another. Alternatively, they can consider the principles of military-medical necessity and proportionality during armed conflict.

Force Feeding and Armed Conflict

During armed conflict, two reasons may permit force feeding hunger strikers. Appealing to the lesser evil, a state may infringe on a person's right to medical self-determination to guarantee public order. Second, invoking the right of self-defense to disable a nonviolent but hostile adversary permits a state to reject a detainee's right to refuse food. In the first case, the state overrides a detainee's right to hunger strike. In the second, detainees forfeit their right to hunger strike. In both cases, force feeding must satisfy the conditions of necessity, proportionality, and humanity. But first, states can seek accommodation to avoid force feeding altogether.

Hunger Striking and Accommodation
When insurgents opt to continue their struggle by hunger striking, states have three choices: let them die, accommodate their demands, or force feed them. As the British learned in Northern Ireland in 1981, letting prisoners die is the worst possible outcome. There, the deaths of 10 Irish Republican Army (IRA) prisoners galvanized support for the IRA, aggravated terrorism

for the next decade, saw the successful entry of the Sein Fein into British politics, and brought resounding condemnation of the British government (English 2003: 263–274; 280–283). In contrast, accommodation is a successful strategy when strikers make modest and feasible demands. In Israel, for example, Palestinian political detainees struck for shorter prison terms in 2013 and 2015 (Weingarten 2017). Fearing widespread riots, Israel acceded to these demands (Khoury 2013). In 2012, imprisoned members of the Kurdish Workers Party (PKK) refused food until Turkey made political concessions to enhance Kurdish autonomy and culture (Krajeski 2012).

Success, however, was short-lived. Fighting erupted between Hamas and Israel in 2014 that killed over 2,000 Palestinians. In Turkey, reconciliation collapsed following an ISIS terror attack against Kurdish and Turkish students in 2016 (UN OHCRH 2018). Blaming the Turkish government for abetting these attacks, the PKK resumed its armed conflict with Turkey until another hunger strike and further negotiations ended that strike in May 2019 (Butler 2019). As these examples show, hunger strikes rarely afford strategic gains alone. Rather they deliver partial and often symbolic gains that incrementally augment broader political objectives.

Against this backdrop, states have a political incentive to seek accommodation. Hunger strikes work best when demands are realistic. States know this, as do savvy strikers. For this reason, few strikes should ever necessitate force feeding. Instead, states should engage hunger strikers from the beginning while reserving their right to force feed well after the strike has begun but well before strikers suffer significant or irreversible harm. The former allows time for negotiation and avoids the specter of inhumane force feeding. The latter prevents the death or incapacitation of hunger strikers. Avoiding these adverse outcomes offers each side an incentive to conclude the strike. Hunger strikers would rather not die, and states would rather not face public and medical opposition to force feeding. Demands for far-reaching concessions, however, present much harder dilemmas. Here, states may have no choice but to consider force feeding if they cannot meet strikers' demands, and if strikers' deaths would significantly undermine public order or national security.

Force Feeding to Maintain Public Order

Appealing to public order to permit force feeding infringes on a person's right to refuse treatment while enabling the state to seek a greater good. However, the lesser evil (rights' infringement), must be not only less harmful than the greater evil (public disorder), but the least of all harmful actions. Considering the appropriate manner of force feeding, a US court, for example, encouraged officials at Guantanamo Bay to feed a hunger-striking inmate enterally in a hospital setting to spare him "the agony of having a feeding tube inserted and removed for each feeding" and "the pain and discomfort of the restraint chair" while he pursued his lawsuit against the US government (Dhiab v Obama 2014).

Although relatively humane, enteral feeding constitutes no trivial rights' infringement and, therefore, requires a substantially greater good to offset the harm and humiliation of force feeding. The greater good does not address the benefit of saving the strikers' lives per se (as vitalism suggests) but the advantage of preserving their lives to maintain public order and prevent political conflict from escalating dangerously following the deaths of hunger strikers (as it did in Britain). But Britain made no prior attempt at accommodation. Similarly, there was no apparent reason that US authorities could not satisfy detainee demands for better conditions at Guantanamo or speedier repatriation, thereby avoiding force feeding and the subsequent outcry. Preponderant security interests that excuse force feeding are rare and only occur when allowing prisoners to die or acceding to their demands carry intolerable costs. States will ultimately make this decision guided by security interests, military necessity, and the lessons of history.

When a lesser evil defense excuses forced feeding, it acknowledges the right of patient self-determination before infringing upon it. In contrast, Yechiel Barilan (2017: 357) considers the military-political context of hunger striking to *deny* hunger strikers this right because, "nobody has the duty to respect the autonomy of the enemy who chooses to kill in the promotion of a political goal." This argument deserves scrutiny because it moves force feeding away from medical ethics entirely.

Hunger Striking and Armed Conflict

When states go to war, they have one overriding goal: to substantially weaken the enemy's military forces. For the most part, these efforts are armed and violent; nonviolence is usually the purview of the weak and unarmed. But as contemporary cases demonstrate, nonstate actors—Hamas, PKK, IRA, or al Qaeda—may find nonviolent tactics, particularly hunger strikes, particularly effective as they continue their struggles (Chenoweth and Stephan 2011). Unlike many nonviolent resisters, nonstate actors employ violence and nonviolence simultaneously (Gross 2015). Nonviolent, hunger striking insurgents are merely continuing to fight by other means. Upon capture, a detainee's right to prisoner of war (POW) status is wholly contingent on maintaining his noncombatant, nonthreatening status. To characterize all hunger strikers as political actors determined to "modify oligarchic concentrations of power" (Filc et al. 2014: 8) and, therefore, entitled to forbearance is misleading. When domestic protesters struggle to transform prevailing political structures, they are not former combatants but citizens exercising their political rights. Formerly armed adversaries, on the other hand, continue to pursue a military agenda and, therefore, enjoy few rights of political expression upon capture.

In this context, humane force feeding in response to hunger striking detainees moves away from questions of patient self-determination to focus on a detainee's right to strike. In its summary of Common Article 3, the ICRC (2010a) explains: "[D]etention is not a form of punishment, but only aims to prevent further participation in the conflict." A POW, in turn, may endeavor to escape, but in-camp resistance is limited to instances of "captor exploitation" that violate the Geneva Convention. Absent exploitation or abuse, resistance may invite "punishment by the captor for order and discipline violations" (DoD 2001: E2.2.3.221). On this interpretation, an inmate or detainee may hunger strike to protest harsh or inhumane living conditions, but not to force political or military concessions from an adversary.

Force feeding is not punishment. But when detainees continue to take part in a conflict by nonviolent means, force feeding hunger strikers is a proportionate self-defensive measure that does not require the enemy's consent to accept or refuse. The forfeited right, however, is construed very narrowly. Detainees do not lose their right to consent to standard treatments for injury or disease. Rather, detainees, like combatants who continue their aggression, however nonviolent it may be, have no right to object to humane and proportionate self-defensive measures. This is the moral basis of any defensive war.

Force Feeding Hunger Striking Detainees

Force feeding hunger striking detainees presents a stark conflict between prevailing norms and practice. "While enteral feeding is solidly supported under US federal law and policy," notes an internal military memo in 2013, "international law and certain medical ethical standards holds that the 'force feeding' of a mentally competent person capable of making an informed decision is never acceptable" (JTF 2013b). Addressing this tension, the preceding discussion casts force feeding as a last resort measure consistent with the logic of defensive war. At the same time, it is clear that medical professionals are reluctant to let otherwise healthy patients die. Despite efforts to frame permissible force feeding in terms of defective autonomy, the rationale driving the *medical* management of hunger strikers is vitalism.

The rationale driving *military* management must similarly avoid the deaths of hunger strikers. Management decisions turn on the military and political costs of three choices: accommodation, force feeding, or letting hunger strikers die. Hunger striking is brinksmanship. Authorities will want to respect the strike long enough to leave room for negotiation, but not so long as permanent injury is imminent. Hunger strikers manage time similarly. Many consume sufficient water, fluids, electrolytes, and vitamins to stay alive and reach their aims (Lederman 2018). States do well to respect an extended timetable and repudiate the American practice of force feeding within days of striking. There are no medical grounds to force feed because death is not imminent, and no political grounds until negotiations have run their course. Under no circumstances is death an option—medical and political accommodation, whether vitamin injections or reasonable concessions are the strategies of choice. Force feeding remains permissible only in rare and extenuating circumstances.

Detainee Care in Contemporary Armed Conflict

The preceding sections cover three central issues of detainee care in war. The chapter opens with quotidian care because this is the norm. By and large, detainees in Iraq and Afghanistan enjoyed competent medical care. In this regard, the United States and its Coalition allies followed the Geneva Convention regulations governing medical attention for wounded adversaries. This policy was not contentious but should be. Despite the convention of treating all *adversaries* equally, equality is morally indefensible unless all belligerents, including host-nation allies, receive the same level of medical attention. Most often, insufficient resources make this impossible. In these circumstances, typical of the wars in Iraq and Afghanistan, detainees can only claim a level of health care equal to that local allies and civilians receive, not the same standard that multinational forces enjoy. Revised along these lines, such a protocol, along with strenuous efforts to improve the local healthcare system so inhabitants can enjoy a dignified life, should guide intervening forces in the future.

Charges of abuse—interrogation and force feeding—dominate discussions of detainee care and, indeed, of military medical ethics. The debate surrounding enhanced interrogation turned on its defense in extreme conditions. This chapter does not settle this debate but explains how it met many of the requirements of deliberative democracy and discourse ethics despite misinformation about the effectiveness of enhanced interrogation. In this environment, a reasonable person will weigh the considered opinions of government, political, and academic authorities. And although flawed for lack of reliable data, the decision he or she reaches to comply with superior orders does not afford grounds for impeachable crimes of war.

The controversy surrounding force feeding, too, is part of a larger discussion about how to wage asymmetric war. Confronted with hunger striking detainees, political and medical interests collide. Framed as medical ethics dilemma, force feeding asks whether a person's best interest trumps respect for autonomy. And although many favor the latter, a robust vitalist argument for preserving the life of a healthy patient guides many practices. Despite respect for autonomy, doctors in the United States and Israel, for example, took pains to prevent the deaths of hunger strikers. But medical ethics comprises only part of the dilemma. Considerations of public order accompanied by stiff custodial duties of care offer a strong case for infringing on patient self-determination when hunger strikers face death. During armed conflict, however, hunger striking assumes an aggressive posture. As detainees fight by nonviolent means, they may no longer claim patient rights to wage their struggle.

Detainee health care imposes enormous challenges that may strain medical ethics. Interposing norms of military ethics push the debate in different directions that alleviate and exacerbate some of these dilemmas. So it also is with health care for local nationals. Their fate is often an afterthought, but the wars in Iraq and Afghanistan saw ad hoc rules of eligibility to tend civilians injured in the crossfire. Concerted efforts to meet the medical needs of civilians in war deserve commendation, but just as preferential treatment for detainees lacks solid grounds, singling out civilian victims of collateral harm infringes on the rights of all who require decent medical attention. The rights of collateral casualties and other civilians are the subject of the following chapter.

7

Care and Compensation for Civilian
Victims of War

Throughout the fighting in Iraq and Afghanistan, multinational forces faced a civilian population ravished by violence and disease. With many sick and injured seeking medical attention at combat support hospitals earmarked for multinational and host-nation security forces, policymakers had to decide how to allocate care for civilians. The first medical rule of eligibility prioritizes treatment for multinational forces while offering emergency care to host-nation allies before they transfer to the local healthcare system (Chapter 5). The first rule, however, says nothing about local civilians, that is, anyone who is not a Coalition soldier, defense contractor, member of the local security forces, or insurgent. A second rule addresses their eligibility for medical attention at Coalition military hospitals:

Local, national civilians qualify for care in multinational medical facilities if,

1. Their injuries pose an imminent threat to "life, limb and eyesight[1]" *and*
2. Their injuries are the direct result of Coalition military action (UK MoD 2014: §2.6–2.8; FM 4-02 2013: §1–43.)

This rule is subordinate to Rule 1, that is, bed space must remain available for multinational forces (e.g., Causey et al. 2012; Pannell et al. 2015).

The medical rules of eligibility for local civilians pose two perplexing ethical questions. First, may military medical facilities prioritize the order of treatment on anything but urgent medical need? If so, why do collateral casualties enjoy an exclusive right to medical attention that other civilians do not? The short answer to the first question is, "Yes," it is permissible to treat civilians using criteria other than medical urgency and subordinate civilian health care to military necessities. The answer to the second question is, "No," collateral casualties enjoy no special rights to *medical care*. Depending on the kind of harm they suffer, civilians may deserve compensation. Money, not scarce medical resources, is the proper coin of restitution. The following sections address each question in turn.

Civilian Medical Management in Wartime

Before 1977, the Geneva Conventions articulated two standards of care, one for wounded and sick combatants, and one for wounded and sick civilians. As Chapters 5 and 6 describe, compatriot and enemy wounded enjoy equal access to medical care by whichever side is dispensing treatment. This view, enshrined in the First Geneva Convention, Article 12 (1949) remains unaltered in subsequent interpretations (ICRC, 1987, Commentary Article 16 §660).

In contrast, the duty to extend impartial care to sick and injured civilians is ambiguous. The First Geneva Convention only pertains to wounded and ill in "armed forces." Nevertheless, Additional Protocol I (1977: Art. 8) stipulates that all references to "wounded and sick" refer to military or civilian persons. As a result, customary international humanitarian law formulates two rules. Rule 110, *Treatment and Care of the Wounded, Sick and Shipwrecked*, reiterates the principle of delivering impartial, need-based medical care to the wounded, sick, and shipwrecked without delay. Rule 88, *Non-Discrimination*, ensures that Rule 110 applies to any sick and wounded, including civilians. Both the World Medical Association and the International Committee of the Red Cross commend these rules to their members (Giannou and Baldan 2010; WMA 2017a).

Despite these rules, occupying forces retain the right to deliver medical care subject to available resources and military requirements. The 1949 Fourth Geneva Convention (ICRC 1949b: Art. 55) requires occupying forces to provide the civilian population with adequate food and medical supplies "to the fullest extent of the means available." "The inclusion of this phrase," reads the accompanying commentary, "shows that the authors of the Convention did not wish to disregard the material difficulties with which the Occupying Power might be faced in wartime (financial and transport problems, etc.)" (ICRC 1958: Art 55, §1). The same article permits occupying forces to requisition medical supplies for use by occupation forces and administrative personnel after "the requirements of the civilian population have been *taken into account*." Attempts to replace this caveat with the positive duty to ensure that "the needs of the civilian population *are sufficiently covered*" were soundly defeated out of fears that such a legal duty might "invite violations of the Convention by laying down conditions which the circumstances of war might frequently prove to be impracticable" (ICRC 1949c: 829–830).

The tension between a norm specifying impartial, technologically sophisticated care, and the necessity of offering limited care to civilians is unavoidable (Bernthal et al. 2014; Mehring 2015: 287–290). By one estimate, multinational forces provided emergency treatment to approximately 10,000 Iraqi soldiers and civilians per year (Donaldson et al. 2010) while in Afghanistan, US forces delivered surgical care to 5,786 Afghan civilians from 2002 to 2013 (Weeks et al. 2018). These numbers are not large. Given the disparity between what a modern army brings for itself and what it finds in a war-torn nation, no occupying or humanitarian force can reasonably offer identical care to combatants and civilians. *Ethical Guidelines and Practices for US Military Medical Professionals* (Defense Health Board 2015: §4.4) are succinct:

> Medics should apply US medical standards when treating American forces. Medical interventions [for host-nation patients] typically are limited to procedures and therapies that are low risk, can be performed quickly, require limited follow-up, and do not undermine the host nation medical system.

In practice, this directive means to forego such lifesaving interventions as controlled airway management (e.g., mechanical ventilation) or aggressive treatment for severe burns or neurotrauma because local hospitals lacked the necessary critical care resources to sustain follow-up treatment (Martin et al. 2010; Sokol 2011; Spinella, Martin, and Azarow 2012).

Regularly offering civilians the care to save life, limb, and eyesight would strain Coalition resources. Rather than prioritize care based on urgent medical needs, the solution was to assume liability for collateral casualties. As a result, the emerging rule of eligibility restricted access to civilians suffering combat-related injuries caused solely by multinational forces and excluded civilians suffering the loss of life, limb, or eyesight from disease, accidents, or injuries sustained at the hands of insurgents. American and international law, however, exempt governments from liability for harm befalling civilians as the result of lawful combat operations (Tracy 2007; Walerstein 2009). Specifically, no claim for injury, death, or loss of property of any inhabitant of a foreign country is compensable if it arises "from action by an enemy or results directly or indirectly from an act of the armed forces of the United States in combat" (10 US Code 2006: §2734). The statute denies liability and monetary compensation. By referring specifically to collateral harm, the medical rules of eligibility contradict the legal statute by reinstating liability and medical compensation for injuries resulting from combat operations. Are the rules defensible nonetheless?

Justifying the Second Rule of Medical Eligibility

To work through an army's obligation to civilians, clarifying moral culpability during war can help explain the reach of financial or medical compensation for injuries. To establish culpability, the first step is to distinguish between accidental and collateral harm. Civilians may suffer one or both during war. Accidental harm is avoidable, unnecessary, unforeseen, and entirely unjustified if the injurer, that is, the combat soldier, is negligent. Alternatively, accidental harm may be excused if the injurer can point to mitigating circumstances. In both cases, the victim is wronged and entitled to compensation. Collateral harm is much more perplexing. Unlike accidental injury, collateral harm is foreseen but unavoidable. As a byproduct of war, collateral casualties are incidental, that is, bereft of any military benefit, yet tightly constrained by necessity and proportionality. Meeting these conditions, collateral harm is a permissible artifact of war. It is not clear, then, that its victims are wronged or entitled to restitution or medical care.

Accidental and Negligent Harm in War

When shells go astray or intelligence misidentifies a private residence as an insurgent command post, innocent people die. These casualties are not collateral but accidental, and, like accidents, may demand compensation. Consider these cases:

Case 1: 4 September 2009. Responding to a call by German forces, an American F-15E fighter jet struck two fuel tankers captured by Taliban insurgents, killing over 90 civilians in the attack. German forces stated that the strike took place after an unmanned surveillance aircraft had determined that there were no civilians in the area . . . but one eyewitness claims that up to 500 people from surrounding villages swarmed the tankers for free fuel. NATO has said its commanders had believed that only insurgents were in the vicinity. (Daily Mail 2009)

Case 2: 29 August 2008. An Afghan woman and two children were killed, and four other children injured as German soldiers opened fire on a civilian vehicle in the northern province of Kunduz. Two civilian vehicles approaching the checkpoint failed to heed clear signals from the troops staffing the checkpoint and the security forces then opened fire . . . First, a vehicle approached the checkpoint but escaped when the forces tried to stop it. The forces [then] opened fire at the second vehicle, which was driving behind the first one and did not heed repeated signals by the forces. When the forces later checked the vehicle, they found two children and a woman dead and four other children wounded in the vehicle. (Deutsche Welle 2008)

Case 3: 3 October 2015. The Pentagon maintained that the deadly US strike on a Médecins Sans Frontières (MSF) hospital in Kunduz, Afghanistan (10/2016), that killed 42 people resulted from unintentional human error and equipment failure. (USCC 2016)

Case 4: 11 August 2006. The Israel Defense Force is investigating Wednesday's north Gaza shelling incident that left 18 Palestinians dead. Southern Command Chief Maj.-Gen. Yoav Galant told reporters that "one possibility is that there was a malfunction in one of our targeting devices." (Greenberg 2006)

In the first three cases, US and German forces agreed to make ex gratia "condolence" or "solatia" payments to the civilian casualties. These include a $2,500 cash payment (and in exceptional circumstances up to $10,000) for loss of life or property, and medical treatment for the injured (MNC-I 2009: B-11). Careful to disclaim liability, support for condolence payments often draws on military necessity. Condolence payments and accompanying medical care are a "politically prudent step to avoid alienating the population from troops" and are "designed primarily to quell anger among the local population" in a culture that accepts payment for accidental or unintentional loss of life (CIVIC 2009:75-77; FM 3-24 2006: §D-37; Holewinski 2012). Following mishaps, military planners expect that payments will hinder insurgents' efforts to gain support and recruit fighters from among the local population (MNC-1(2009): i,1). Condolence payments by US forces, for example, totaled $21M in 2005 and $7M in 2006 in Iraq, and $210,000 in Afghanistan in 2006 (GAO 2007).

Military necessity, however, fails to anchor a firm duty of compensation. First, the appeal to military necessity invokes the benefits that compensation affords the *injuring* party. It is, therefore, situationally dependent. Israel, for example, has little reason to think that any form of compensation will quell resentment or avoid alienating Palestinians. In contrast, Coalition forces might think compensation improves their chances against insurgents. Second, there is insufficient evidence to determine whether and how condolence payments or medical attention shore up a counterinsurgency. Medical care (and pharmaceuticals) are precious assets in conflict areas. They may indeed buy loyalty, support, cooperation, and gratitude. These outcomes, however, are unrelated to liability or accidental harm. Instead, such benefits are attainable anywhere anyone appreciates superb medical care. As such, multinational forces might do better to direct medical attention and compensation where it realizes the greatest military or political benefit rather than only offering it to collateral casualties. To attain maximum benefit, financial or medical resources might be better spent in areas where the Coalition's hold is precarious or on well-connected families or political parties who can mobilize support for the government. In this view, the second rule of medical eligibility should eschew liability entirely and treat civilians to gain the highest military advantage. Yet it does not. Liability still nags because multinational forces remain at fault for accidental harm.

Accidental and Negligent Harm: Fault and Liability

"To be at fault," writes Jules Coleman (1976: 270), "an actor (1) must fail to satisfy a standard of reasonable conduct, and (2) in some sense that failure must be imputable to him as his doing" (also Greenawalt 1984). The first condition of fault is wrongdoing, and the second is responsibility. Both are necessary. Fault is to attribute an inappropriate act to a specific agent and causally link that act with harmful outcomes. Negligent harm comprises both wrongdoing and responsibility. It generates substantial liability and the duty to recompense. In some cases, negligence also demands punishment. In contrast, accidental harm may be excused. Excused harm acknowledges wrongdoing but denies responsibility if the injurer can appeal to circumstances beyond his control. Here the injurer can claim: "It was not my fault." And although excused harm may not entail punishment, it does not extinguish liability or the obligation to compensate victims.

It is difficult to know whether the harm described in the cases above is negligent or accidental. US and German authorities denied liability. Although individual service personnel in Case 3 (US attack on MSF hospital) were punished with "administrative actions" (e.g., suspension, removal from command, and letters of reprimand), none faced criminal charges because their actions were not intentional but the product of human error and the "fog of war" (US Central Command 2016). In Case 1 (German attack on fuel tankers), the German courts approved condolence payments. Still, they did not find the commander liable because he "acted reasonably according to the information available to him at the time." Rejecting any legal liability, the German court concluded, "later findings about the true situation (namely the presence of civilians) could not make the action illegal in retrospect" (Landgericht Bonn 2013: §77,81).

In neither case, however, was the loss of life *morally* justified. Either the injurers were unjustifiably negligent so that better planning, intelligence, or system maintenance might have avoided the tragic outcome, or morally excused if random events and the fog of war overcame their best intentions. In either case, their victims merit compensation for the undeserved harm they suffer. Whether with money or medicine is a question I will consider soon. First, I want to ask whether collateral harm incurs the same liability as accidental or negligent harm.

Collateral Harm: Liability and Compensation

Consider the following case:

> Preplanned targets primarily included leadership buildings, government buildings, and security buildings. These attacks, carried out by the United States solely with precision-guided munitions, led to few known civilian casualties. In addition to the accuracy of such weapons, thorough collateral damage estimates helped minimize the civilian toll . . . Weapon choice and fusing contributed to the low casualty rate from bombing. (HRW 2003: 50)

Human Rights Watch describes the gold standard of collateral harm during war: high-value targets, meticulous planning, weapons choice, and proportionate but unavoidable harm to the civilian population. Collateral harm is not a mistake. Instead, it is unavoidable, foreseen, and closely reckoned as its architects calculate proportionality. Planners forecast collateral casualties through computer simulations before the advent of hostilities (HRW 2003: 19) to conclude that civilian casualties were not excessive "relative to the anticipated military advantage" (ICRC 1977a: 51.5). This calculation is precisely what international humanitarian law and ethics prescribe (Chapter 1). As such, collateral casualties are an integral part of the war project, without which it is all but impossible to wage just war.

Collateral harm does not hint of negligence or of causing damage that greater diligence might have avoided. The injurers commit no wrong, and without wrongdoing, there is no fault. Therefore, based on liability alone the second rule of medical eligibility is too broad. Although the rule justifies care and compensation for those who suffer accidental or negligent harm, the case for compensation seems much weaker for collateral casualties.

Nevertheless, a broader reading of collateral harm can reinforce the grounds for compensation. In the wake of a casualty-heavy military mission, one often hears about "disproportionate" collateral harm. Technically, this description is incorrect. By definition, collateral losses must be proportionate. Disproportionate casualties exceed those necessary to accomplish the mission's goal and are, in principle, compensable. Establishing disproportionality, however, is exceptionally difficult. Commanders in the field assess proportionality ex-ante, based on an operation's expected costs and benefits. Proportionality is not a retrospective assessment but a good faith judgment based on available evidence that few are in a position to question after the fact.

In response, however, Neta Crawford (2013) looks to systemic liability for collateral harm and asks, "Are institutions doing all they can to minimize harm to civilians?" "Do defense officials search for alternative rules of engagement that will reduce harm to civilians without sacrificing military advantage?" "Is the military developing adequate methods to assess collateral harm accurately before conducting strikes?" The answer, concludes Crawford, is only sometimes. Norms protecting civilians are changing but insufficiently developed and internalized. States do not incur liability because they cause collateral harm, but because nations fail to diminish the level of collateral damage when they can. In these circumstances, collateral harm is unnecessary, wrong, and inexcusable. Condolence payments and medical treatment for collateral casualties are ways for states to meet their responsibilities to civilians injured in war. Formulated in this way, however, collateral harm is only *sometimes* wrong and only sometimes compensable.

Collateral harm is wrong when systemic oversight fails. But if such deficiencies are curable, then collateral harm might be justifiable. If so, grounds for medical or monetary compensation are difficult to sustain.

Nevertheless, collateral casualties still trigger some degree of responsibility. "We hurt them, we fix them" is an adage attributed to American troops that captures this perspective concisely (Hodgetts et al. 2005: 6). In a similar vein, Dutch authorities repudiate legal liability but endorse condolence payments as an "expression of the moral obligation to families unintentionally harmed" (CIVIC 2009: 77). There is no hint that American, German, or Dutch soldiers were necessarily at fault or could have done anything more to avoid collateral harm. The impulse toward compensation or medical aid is a measure of the responsibility they feel for the undeserved injuries they cause, however permissible they may be. Nevertheless, the obligation to compensate collateral casualties is weaker than that due to victims of negligent or accidental harm.

To understand the relatively weak reach of collateral harm, consider how a person running to save a small child about to step into traffic, knocks down and injures a bystander. Analyzing this case, David Rodin (2011: 86) concludes:

> although lesser evil justification defeats liability to punishment, it does not defeat many other significant forms of liability, for example, the liability to pay back debts or the liability to compensate for harm. . . . [A]ffirming that the rescuer was all-things-considered justified in bruising the ribs of the bystander is consistent with believing that he is liable to make good the harm he has inflicted in some way—perhaps by apologizing, tending to him in the hospital, or making a financial contribution.

Here, the rescuer derives no benefit from injuring the bystander. The rescuer, moreover, commits no wrong in the sense of violating a "standard of reasonable conduct." In these ways, Rodin's description mirrors the intuitions underlying medical rules of eligibility and the impulse to fix those we hurt. Compensation recognizes that despite any reasonable excuse or justification for infringing on one's right to life or bodily integrity, the victim is undeserving of the harm he or she suffers. This suffering, even at the hands of a rescuer, is the moral basis of compensation for innocent collateral casualties in war. Absent wrongdoing, however, the weight of compensation—an apology or financial assistance—is not as substantial as the compensation due to victims of accidental, negligent, or dispropor-tionate harm.

Accepting an obligation to compensate collateral casualties, however modest it is, is a sea change in the conduct of war, particularly during defen-sive wars. In the best case, belligerents take no notice of the civilian popula-tion beyond trying to avoid direct or disproportionate casualties. In Israel's recent wars against Hamas (2008, 2014) and Hezbollah (2006), for example, there was no thought of compensation for the families of the civilian dead or the injured of either party. Claiming self-defense, each side tars the other with aggression. Again, the thinking turns on liability. In a defensive war, the aggressor should assume responsibility for war's devastation, not the nation compelled to take up arms to defend itself. This view, reinforced by the combat exclusions of liability, typifies modern war. But legal forbear-ance does not entirely wash out the moral claims of its innocent victims who nonetheless suffer death and disability at the hands of armed forces.

At this point, several moral obligations to compensate civilians converge. First, there is a strong but narrowly defined obligation to compensate victims of negligent, accidental, unnecessary, and disproportionate harm. None of these harms is trivial and may equal or exceed collateral harm in their se-verity during armed conflict. In each instance, the obligation to pay compen-sation or provide medical attention falls on the forces directly responsible despite the exemptions from liability states allow themselves. Second, lia-bility for collateral harm turns on a nation's culpability. Aggressor nations are criminally responsible for war and, thereby, assume weighty obligations to compensate victims of any collateral harm. Conversely, nations compelled to fight in self-defense incur significantly weaker obligations. While there is sometimes a strong inclination to meet these debts with medical care, mone-tary restitution is the better alternative.

Compensating Civilians in Wartime: Money or Medicine?

The intuition to fix those we hurt is not misplaced, but money, not medicine, is the proper tool. It is a fundamental principle of medical ethics that ante-cedent causes of injury or disease are irrelevant when providing treatment. The victims of an automobile accident, for example, merit medical attention based on the severity of their injures, whether one driver was intoxicated, another the victim of a mechanical malfunction, and the third a pedestrian who walked into traffic because the lights were out. In each case, a different agent is liable—the victim, the car manufacturer, and the city—yet none of this is relevant in the emergency room. For one, any effort to determine, much less rank, antecedent conditions is usually beyond the ken of the medical staff. Whether war or a busy Saturday night, there are insufficient time and information to ferret out, much less rank, antecedent conditions. Second, the right to medical care is a fundamental human right to be free of unnecessary suffering. It is a claim right that the sick and injured have against those who can provide aid. As a fundamental human right, its weight depends solely on the degree of suffering, irrespective of such antecedent conditions as a person's moral failings, bad luck, or the actions of others. But if this is true, why do military-medical necessity or associative duties temper the demands of medical urgency, but liability does not? Recall the previous arguments: soldiers capable of a rapid return to duty receive medical attention before the seriously wounded, while compatriots receive significantly better care than host-nation allies regardless of the severity of their wounds. Why then does not liability, even weak liability, afford preferential treatment to collateral casualties?

When fundamental moral obligations conflict, the force of one duty can outweigh another. I have already described how rules of mass casualty triage can override the duties of impartial care and obligate military medical workers to return soldiers to battle before treating those more critically wounded (Chapter 5). Underlying these priorities is an appeal to utilitarianism. In public emergencies, the greater good is served when soldiers or first responders receive prior attention so they can preserve the security and lives of all. In this way, preferential treatment for some enhances the rights of all.

Associative duties of comradery and contractual obligations to provide warfighters with the best possible care lean in a different direction. These principles obligate medical personnel to attend to compatriots before enemy soldiers or civilians (Chapters 2 and 5). The medical rules of eligibility endorse a compatriot's blanket entitlement to receive prior attention in any circumstance and regardless of another's needs. This entitlement does not draw on a utilitarian calculus as much as a special obligation of care. I emphasize *care*. Although financial compensation can satisfy liability, it cannot meet the burden associative duties place on those best situated to offer medical *attention*. Liable harm does not afford a superior right to receive medical care before others. In contrast, associative duties of care require hands-on nurturing and support. Money cannot satisfy these obligations. Therefore, associative duties, like the dictates of mass casualty triage, override obligations of impartial medical care when resources are scarce.

There are good reasons, then, to avoid using medical care to compensate the accidental, unnecessary, disproportionate, and collateral casualties of war. This leaves multinational forces to consider financial restitution. Whether Coalition payments of $2,500 per person are sufficient compensation for liable harms depends on how likely civilians are to accept it and whether it covers civilian losses. Iraq and Afghanistan are poor countries, and the sums are usually acceptable. Whether money or medicine eased resentment or swayed civilians to support their government is an empirical question I will take up in Chapter 10 as the discussion turns to utilizing medicine to win hearts and minds.

Beyond compensation, however, is a more substantial duty that humanitarian forces, in particular, owe the people they are fighting to protect irrespective of liability. Compensation for accidental, negligent, or collateral harm is a useful adjunct to just war. Still, it does not address the debilitating effects of noncombat accidents and disease, nor does it offer a firm rationale to determine the appropriate level of aid. Coalition payments only meet some vague demand of local custom. Looking past liability to the good of the entire civilian population, however, the principle of broad beneficence defines the obligation to render aid. At this juncture, medical care assumes a central role during and after the fighting. The moral demands of humanitarian war compel us to consider an alternative second rule of medical eligibility.

The Second Rule of Medical Eligibility Reconsidered

As it stands, a rule that bases medical eligibility on liability for collateral harm satisfies no one. In a defensive war, a defending nation does no wrong when it harms civilians insofar as their injuries are, in fact, collateral, and not negligent, accidental, or disproportionate. Assuming collateral damage is not excessive, there are usually no grounds to reduce harm any further by obligating an occupying power to evacuate and tend injured civilians beyond what the "means available to it" permit (ICRC 1949b: Article 55). To do so would either divert resources from the war effort or require such significant assets as to make defensive wars unfeasible. The same argument constrains postwar reconstruction in a defensive war. Unless necessary for some strategic purpose—strengthening regional security or preventing anarchy—the grounds for reconstructing a war-torn enemy nation are weak. Failure to aid reconstruction in postwar Gaza (2014) or South Lebanon (2006), for example, might destabilize the region. If not, Israel disregards no duty for failing to pursue postwar reconstruction in these regions. The second medical rule of eligibility, therefore, has no place in defensive war. The first rule alone suffices. Humanitarian wars, on the other hand, require a second rule far broader than the current formulation provides.

In humanitarian wars, the civilian population deserves special attention. Chapter 1 introduced the concept of "broad" beneficence to distinguish the duty to tend an individual patient (narrow beneficence) from the wider responsibility to attend to the welfare of a political community. In defensive wars, the political community comprises compatriots; in humanitarian war, the affected community spreads further to embrace the beneficiaries of intervention. This substantial difference generates a duty of beneficence absent from defensive wars, namely, to realize a greater good for the target population. Therefore, while defensive wars measure proportionality by comparing civilian casualties to military advantage, humanitarian wars weigh civilians killed or injured against civilians saved.

Infused with the obligation to rescue the local population and ensure their welfare, humanitarian wars generate far greater concern for the victims of war than defensive wars do. The victims of humanitarian war push well beyond those harmed directly by military operations to include those suffering the effects of wartime malnutrition, disease, or injury, irrespective of when and how they were wounded or sickened. The downstream and indirect effects of war are significant, four to ten times greater than direct, violent deaths (Geneva Declaration 2015: 34, 43 n.19; also Hagopian et al. 2013; Wise 2017). The obligation to attend to the welfare of the civilian population does not stem from liability, but from the comprehensive duty of broad beneficence and rescue that the responsibility to protect entails. Therefore, the revised second rule of medical eligibility in humanitarian wars encompasses the short- and long-term welfare of the civilian population. Following the first rule that distributes medical resources to compatriot and allied warfighters, the second rule distributes whatever resources remain based on medical urgency or clinical-medical necessity.

By addressing the welfare of the entire civilian population, the revised rule remedies two functional deficiencies of the existing guideline. First, it overcomes the disparate standards of liability by offering a single category of eligible recipients, namely, the whole civilian population. In contrast, any rule subject to liability must distinguish among different types of injuries and harm to award care and compensation appropriately. Navigating this labyrinth in the field is daunting and renders any liability-based rule of eligibility impractical. Although caregivers might readily see that a patient is a soldier or civilian, compatriot or local national, there seems no practical method to determine whether their wounds are military or civilian in origin or, if military, the result of humanitarian or insurgent operations or, if at the hand of humanitarian forces, accidental, negligent, or collateral. In contrast, a broad beneficence-based rule does not require any finer distinction than distinguishing compatriots from local nationals, a permissible criterion of medical eligibility that characterizes its first rule (Chapter 5).

Second, beneficence offers a single medical principle for distributing care within this group, namely, medical urgency. Medical urgency speaks to *clinical* rather than *military*-medical necessity (Chapter 1) and reflects the imperative to save as many lives and limbs as possible by treating dire cases first. Evaluating these medical needs is what doctors do best. Adopting an undifferentiated civilian patient group and the principle of medical urgency broadens the existing rule of eligibility. Broad beneficence directs military medical practitioners to save any local national's life, limb, or eyesight, whether caused by injury, disease, friend, or foe.

Saving every civilian's life, limb, or eyesight is a costly undertaking. Earlier, I explained how a revised second rule turns to medical urgency to distribute *remaining resources*. But the rule must push further. If the resources remaining after fulfilling the first rule are insufficient to save life, limb, and eyesight across the civilian population, then humanitarian forces must provide them. The revised second rule establishes a floor of morally minimal medical care, an obligation that entails significantly greater resources than intervening nations have allocated in previous conflicts. To avoid obstructing military operations, obligations of beneficence may play out over time as the pool of available resources grows. During the combat phases of humanitarian intervention, multinational forces will provide emergency medical relief, while deferring the balance of their obligation to postwar reconstruction (Chapter 11).

In the meantime, medical providers will ask how to distribute whatever medical assets remain after attending to compatriot and host-nation military personnel. I suggested earlier that clinical medical urgency is the most practical distributive standard to utilize. Nevertheless, one may imagine instances where care for specific civilians may offer considerable military benefits. In Chapter 10, I describe how attention to grateful civilians may deliver intelligence or other aid following medical care. Two situations warrant attention to military necessity. First, military necessity may function as a tiebreaker when two or more patients are equally needy and resources are scarce. Second, military officials may think to single out a promising patient who may collaborate in exchange for medical attention (Chapter 10). Each case is problematic. In the first case, trying to break ties puts inordinate pressure on healthcare providers ill-equipped to evaluate military benefits. In the second and for the reasons described throughout this chapter, financial remuneration is a far more reasonable vehicle for enlisting civilian support.

Civilians round out the wartime sick and injured military medicine must attend. To put their rights to healthcare in perspective, it is useful to integrate the preceding chapters and summarize the medical rules of eligibility for warfighters, detainees, and civilians.

Summing Up: Medical Rules of Eligibility for Warfighters, Detainees, and Civilians

The medical rules of eligibility described in this and the preceding chapters are lexically ordered. Only after fulfilling the first rule to attend to compatriots and warfighters may military medical providers fulfill the second rule and care for local civilians. The medical rules of eligibility incorporate five important distributive principles: associative duties, military-medical necessity, liability, beneficence, and medical urgency. Each principle generates a responsibility to treat certain classes of the wounded, but not all. Together, they govern casualty care in wartime.

Military-medical necessity allows multinational facilities to tend allied soldiers who can return to duty and some wounded civilians who might aid their war effort. Except for compatriots, all other wounded, including detainees, must seek attention at local healthcare facilities whose level of care may be inferior. For compatriots, associative duties offer priority treatment regardless of the severity of their wounds. Military-medical necessity and associative duties drive the first rule of eligibility. Moral liability affords preferential attention to civilians harmed accidentally or negligently and, to a lesser degree, collaterally. Liability, however, is best satisfied by financial compensation, not medical care. Beneficence, a feature of humanitarian rather than defensive war, pushes further and generates a broad-based obligation toward the entire civilian population. Beneficence, not liability, underlies the revised second rule of eligibility. Medical urgency or clinical-medical necessity is a subsidiary principle. Once patients move into one category or another, urgent medical reasons determine the order or treatment within each group. The principle of impartiality, that is, the duty to provide needs-based care without regard for sex, race, nationality, or religion, dominates within groups, but not between them.

International humanitarian law neither embraces nor repudiates military-medical necessity and associative duties but continues to wrestle with each. In this chapter, I explained how military necessity permits an occupying force only to take the needs of the civilian population "into account" and provide care "to the fullest extent of the means available to it." "Occupying force" connotes a defensive war, one where one nation exercises its right to self-defense to defeat and subjugate an aggressor. During and after a defensive war, the occupier's geopolitical interests and disposable resources frame its responsibilities to rebuild medical and other essential infrastructures. For the most part, military-medical necessity governs the provision of medical care in defensive wars. Military-medical necessity speaks directly to the medical means required to prosecute just war, without which no nation can defend itself or undertake humanitarian intervention. Hence, as a distributive principle, military-medical necessity is a necessary condition of ethically based medical management in war. And in defensive war, where states incur little liability and have no overriding obligation to any civilians but their own, the principle of military-medical necessity is probably sufficient to regulate combat casualty care of all kinds. In the absence of host-nation allies, there is rarely any need to invoke associative duties of preferential treatment. Therefore, the medical rule of eligibility in defensive wars is parsimonious. Put simply, it requires medical personnel to deliver the care necessary to maintain unit readiness and conserve force capabilities.

Humanitarian wars, or wars that pair multinational and host-nation forces to oust a rights-violating regime and restore governance, introduce many more actors with competing healthcare rights. Military-medical necessity remains a necessary condition of delivering health care during humanitarian wars, but it is not sufficient. Host-nation allies present the first challenge. On the one hand, they enjoy the same medical rights as everyone else. On the other hand, intervening forces have special and sometimes overriding obligations to compatriots that put host-nation allies in a subordinate position. Struggling to reconcile these competing obligations, international law recognizes that superior medical care for multinational forces is permissible as long as Iraqi or Afghan soldiers, for example, receive the same standard of medical care as multinational soldiers treated in Iraq or Afghanistan (Chapter 5). The result is the same two-tiered system that associative duties justify. Every injured soldier receives similar in-theater care, but multinational forces enjoy the exclusive right to continuing care in Europe or the United States. Continuing care is no trivial issue. When host-nation wounded cannot benefit from adequate follow-up care in local facilities, their initial treatment may differ substantially from what Coalition casualties receive at the point of injury.

Detainees are in a similar situation. International humanitarian law embraces a single rule of medical eligibility for detainees, namely, to treat adversaries as one's own. In a defensive war, the rule is sensible. For one, each nation is keenly wedded to reciprocity. Comparable care for prisoners of war serves each side's mutual interest to protect its own and preserve morale. At the same time, each side also houses one another's prisoners. There is no opportunity to offload prisoners to facilities run by the local government. In humanitarian wars, the rule of comparable care for detainees is not relevant. In many cases, multinational forces lose few soldiers to insurgent captors, leaving little incentive for reciprocity. As the fighting progresses and the new government gains a foothold, moreover, multinational forces transfer detainees to local prison and medical facilities. There they should enjoy the same level of care that host-nation allies receive, and the same rule of medical eligibility applies.

To this point, the principles of medical-military necessity and associative duties guide medical management in humanitarian war. What of civilians? Restricting military-provided, civilian care to available resources, international humanitarian law does not offer much. A liability-based rule affords preferential care to some civilians, namely, collateral casualties, but the rule is indefensible and unworkable. A broad-based duty of beneficent care for the beneficiaries of intervention recognizes how sustainable medical care is inseparable from the humanitarian mission. The responsibilities to protect and rebuild grasp this obligation. It is not yet law, but as I argue in Chapter 11, these responsibilities dovetail with the duty of broad beneficence that guides humanitarian war. In the combat phase of operations, armed forces can meet their obligations as they bolster human security and improve medical care. But if defensive wars end with the satisfaction of the defender's security interests, humanitarian wars do not. Duties of beneficence draw humanitarian forces into the postwar period and impose the responsibility to rebuild. The result is a second rule of eligibility for civilian medical care in humanitarian war that slowly grows more expansive as the fighting winds down. Until it does, clinical-medical necessity mostly guides practitioners as they utilize surplus resources for sick and injured civilians.

Eligibility rules driven by associative duties and military-medical necessity will inevitably encounter many difficulties during war when resources are scarce. Managing assets differently from civilian distribution schemes, medical rules of eligibility are limited to wartime military facilities. They have little to say about the priority of care during postwar reconstruction. Once the fighting ends, the principle of military-medical necessity drops into the background and associative duties turn their attention to delivering veteran care. Fledgling healthcare systems should serve the entire population without distinction, and their rebuilding is a major undertaking for which the international community should assume a significant part. Associative duties and military-medical necessity are temporary expedients that ultimately pave the way for the principle of clinical-medical necessity that dominates peacetime bioethics and health care.

Combat casualty care, as described in these chapters, is inseparable from medical research. Combat casualty care looks backward. Attending to sickness and injury, its role is therapeutic and curative. In the best cases, it returns soldiers to duty. But often it cannot. Medical research is forward-looking. Its role is preventive. By forestalling debilitation, more warfighters fight better. Pushing further ahead, medical research abandons its therapeutic role to build stronger and faster soldiers. At the same time, military medicine assumes a political role as planners deploy medical care to win backing from the local population. In each case, medicine becomes a weapon of war and a tool of counterinsurgency.

PART III

OFF THE BATTLEFIELD: MEDICINE AS WEAPON OF WAR

8

Military Medical Research
and Experimentation

Throughout history, armed conflict has proved a catalyst for critical and innovative medical technology. The Romans were among the first to discover the benefits of wound debridement and public hygiene (Broughton, Janis, and Attinger 2006). Ambrose Paré (1510–1590), a pioneer of military medicine, confronted unprecedented injuries and burns that he could only treat by trial and error (Paré 1968). Dominque Larrey experimented with surgical techniques to amputate limbs and treat gunshot wounds during the Napoleonic Wars ([1814] 1987; Baker and Strosberg 1992). The US Civil War saw the introduction of anesthesia and early efforts to build dedicated units to evacuate the wounded from the field of battle (Ginn 1977). Antiseptics saved lives during the Franco-Prussian War (Cope 1941), while the British experimented with a vaccine for typhoid fever during the Boer War (Pagaard 1986). World War I introduced bacteriological monitoring of wounds, maxillofacial reconstruction, and care for post-traumatic stress disorder (PTSD; "shell shock"). With these and other innovations, deaths from infection and disease drew even with deaths on the battlefield for the first time in modern history (Gabriel and Metz 1992 II: 239–252). World War II witnessed the rapid development of penicillin on a scale sufficient to save the lives of Allied soldiers and change the face of modern medicine (Adams 1991; Sheehan 1992).

World War II, however, also saw Japanese and German physicians conduct brutal medical experiments. Addressing these abuses, the 1947 Nuremberg Code codified 10 ethical principles to regulate human research. Voluntary, informed consent leads the list followed by necessity, social utility, reasonable risk, and constant concern for the subject's welfare. Nevertheless, American and British scientists experimented on service personnel with nerve gas and mind-altering drugs despite the laws and regulations that should have blocked these experiments (Lederer 2003; Moreno 2013; Schmidt 2015). At the same time, medical professionals aided US and British efforts to develop, and defend against, chemical and biological weapons (Gross 2008b).

Despite these dark cases, military medical research and experimentation can serve the ends of just war as they maintain force capabilities. The salient issues turn on proper research protocols that respect the military subject's rights, promote broad beneficence, and adhere to the constraints of military-medical necessity. To clarify these matters, this chapter and the next distinguish between therapeutic and enhancement research. Medical therapies are preventive, curative, or rehabilitative. Preventive therapies impede physical or mental degradation and include vaccinations and other prophylactic measures. Curative therapies might be surgical or pharmacological; their purpose is to restore normal functioning. On the other hand, rehabilitative therapies, such as prosthetic devices, hope to restore functioning to the highest degree possible.

Medical enhancements, in contrast, are not therapeutic. They neither prevent nor cure any disease but afford a military organization the means to increase its chances of prevailing in armed conflict. Enhancement pushes healthy warfighters beyond the range of normal cognitive and physical capabilities. Emerging technologies may be pharmacological (e.g., nootropic or "memory" pills), surgical (brain-computer interfaces), genetic (gene editing), or mechanical (exoskeletons). Enhancement research, the subject of the following chapter, raises unique ethical challenges that differ from therapeutic research.

This chapter highlights the ethical issues attending therapeutic research during the wars in Iraq and Afghanistan, the crucible of military medical research in this century so far. Over the years, American and British authorities codified human research regulations to meet concerns that military service personnel are a unique, vulnerable patient population. More stringent than the rules governing civilian medical research, these regulations tighten requirements for informed consent that hampered clinical studies of emerging technologies. In response, two policy proposals broaden the scope and efficacy of military medical research. The first eases the rules regulating clinical research to afford military research subjects the same safeguards that civilian research subjects enjoy. The second enlists the civilian population when service personnel cannot provide the critical mass of clinical research subjects for military medical science.

Therapeutic Military Medical Research and Experimentation

Between the Vietnam War and the wars in Iraq and Afghanistan, the ethical and legal landscape of clinical research changed rapidly. In response to a growing awareness of patient rights among bioethicists and revelations of research abuses, the (US) Commission for the Protection of Human Subjects of Biomedical and Behavioral Research (1974–1978) set new standards for human research. Emerging regulations emphasized respect for persons, informed consent, protection of immature and incapacitated test subjects, and the fair distribution of costs and benefits among subjects and their communities (Belmont Report 1979; Jonsen 1998: 99–106). As the United States returned to war in the Middle East, two challenges engaged research ethics: administering investigational drugs on the battlefield and conducting clinical studies in-theater.

Investigational Drugs and Military Medical Experimentation

In 1990, concerns about informed consent and vulnerable military populations ignited a public debate over the administration of investigational drugs in the US military. An investigational drug is one the US Food and Drug Administration (FDA) has approved for testing in humans but not for sale to patients (NIH 2019). When investigational drugs hold particular promise, the military may administer them to troops to assure their health and to maintain operational readiness. During the First Gulf War (1991), for example, American authorities considered investigational drugs to protect soldiers against nerve gas and botulism. The vaccinations were unproved and under investigation, but offered significant military benefits. Ordinarily, a medical provider must obtain informed consent before administering any drug. As outlined in Chapter 2, however, military service limits a person's right to refuse treatment. As such, many standard treatments are mandatory for service members. Investigational drugs, however, are neither standard nor proven. Military authorities seeking compulsory vaccination must acquire a waiver of informed consent when battlefield conditions make it infeasible to acquire soldiers' agreement. Following vigorous public debate, new guidelines invested the US president alone with the authority to issue the appropriate waivers (Chapter 3).

Controversy flared again in 1998 when the US Army wanted to inoculate troops against airborne anthrax using a vaccine approved for subcutaneous anthrax. Critics maintained that the US Department of Defense (DoD) required a waiver of informed consent because the drug was investigational. In response, the DoD argued that the vaccine was a standard treatment (Cummings 2002; FitzPatrick and Zwangziger 2003). The DoD prevailed, leaving dissenting American soldiers to resign from service if they declined vaccination. The dispute resurfaced again in 2005 when the DoD successfully secured an Emergency Use Authorization (EUA) to continue mandatory anthrax vaccinations (Nightingale, Prasher, and Simonson 2007). Well into the war in Iraq, 300–500 service members refused inoculation, and nearly 40 faced court-martial (AP 2003; Parasidis 2015). In the United Kingdom, on the other hand, anthrax vaccinations were voluntary. The refusal rate varied from 22% early in the war when the threat of biological weapons was high, to 59% when this threat subsided later (Murphy et al. 2008).

At first glance, mandatory investigational drugs are treatment, not research. Under the circumstances, they offered US authorities the best hope to shield troops from the threat of biological and chemical warfare. But "hope" is the operative word. Drawn on imprecise data, the efficacy of investigational drugs remains uncertain so that prescribing them in novel circumstances constitutes experimental research. Were the drugs useless or dangerous, research norms would demand cessation. Were they efficacious but highly risky, military necessity may permit their continued use if required to keep soldiers fit for duty. Service personnel may still refuse treatment but face sanctions if they do.

The evolving practice of administering investigational drugs suggests a model of permissible military medical research that differs significantly from civilian medical research. Civilian research is directly curative or rehabilitative; its goal is to help a particular patient or patient class such as diabetics or lung cancer patients. The principle guiding medical research is each individual's right to health care consistent with maximizing utility and providing the state of health required for a dignified life. The devil is in the details, particularly when health officials must balance therapies that save lives against those that improve their quality. But the principles of utility and patient rights are not controversial.

In contrast, military medical research serves two goals. Like civilian medicine, military medicine is curative or rehabilitative. But unlike its civilian counterpart, military medical research searches for therapies to prevent troop degradation, return warfighters to duty, and maintain unit readiness. Research to prevent and treat traumatic brain injury and severe hemorrhaging top the list. Second, but subordinately, military medical research invests in the curative and rehabilitative therapies required to maintain a dignified life: advanced prosthetics, mental health care, and rehabilitation. Each goal drove subsequent research as multinational forces moved into the Mideast.

Military Medical Research during the Iraq and Afghanistan Wars

Novel injuries and diseases coupled with urgent demands to maintain force capability propel medical research during war. In Iraq and Afghanistan, improvised explosive devices (IEDs) were the leading cause of death, accounting for 60% to 70% of all Coalition fatalities and dwarfing the gunshot and fragmentation wounds of earlier conflicts (Kelly et al. 2008; Penn-Barwell et al. 2015). Massive hemorrhage and catastrophic brain injury were the most common cause of death (Eastridge et al. 2012b). Severe injuries among survivors included PTSD, traumatic brain injury, musculoskeletal injuries, and limb amputation (Baker 2014; Warden 2006).

While technological innovations, body armor, and explosion-resistant vehicles significantly reduced the number and intensity of IED attacks, it remained for military medicine to tend the injured. Ultimately, military medicine achieved unprecedented survival rates of over 90% during the wars in Iraq and Afghanistan (Goldberg 2016). To meet its responsibilities, military medicine requires urgent research to control bleeding under battlefield conditions (tourniquets, hemostatic agents, and transfusion protocols), optimize field surgery, treat brain injury, develop limb prosthetics, and mitigate PTSD (Bridges and Biever 2010; Eastridge et al. 2012a).

Military medical research, like other medical research, takes several forms. In retrospective studies, investigators mine military databases and trauma registries for a specific injury or illness and follow anonymized, past-patient progress from the date of injury and through care and rehabilitation to track the efficacy of various treatments (Brosch et al. 2008). Researchers do not choose the treatments but compare various protocols that medical units select from available standards of care. To facilitate retrospective studies, the United States, Great Britain, and NATO developed trauma registries to collect the data from all combat casualty care during military operations in Iraq and Afghanistan (Balazs 2019). Retrospective studies permit analyses of large numbers of subjects. As evidence accumulates, practitioners can enhance patient safety, adopt better protocols for airway management, resuscitation, and trauma, and improve training (Costanz and Spott 2010; Eastridge et al. 2009; O'Connell et al. 2012).

Prospective observational studies follow (observe) patients who receive treatment before the commencement of research and track their progress over time. Observational studies "identify and evaluate causes or risk factors of diseases or health-related events . . . and [assess] the strength of the relationship between an exposure and disease variable" (Song and Chung 2010). Research subjects are patients whom investigators confront at the point of injury or illness, often in combat support hospitals. Like retrospective studies, observational studies track a predetermined course of treatment that the researcher does not control. For example, researchers exploring in-theater management of traumatic brain injury followed the treatment course of 99 patients at an Echelon III medical facility for 72 hours following injury (Fang et al. 2015). Their goal was to identify predictors of mortality to improve outcomes for patients. In another study, investigators observed the course and outcome of prehospital medical interventions among 2,000 combat casualties over six years to conclude, "the most common incorrectly performed and missed interventions were airway interventions and chest procedures respectively" (Lairet et al. 2019: 133). Observational studies also include clinical surveys. Among healthcare professionals, clinical surveys measure attitudes or healthcare practices related to military medicine. Among patients, clinical surveys may be noninvasive or invasive. Clinical surveys track such patient behavior as sleep habits or exercise. An invasive survey, in turn, may look for correlations between biomarkers or neuroimaging data and subsequent psychological behavior (e.g., Isaac et al. 2015).

Unlike retrospective and observational studies, controlled clinical trials introduce an experimental intervention to evaluate new drugs, surgical treatments, or medical devices. Investigators randomly divide research subjects into different groups or arms. One arm administers the experimental intervention, while another offers patients an existing protocol or a placebo. Controlled clinical trials put subjects at risk because those in the experimental arm receive a treatment whose efficacy and safety remain unknown, while those in the placebo arm receive no treatment at all. Studies are double-blind so that neither researchers nor subjects know the arm to which they are assigned. For many researchers, randomized controlled trials are the gold standard of medical science (Kirstin Borgerson 2020).

Prehospital research is an essential category of a controlled clinical trial. In a prehospital study, investigators engage research subjects immediately following traumatic injury but prior to hospital admission. Research transpires in the field, whether on the street after an automobile accident or the battlefield following a military operation. Having yet to reach a hospital, the injured must receive experimental care on the spot or in transit to a medical facility. Effective prehospital care is especially critical during armed conflict when the time required to evacuate combat injuries to a hospital is protracted (Mabry and Kotwal 2017). Under these conditions, patients are incompetent, that is, unconscious or significantly impaired and unable to agree to experimental treatment. Nor are family representatives available in-theater to consent on a patient's behalf. In these circumstances, formulating feasible rules for military medical research is especially challenging, particularly if military enrollees comprise a vulnerable population.

Military Medical Research: Vulnerable Populations and Informed Consent

American statutes define vulnerable populations as those "likely to be vulnerable to coercion or undue influence, such as children, prisoners, mentally disabled persons, or economically or educationally disadvantaged persons" (45 CFR 2019: §46.111[a][3]). These are different categories. Children, the mentally disabled, and, perhaps, the uneducated, lack the cognitive facility to avoid coercion or undue influence from those they trust uncritically. In contrast, prisoners and the economically disadvantaged are prime targets of coercion at the hands of those who may withhold the liberties and goods they require for a dignified life.

Military service personnel do not appear in the list of vulnerable populations. Nevertheless, there is legitimate apprehension about coercion and undue influence that come from "institutional or hierarchical dependency" (European Parliament 2014: para. 31). Although soldiers sign consent forms to participate in clinical studies, concerns arising from rank disparity, fears of offending one's superiors, and peer pressure can undermine informed consent when soldiers are asked to accept investigational drugs or participate in medical experiments.

To protect a patient's right to self-determination, US authorities enacted regulations to oversee clinical research and protect the rights of military subjects. The DoD *Human Subjects Protection Regulatory Requirements* require informed consent, medical supervision, a research subject's right to end an experiment, and an independent ombudsman or research monitor (DoD 2011: 24–25) to oversee recruitment and experimentation (US Army 2017). Further requirements forbid involvement of superior officers during the solicitation of research subjects (Spence 2007).

These conditions facilitate the fully informed consent research subjects must provide when participating in medical experiments and clinical trials. When subjects are unconscious, incapacitated, or otherwise incompetent to give consent, family members may act as surrogate or proxy decision-makers and tender consent on a patient's behalf. When neither the research subject nor his proxy can provide consent, investigators may request waivers of informed consent. Additionally, US research guidelines require public consultation with the communities from which investigators draw and conduct medical studies. These rules protect vulnerable ethnic, racial, or religious communities from exploitation and assure that the fruits of research benefit the community that assumed its risk. Community consultation might be less applicable in the military setting but may usefully shed light on military service personnel and their families' interests.

British regulations also demand a research subject's consent, but unlike US practice, British bioethics and medical law do not recognize waivers of informed consent. When a family member is unavailable, UK regulations permit a "professional" legal representative to give consent based on the patient's "presumed will" (National Health Authority 2008: 15). The professional representative may be the patient's primary physician or a person nominated by a local NHS provider or Health Board to determine the patient/research subject's wishes and best interests. As in the United States, research must benefit the patient and mitigate risk. No community consultation is required in the United Kingdom. Instead, researchers must ensure that the "interests of the patient always prevail over those of science and society" (Health Research Authority [UK] 2008: 15). To ensure patient safety, British military officials, like their American counterparts, appoint an independent medical officer (IMO) and Volunteer Champion to "safeguard the health, safety, and well-being of the participants" (Ministry of Defence [UK] 2014: 8; Linton 2008).

To ensure that investigators meet statutory and ethical guidelines, independent and multidisciplinary Institutional Review Boards (IRB) in the

United States (DoD 2011: 11–29), and Ministry of Defence Research Ethics Committees (MODREC) in the United Kingdom (UK MoD 2020a), oversee research approval and compliance. Research oversight is complicated and time-consuming. Charged with what British officials term "proportionate scrutiny" (UK MoD 2020a: 5-2), committee members seek a balance between outcomes and rights. Outcomes comprise benefits net of cost; rights speak to respect for dignity and autonomous decision-making, informed consent, and permissible risk.

Two Decades of Military Medical Research

The American and British rules and regulations guided two decades of military medical research since 9/11. To paint a fuller picture, Table 8.1 describes a sample of research articles drawn from PUBMED, the Joint Combat Casualty Research Team (JC2RT),[1] and Butler, Hagmann, and Butler's 1996 review of combat casualty care in special operations. The PUBMED sample drew 220 abstracted articles from a total of 4,324 that met the search criteria "(military or army) and (Iraq or Afghanistan)" since 2003. Organized by the US Army Institute of Surgical Research in 2006 to conduct combat-relevant medical research in-theater, the Joint Combat Casualty Research Team focused on hemorrhage/acute care, prehospital care, traumatic brain injury, and PTSD (Dukes et al. 2015). Before hostilities in Iraq and Afghanistan, Butler, Hagmann, and Butler (1996) surveyed the existing literature to formulate new guidelines for combat casualty care that were widely adopted in the next decade's fighting.

During the war years, published research focused on reports (26%), retrospective studies (27%–43%), clinical surveys, observational studies (26%–34%), and case studies (9%). Controlled clinical studies were infrequent. The random PUBMED sample of 220 publications returned 10 controlled studies (5%). For a closer look, a further search of all 4,324 publications returned 80 abstracted articles matching the filters "randomized controlled trial (RCT)" or "controlled clinical trial (CCT)." Of these, six did not meet RCT or CCT criteria.

The remaining 74 clinical trials recruited a diverse research population, comprising active duty service personnel (43%), veterans (36%), and military families (9%). Issues of greatest interest were post-traumatic stress disorder (PTSD) and related mental health issues (57%), traumatic brain

Table 8.1. Distribution of Research Articles in Military Medical Journals, Research Team Studies, and Literature Reviews

ITEM	PUBMED 2003–2020	Joint Combat Casualty Research Team (JC2RT) 2011–2018	Butler, Hagmann, and Butler 1996 1970–1995
Report Literature review; lessons learned; new technologies; current practice; doctrine; handbooks, medical history; conference proceedings	58 (26%)	12 (26%)	25 (36%)
Retrospective Study Data drawn from UK, US, and other multinational trauma registries	60 (27%)	20 (43%)	10 (14%)
Case Study	9 (4%)	0	4 (6%)
Clinical Survey/Observational Study One-time or longitudinal questionnaire or clinical survey among healthcare professionals (e.g., health care practice, attitudinal studies) or patients (e.g., sleep habits, exercise, biomarkers, or pain management); prospective observational study of the progress and outcomes of preexisting treatment protocols.	75 (34%)	12 (26%)	7 (10%)
Controlled Clinical Trial/Experimental Intervention Prospective studies introducing an experimental manipulation or intervention with or without randomized control groups.	10 (5%)	2 (5%)	8 (11%)[1]
Nonhuman Study Animal, mannequin, simulation, or equipment	8 (4%)	0	13 (19%)
Insufficient information to identify			3 (4%)
Total	220	46	70
n (margin of error)	4,324 (6%)	46 (0%)	141 (8%)

[1]These eight studies only recruited civilian research subjects.

injury (TBI) (12%), and equipment (7%). Other research areas covered pain management, alcohol abuse, and parenting protocols. Of the experimental interventions studied, 73% were noninvasive psychological therapies, such as virtual reality, mindfulness training, cognitive therapy, meditation, and expressive writing. Nineteen percent of the studies utilized invasive interventions including pharmacological or nonsurgical therapies such as analgesics, antidepressants, hyperbaric oxygen, and electric stimulation. Only four controlled clinical trials enrolled active duty personnel from the Iraq or Afghanistan theater. These studies introduced medication for mild TBI and diarrhea, a dietary supplement, and yoga exercises.

The publication survey data paint a very narrow picture of clinically controlled military medical studies since 2003. None introduced more than minimally invasive experimental interventions. Research subjects were sufficiently competent to understand the experimental trial, participate voluntarily, and tender informed consent. None of the studies, therefore, required approval from patient family members or representatives, or waivers of informed consent. None of the clinical trials conducted prehospital research in-theater or enrolled incompetent patients to test surgical procedures, medical devices, or other invasive technologies. And although military medical research provided crucial lifesaving data, the paucity of controlled experimental research adversely affects its contribution to medical science. Rigorous rules of informed consent sometimes stood in the way.

Military Medical Research Falters

On their face, safeguards to ensure service members' rights to fully informed consent are not so onerous that they impede military medical research. Retrospective studies do not require informed consent or qualify easily for waivers because they are anonymized and pose no risk to research subjects. Observational studies, on the other hand, follow specific patients in real time and, therefore, require a subject's consent or that of their representative. Because observational studies introduce no additional risk of harm, Institutional Review Boards (IRB) or supervising ethics committees may waive consent if patients are not conscious and a legal representative is unavailable. Clinical studies, too, require informed consent from research subjects or their representatives. Because controlled clinical studies pose risks and uncertainty, the subject's representative must judiciously weigh the trial's risk and benefits as well as the subject's wishes. In-theater, research patients are unconscious while representatives or family members are unavailable to approve prehospital research (Dutton et al. 2008). In these cases, US regulations permit waivers of informed consent if research is necessary for the military, benefits the patient, and presents reasonable or minimal risks (DoD 3216.02 2018: §3.9; FDA Guidance 2013:§20–21). UK regulations make no room for waivers but allow a third party to serve as a research subject's representative.

Notwithstanding regulations that should facilitate research, approval for controlled randomized studies to test surgical or pharmacological interventions or promising medical devices faltered. Another look at Table 8.1 highlights the preponderance of retrospective, observational, and survey studies that do not require informed consent, or wherein subjects or their proxies readily provide consent, or waivers are available because the studies pose no added risk of harm. In contrast, randomized controlled experimental studies are in very short supply. In no US sample was research undertaken with waivers of informed consent, although these are technically available. In none of the controlled clinical studies sampled did researchers turn to representatives to collect data from patients who could not give consent.

Despite the urgency of randomized prehospital research, investigators describe how disagreement among US government agencies about ethically permissible protocols and stringent demands for informed consent hindered research as early as 2005 (McManus et al. 2005). And although UK protocols were comparatively streamlined, the result was to shift military medical research from the standards of randomized controlled studies to retrospective and observational studies and the limitations these entail. In 2013, the US Government Accountability Office (GAO 2013: 2) reported DoD estimates "that about 24 percent of service members who die in combat could have survived if improved and more timely medical care could be made available." Research gaps in diagnosing, resuscitating, and tending casualties with survivable wounds persisted. By 2008, medical defense officials could resolve only 9% of these gaps. And although this figured improved by 2014, only 39% of the high-priority research gaps in military combat casualty care, including research to control bleeding, replace blood, and perform damage control surgery were closed (Rasmussen, Rauch, and Hack 2014: S55; also Rasmussen et al. 2015). Why was this gap so persistently wide? Lack of funding and interagency communication were undoubtedly two obstacles (GAO 2013). But concerns about gaining informed consent from service personnel hindered approval of controlled studies in particular and military medical research more generally.

Conflicting Rules of Informed Consent

In the United States, conflicting rules regulating informed consent contributed to the slow pace of clinical studies. The US Code of Federal Regulations (45 CFR 2019: §46.116) regulates most clinical research conducted or supported by civilian or military agencies. If a person or his agent cannot give informed consent, waivers of consent are available when research is essential and involves no more than minimal risk. At the same time, however, the US Food and Drug Administration (FDA) adopted stricter rules that made it difficult to obtain waivers for minimal-risk research to experiment with FDA-regulated products. One outcome was to hamper studies of unapproved but promising investigational medical devices to monitor wounded and incapacitated warfighters on the battlefield even when these devices posed no risk (Bohannon 2011). Such obstacles led American researchers to complain:

> FDA and DoD requirements for informed consent meant to protect individuals enrolled in research can have the untoward effect of impeding research necessary to provide evidentiary standards for advances in therapeutic, diagnostic, and preventive clinical interventions ... these requirements ironically make the most innocuous research (from a subject's perspective) the most difficult to approve. (Berwick, Downey, and Cornett 2015: 198–199)

Although subsequent regulations relaxed some constraints on minimal risk studies (21st Century Cures Act 2016: §3024; 45 CFR 46 2019), severe limitations plagued American research during the war years.

Prehospital trauma research (e.g., fluid resuscitation or intubation) was especially affected (Osborne, Knudson, and Holcomb 2017). Critically wounded soldiers cannot give consent, nor are representatives available on the battlefield. Requests for waivers of informed consent faced severe headwinds. Noting that controlled clinical research must benefit the research subject, a 2016 US study explained: "The Secretary of Defense or his/her designee has the authority under 10 USC. §980 to waive the requirement for informed consent for a specific research study if it is deemed necessary to the armed forces and may directly benefit the subjects (*notably including subjects in control groups*)" (Berwick, Downey, and Cornett 2016: 198, emphasis added). Because control group subjects do not always benefit, particularly those receiving placebos, this interpretation, coupled with restrictions on permissible risk, effectively prohibited controlled experimental studies of severely injured service members (Hatzfeld et al. 2013: 117; Perkins et al. 2012).

In the United Kingdom, the problem was less critical. While UK regulations greatly expanded the role of legal representatives to permit personal and professional representatives to give consent, these rules could not accommodate research if no representative was available in deployed settings. Addressing these lacunae in 2005 and 2006, UK lawmakers modified their regulations to allow researchers to defer informed consent until a subject was competent or a legal representative available. In the meantime, researchers could recruit incapacitated subjects for randomized controlled emergency studies with the preapproval of the ethics oversight committee (Health Research Authority [UK] 2008: 9; also Hodgetts 2014; Davies et al. 2014). Examples of pertinent research include the emergency use of tranexamic acid in severe trauma (Perry et al. 2014), expedited treatment for traumatic hemorrhage, and prospective observational studies requiring blood samples and cardiographic imaging from severely injured soldiers (Nordmann et al. 2014). Strict European Union regulations (EU 2014: §31), on the other hand, required immediate consent of the patient/research subject or her representative, thereby rendering any prehospital research involving EU service personnel impossible.

Alternative Research Protocols

Does the lack of controlled clinical studies impede military medical research? The US Government Accountability Office (2013) noted significant, unresolved gaps in casualty care research. To close these gaps, investigators turned to alternative, noninterventional research models termed "focused empiricism" (Rasmussen and Kellerman 2016) or "clinical innovation" (Hodgetts 2014). Each model encourages American and British researchers to integrate clinical surveys, retrospective data, and emerging evidence to develop the best possible treatment protocols when "high-quality data are not available to inform clinical practice changes [and] there is extreme urgency to improve outcomes" (Berwick, Downey, and Cornett 2016: xxxvi). These data sources obviate the need for informed consent from incapacitated research subjects and, for example, comprise most of Butler, Hagmann, and Butler's (1996) study of combat casualty care in the mid-1990s. Until then, combat casualty care drew mostly on civilian trauma protocols. But the pressure of treating severe injuries under fire, securing rapid evacuation, and administering pre-hospital care rendered many civilian protocols unsuitable. Changing course, Special Operation Forces medicine turned to field experience, interviews and focus sessions, literature reviews, animal studies, retrospective studies, and civilian clinical studies to formulate new guidelines (Butler, Hagmann, and Butler 1996; Table 8.1 column 4). Subsequent large-scale fighting in Iraq and Afghanistan proved the efficacy of these innovations (Butler and Blackbourne 2012; Butler 2017).

Nevertheless, retrospective studies are inherently limited to existing protocols and do not make room to test entirely novel approaches. Nor does focused empiricism alone overcome the legal and ethical impediments that restrict trauma research when consent is unavailable. Focused empir-icism and clinical innovation, despite their achievements, only make the best of an adverse research environment. Closing the research gap to afford better trauma care requires some fundamental changes in military medical research.

Honing the Ethics of Military Medical Research

Two avenues—consistent implementation of informed consent requirements for service personnel and aggressively recruiting civilians—can increase the pool of research subjects to facilitate combat care research wherein neither the patient nor a representative can consent. Neither is without difficulties. If service personal are a vulnerable population, they require tighter, not weaker protection. Civilians, in turn, may find that they do not benefit directly from military medical research. If so, why should they consent to participate?

Vulnerability and Informed Consent

Prompted by past abuses of experimental subjects in the military, American and British research protocols help ensure that service personnel can make informed choices about research participation and that military authorities will respect those decisions. However, it would be a mistake, as some sug-gest, to see military personnel as a vulnerable population on par with minors, prisoners, or the economically or educationally disadvantaged who require special protection (McManus et al. 2007; Parasidis 2016). Service personnel do not lack sound decision-making capacity nor suffer from socially inflicted disabilities. There are no a priori reasons that make them incapable of making informed choices about participating in medical research.

Coercion, Undue Influence, and Informed Consent
It is essential to distinguish concerns about coercion from the central role of social norms and authority figures in medical decision-making. As a person or his proxy deliberates, healthcare professionals are right to protect research subjects from those with competing interests. But protection from coercion and undue influence does not prohibit anyone from taking counsel. It is an exceptionally rarified and atomized view of autonomous decision-making to think that any person, much less someone who is ill, judiciously collects information alone and deliberates in isolation. In Chapter 6, I explain how consent is a social construct when individuals agree to participate in hunger strikes or some other act of political defiance. In their deliberations, they weigh individual and collective interests as they respond to norms of fidelity, mutual responsibility, and duty. Individual interests speak to personal health and well-being. Collective interests call attention to public and political welfare, and shared security. As they weigh their concerns, prospective research subjects may solicit the opinions of others to guide their decisions. Heteronomous appeals to external authorities do not impair decision-making but are integral to robust consent.

In the same vein, any decision to participate in military medical research legitimately reflects many social, communal, and cultural influences. These include deference to moral authorities (whose opinion one values highly), to organizational authorities (who train and supervise subordinates), and to communal norms that orient personal behavior. Like many organizations, the military is hierarchical. But to suggest that a military community is excessively coercive and seriously abridges personal autonomy is to misunderstand the fundamental role communities and their members play in individual decision-making. While close-knit friendship and professional bonds tightly bind some military communities, the military remains a voluntary organization that prizes both compliance and initiative. Each is an essential component of individual decision-making.

The military does not undermine autonomy any more than any ethnic or religious community that participates in medical research. In both cases, community authorities are legitimate sources of guidance. As such, it is reasonable to allow soldiers to consult with their commanders as long as superiors recognize their obligation to provide sound advice about a person's interests and those of the institution. For the same reasons, legal representatives of military personnel deserve the same decisional discretion accorded representatives of incapacitated civilian research subjects. There is no reason to think that a person's or his proxy's decision to participate in medical research is not free and informed unless accompanied by *overt* coercion, that is, by the threat of physical or psychological harm.

Unquestionably, military organizations are coercive. When protocols demand the resignation of service personnel who decline investigational drugs, coercion incentivizes consent. In this case, the proper response is to invoke the public health paradigm that permits sanctions to guarantee compliance to prevent or stem a health emergency (Chapter 1). Service personnel must accept investigational treatments to keep them fit for duty and ensure mission integrity. Compliance must be widespread, if not universal, to effectively sustain a fighting force, just as it must be to avert a pandemic. Under these circumstances, sanctions are permissible insofar they do not deny service members the option of refusing investigational drugs as some reasonable albeit high cost.

Military medical research, however, is not the same as mandatory treatment. Although both offer therapeutic benefits to individual patients and, more generally, to the community of warfighters and civilians they serve, medical research is riskier and its outcome far less certain. Having approached the threshold of acceptable risk, investigational drugs permit a reasonable assessment of their costs and benefits. When the benefits are significant and the cost proportionate, treatment is mandatory. In contrast, medical research investigates therapies of unknown efficacy or value. Participation carries a substantial and undetermined risk that does not permit any reasonable assessment of proportionate harm and military advantage. Soldiers, therefore, may refuse. Risk assessment, therefore, is at the heart of military medical research. How much risk should a soldier bear in the service of medical science?

Acceptable Risk for Military Medical Research
To determine the criteria for reasonable risk, it is important to distinguish between clinical care and clinical research. While clinical care offers therapeutic benefits to a patient at some cost, research experiments afford therapeutic benefits to future patients but may not necessarily aid research subjects. Research subjects falling into the placebo arm of a randomized

clinical study, for example, do not benefit when the experimental treatment could have effectively cured their illness or injury. To reduce the hazards of research, some researchers adopt the principle of "clinical equipoise." Clinical equipoise requires investigators to compare the risks of each arm of a randomized study and ensure that neither puts the subject in greater jeopardy (Weijer and Miller 2004). When a current treatment offers only a poor outcome, and the experimental intervention is yet untested, clinical equipoise demands that "no patient will receive a treatment known to be less effective or more dangerous than the alternative" (Beauchamp and Childress 2009: 321–322). "Known" is probably too strong a condition. Researchers can only *expect* the experimental treatment to be more effective and less dangerous than the alternative.

DoD guidelines requiring that clinical research "intend to benefit each subject enrolled in the study, [including] subjects enrolled in study placebo arms" (US Army 2017: 3) refer specifically to incompetent patients who cannot provide informed consent. The provision is onerous unless interpreted to mean that research should not be *expected* to impose higher risk on subjects in control groups than on experimental subjects. This interpretation is consistent with the principle of clinical equipoise. Does defaulting DoD regulations to clinical equipoise increase the likelihood that researchers will conduct randomized controlled studies? The answer is not clear. As critics point out, clinical equipoise sets a very high bar for acceptable risk that jeopardizes experimental controls (i.e., placebo arms). By failing to distinguish between clinical medical ethics and research ethics, proponents of equipoise require medical scientists to attend to research subjects in the same way physicians attend to their patients (Miller and Brody 2003, 2007). On the other hand, proposals for randomized clinical studies among service members rarely moved past the obstacles of attaining waivers of informed consent. As a result, clinical equipoise remains unassessed.

Military medical research in the United States and the United Kingdom seems caught between conflicting forces. On the one hand, the military mission requires controlled clinical studies to develop medical care needed to maintain unit readiness and, more generally, serve the welfare of the political community. On the other hand, military organizations remain sensitive, perhaps excessively so, to the vulnerability of enlisted service personnel. The results are tighter controls on military than civilian medical research (Gillenwater 2008). Despite provisions that permit American and British researchers to either waive informed consent (US) or seek it later (UK), neither nation conducted much, if any, in-hospital or prehospital controlled clinical research with subjects who could not provide consent.

Past histories of abuse and exploitation, public distrust and insufficient confidence in existing oversight mechanisms, and an excessively paternal-istic view of soldiers' decision-making capacities account for the lack of con-trolled clinical studies of invasive, experimental therapies. To overcome many of these deficiencies, it is only necessary to equalize the status of military and civilian research subjects while recognizing that each group is equally vul-nerable. Military and civilian research should embrace the same standards of consent, oversight, and community consultation. Granting service personnel and their representatives the same degree of decision-making capacity and protections as civilians would open the door for greater controlled exper-imental military medical research. To this end, US authorities should also consider the British practice permitting professional legal representatives to tender consent if friends or family are unavailable. A larger pool of surrogate decision-makers is, in many ways, superior to waivers of informed consent. Because waivers are approved when a project is first reviewed (or annually thereafter) rather than when conducted, they may grow stale. The participa-tion of professional representatives might help ensure up-to-date ethics com-pliance and subject protection without impeding research.

Properly executed, existing provisions are sufficient if unencumbered by unwarranted fears about soldiers' vulnerability. Nevertheless, and precisely because soldiers are competent decision-makers, medical research belongs on their educational agenda, to explain the vital role of the many research protocols, their rights as test subjects, the benefits that accrue, and the lessons of past malpractice. None of these suggestions relax existing protocols; they only facilitate their implementation.

Aggressively Recruiting Civilians

Controlled, in-theater clinical research is not only constrained by obstacles to securing informed consent but by logistical difficulties as well: lack of trained research personnel, staff rotation, and the intense pressure of attending to multiple casualties that leave little time for clinical studies. As a result, ci-vilian trials, particularly for prehospital and trauma care, are necessary to inform military medical doctrine (Holcomb and Hoyt 2015; Rasmussen and Baer 2014). Civilian-populated studies led to significant advances in major extremity trauma and rehabilitation (METRC 2019), blood transfusions and damage control resuscitation, and treatment for traumatic brain injury (Berwick, Downey, and Cornett 2016: 184–185). And while the benefits of collaboration are many, military and civilian research is not symmetric. The medical needs of young, healthy men and women operating in an austere environment during armed conflict differ significantly from those of a random sample of civilian trauma victims. As a result, a civilian-based study for military emergency trauma care, for example, may be of great value to the military but of only marginal benefit to the civilians and communities participating in the study. In other instances, civilian and military research may complement each other. Studies have shown, for example, that military casualties with severe TBI are three times more likely to survive than similarly injured civilians (Berwick, Downey, and Cornett 2016: 174). The cause for superior survival rates remains the topic of further investigation, but points to the significant benefits of collaborative research.

Community consultation may help their members better understand military needs and agree to participate in vital clinical studies. It is a peculiar but significant feature of American emergency medical research to solicit community input. Community consultation disseminates pertinent information, collects feedback, and respects communities by "identifying potential community-level concerns" (FDA 2013: paragraph 54). When a person requires an emergency *treatment* of proven benefit but cannot consent, it is reasonable to proceed based on the individual's best interest. But when a person is recruited for emergency *research* and cannot grant permission, calculations of best interest move to future patients and the best interests of the community of which research subjects are members.

Considering the greater social good is a fair topic of community consultation and public discourse. Each permits communities to ask how military research will provide health benefits to their members. The answer is not always clear. Consider military trauma research that requires victims of gunshot wounds or urban violence. Community members may object because the experimental protocol affords far less benefit to urban casualties than to military casualties or because medical research only diverts attention from the root causes of gun violence: poverty, substandard education, or weak law enforcement. The interests of the research community do not always dovetail with military interests or with the interests of other groups that may benefit from the research. The consultation process allows civilian and military communities to understand the politics of medical research and know who benefits and who bears its risks. Given histories of abuse, communities should be wary of exploitation and are right to expect a fair distribution of research benefits and risks (e.g., Katz et al. 2006).

During war, the situation is more complicated. Weapons and injuries are sometimes unprecedented, research needs are urgent, and the learning curve is steep. Ultimately, military medical research improves warfighter health, sustains a fighting force, and serves a nation's war aims. When safeguarding national security or intervening on behalf of a persecuted people, war serves collective interests. Articulating the claims of those affected, whether the local, military, national, or rescued community—is an integral part of community consultation. By pushing the scope of *community* beyond the local group providing research subjects to embrace the body politic, the cost-benefit calculus changes. By taking stock of national interests, a calculation of expected utility permits relatively small benefits for the experimental community if the benefits across the political commonwealth are significant. This is not how community consultation usually works; local communities typically weigh their members' costs and benefits in isolation (Goldkind et al. 2014). But wartime should broaden its perspective considerably. Investigators should approach communities whose particular characteristics are conducive to military medical research. In turn, those communities ought to weigh these requests seriously. Nevertheless, no potential research subject has an absolute obligation to participate. The risk may be too high and benefits too marginal even after weighing the public good. Consideration of the public good, however, is a wartime obligation *if* all society's members benefit from a war effort. From this perspective, UK regulations stating, "The interests of the patient always prevail over those of science and society," require qualification. A patient or a community may, and often should, broaden patient interests to embrace those of their national community, particularly in wartime. In this way, community consultation would also benefit medical research in the United Kingdom.

Looking Forward

To forever forestall the horrific German and Japanese medical experiments of World War II, the Nuremberg Code emphasizes the overwhelming importance of informed consent for all kinds of medical experimentation. The preponderance of benefit over risk and concern for test subjects' welfare afford further guarantees of permissible experimentation. Nevertheless, the Nuremberg Code did not prevent postwar abuses. For this reason, Moreno, Schmidt, and Joffe (2017) call upon the medical profession to collaborate closely with government agencies to protect research participants. It's the right call, but the pendulum may have swung too far, hampering and, perhaps, preventing essential wartime research. The upshot is neither to strengthen nor unacceptably weaken research protections for warfighters, but to place them on par with civilians. Following the experience in Iraq and Afghanistan, focused empiricism, better use of waivers, the universal adoption of legal representatives for incompetent research subjects, and closer military-civilian cooperation also may improve military medical research in the next war.

Nevertheless, one may ask, what about a more conservative approach? As diminishing fatality rates attest, military medicine made considerable progress without enrolling incompetent research subjects. Perhaps the current, cautious approach to military medical research only slows research while protecting the rights of soldiers who may not be a vulnerable audience but are certainly a captive one. There is, however, a disconnect between the rules to protect experimental subjects and their implementation that is difficult to justify. Implementing, rather than obstructing, the regulations designed to protect soldiers can provide the edge needed to prepare for future conflicts. Cross-fertilization is also essential. American research protocols might benefit from the inclusion of professional legal representatives common in the United Kingdom. The United Kingdom would gain a broader perspective of the public good that the transparency and cooperation afforded by community consultation can attain.

These recommendations do not speak directly to enhancement medical research. Informed consent drives ethically sound enhancement research, but test subjects are healthy and alert. They do not require surrogate decision-makers. Nevertheless, informed consent and coercion are at the center of any medical study, particularly one that offers no direct therapeutic benefit to its recipients. The ethical demands of enhancement research are the subject of the next chapter.

9

Warfighter Enhancement:
Research and Technology

Since World War II and throughout the Cold War, physicians have helped develop chemical and biological (CB) weapons (Gross 2006: 245–286). The moral dissonance of doctors building weapons of mass destruction was palpable but remained unresolved until international law banned biological weapons in 1972 and restricted chemical weapons in 1993. Rogue regimes persist, of course, leaving nations to develop defensive measures. And although CB weapons research has waned, the prospect of medically enhancing warfighters raises many issues anew.

In contrast to medical research to treat traumatic brain injury or hemorrhage (Chapter 8), enhancement technologies are not therapeutic: soldiers designated for enhancement are not sick or injured. Instead, commanders seek to improve soldiers' warfighting ability while reducing risk to life and limb. Enhancements may be cognitive or physical; invasive or noninvasive; and pharmacological, genetic, physiological, or mechanical (Table 9.1).

Table 9.1. Military Medical Enhancement Technologies

Targeted Performance	Pharmacological/ Biological Invasive	Physiological Invasive	Mechanical Invasive	Noninvasive
Cognitive	Nootropics (memory pills)	Vagus nerve stimulation	Brain-computer interface	Transcranial magnetic stimulation
	Amphetamines, Modafinil	Genetic editing	Human-assisted neural device	Body- area networks Targeted neuroplasticity training
	Propranolol (beta-blockers)			
Physical	EPO (blood doping) Steroids	Lasik vision enhancement	Robotic exoskeletons	Wearable exoskeletons

Cognitive enhancing pharmaceuticals include nootropics to improve memory, amphetamines and Modafinil to prevent fatigue and enhance alertness (Caldwell and Caldwell 2005; Schermer et al. 2009), and propranolol, a beta-blocker to impede memory consolidation to forestall post-traumatic stress disorder (PTSD) or moral injury (Giordano and Wurzman 2011; Giustino, Fitzgerald, and Maren 2016). To enhance physical performance, erythropoietin (EPO), or "blood doping," stimulates red blood cell production and boosts endurance (Eisenstein et al. 2018; Friedl 2015). A futuristic "pain vaccine" might allow the wounded to soldier on without otherwise debilitating effects (Jacobson 2015). Pharmacological enhancements are invasive; they must be swallowed or injected. Invasive physiological and mechanical enhancements also lift cognitive and physical capabilities. Vagus nerve stimulation (VNS) increases the synaptic plasticity of brain cells to optimize learning, decision-making, and language acquisition (Pellerin 2017). Implanted brain-computer interfaces (BCI) or Human Assisted Neural Devices (HAND) enhance information processing and sensory perception (Evans 2011; Jebari 2013; NRC 2009: 67–77). The US Defense Advanced Research Projects Agency (DARPA 2018: vol. 1–130) funds genetic research to protect warfighters from "accidental or intentional" gene editing (Wegrzyn nd). Future genetic technology may fortify soldiers by modifying their genomes by design (Mehlman and Li 2014). More modestly, physical enhancements such as laser eye surgery can push vision beyond the 20/20 norm (FDA 2018).

Not all enhancements are invasive. Human-computer interfaces couple externally monitored EEG signals with biofeedback (Miranda et al. 2015: 61) or employ sensors, artificial intelligence, and information systems built into body-area networks and wearable displays to optimize human performance (DARPA 2018: vol. 1–98). Targeted neuroplasticity training (TNT) and non-invasive stimulation improves learning and optimizes training (DARPA 2017, 2018: vol. 1–129), while transcranial magnetic brain stimulation (TMS) uses a magnetic field to stimulate nerve cells from without (Bostron and Sandberg 2009; Tennison and Moreno 2012). Finally, wearable exoskeletons increase the speed, endurance, and strength of warfighters (Army Technology 2013; Bogue 2009, DARPA nd.) and incorporate wearable sensors rather than implants.

Although these technologies are promising, the ethics of enhancement focuses entirely on *utilizing* enhancement technologies. Some concerns emphasize the short- and long-term medical or social consequences that enhancement brings to individuals, their unit, and their family during and after military service. Other fears call attention to violations of human dignity, autonomy, informed consent, and cognitive liberty (Annas and Annas 2009; Mehlman 2013, 2019). All are compelling questions, but they are premature pending an assessment of military necessity and the research ethics necessary to develop new technologies.

Addressing the first challenge, the following section asks: "Are medical enhancements militarily necessary?" This sounds like an obvious question but is rarely answered. Military ethics should work through a two-stage process (Gross 2010: 241–252) to first ask whether a military operation or, in this case, a medical technology is worth our while. If so, we can then ask whether and how anyone's rights are violated in the process. All too often, however, ethics jumps to the second question before answering the first. For example, there is often a rush to ask, "Were innocent civilians killed justifiably?" following an attack accompanied by significant collateral casualties. But the first question must be: Was the attack necessary? Did it accomplish an important military goal? Considering enhancements, one must ask the same questions. The answers are far from simple. Many enhancements are unnecessary, and only those of demonstrable value merit researchers' efforts to develop appropriate technology in ethically sustainable ways. After paring this debate to its basics, the subsequent discussion turns to the ethics of developing valuable technologies, civilians' rights to demand enhancements, and the problematic role of medical professionals who enhance warfighters.

Military Medical Enhancement: A Solution Looking for a Problem?

"Today," writes Joel Garreau (2005), "DARPA is in the business of creating better soldiers—not just by equipping them with better gear, but by improving the humans themselves." " 'Soldiers having no physical, physiological, or cognitive limitations will be key to survival and operational dominance in the future,' Michael Goldblatt [Director, Defense Sciences Office, DARPA in 2003] once told a gathering of prospective researchers."

Operational dominance draws on the prowess of the individual warfighter, a "*super soldier,* realizing the Spartan ideal of creating a soldier that can endure more than ever" (Galliott and Lotz 2017: 2) or a "*Jedi knight,* a super-empowered soldier able to perform solo missions and to transmit data back to headquarters" (Malet 2015: 3). Taking stock, the National Research Council (2009: 78) enthused: "A soldier can be trained to set reflexive neurons in a state to pull the trigger without higher neural involvement, decreasing the time between acquiring and engaging the target."

A quick trigger finger might be a good thing, especially when coupled with exoskeletons that boost strength or with helmets that can monitor neuro-states, regulate the flow of information, prioritize tasks, and map terrain. These technologies, however, ignore a more fundamental question: How many soldiers must pull a trigger to fight a modern war? The answer is, not many.

By emphasizing individual performance, enhancement research places the solitary warrior at the center of armed conflict. This view speaks to a *gladiatorial* model of warfare inconsistent with contemporary armed conflict and the revolution in military affairs (RMA). In many respects, RMA is pulling the warfighter away from the immediate theater of operations by developing unmanned drones, autonomous weapons, and precision-guided munitions. At the same time, successful counterinsurgency leans heavily on population-centered initiatives and trust-building measures to encourage local cooperation and joint reconstruction efforts. This process, so essential to conflict resolution, stability, and nation-building, is antithetical to the mindset of "super-empowered soldiers" whose mission is to "run and gun," kill insurgents, and destroy their lines of supply. Is an army of knights or gladiators best equipped to win a modern war?

Considering the potential capabilities of enhanced warfighters, one might expect two benefits from investing in military medical enhancement: force protection and mission success. Making soldiers smarter, faster, stronger, and ever alert might better avoid the harm that befalls warfighters during combat. Ultimately, enhanced soldiers should make such a substantial contribution on the battlefield that their army prevails. The sections below consider each claim.

Force Protection

Force protection comprises measures that minimize exposure to, and the consequences of, deadly harm. In recent wars, improvised explosive devices (IEDs) were the leading cause of death and severe injury (Chapter 4). The first line of defense includes human intelligence, surveillance, and electronic jamming equipment to prevent IED attacks and injuries (Shachtman 2011; Wilson 2007). Technology could not frustrate all IED attacks, however, thereby leaving military planners to mitigate IED injuries they could not prevent. Defensive measures combine armored vehicles, body armor and helmets, fire-resistant clothing, front-line medical facilities, and speedy evacuation. Among the most effective responses were "Mine Resistant, Ambush Protected Vehicles" (MRAP). These replaced the lighter High Mobility Multipurpose Wheeled Vehicle (HUMVEE), and reduced IED casualties from 22% to 6% (Friedman 2013: 62).

None of these force protection measures includes enhancement. There is no enhancement listed in Table 9.1 that can protect forces from IED attacks. Smarter, faster, and stronger troops might avoid some of the dangers of close quarter combat, but guerrillas who utilize IEDs often avoid these confrontations. In what ways, then, can enhanced soldiers help win wars?

Winning a Counterinsurgency

"As impressive as our weapon systems may be," writes Patrick Lin (2012), "one of the weakest links in armed conflicts—as well as one of the most valuable assets—continues to be the warfighters themselves." Enhancement technologies restore warfighters debilitated by hunger, fatigue, fear, and confusion to their full fighting potential. As intuitive as Lin's claim sounds, it takes an exceptionally narrow view of modern warfare to think that hungry, tired, and timorous warfighters are its weakest link, and enhancements are the key to military success. Military personnel are essential, but many factors contribute to a state's failure to prevail in an asymmetric war. Off the field, these are political factors. Overly ambitious military goals that seek the annihilation of a guerrilla army or stable regime change are one example that recent wars in Libya, Iraq, Afghanistan, and Lebanon confirm. In Pakistan, diplomatic and political failures to convince local leaders to withdraw their protection of the Taliban crippled the US counterinsurgency there (Jones 2008). As a result, political leaders and policymakers may be better candidates for cognitive enhancement than combat soldiers are. In the field, successful counterinsurgencies do not depend on the larger body counts enhanced soldiers can provide, but on population-centered measures: human security, public diplomacy, civil affairs, stakeholder cooperation, and reconstruction.

American-led counterinsurgency strategy follows variants of Clear, Hold, and Build measures. Clearing operations deplete enemy forces and take territory during the invasion stage. During the Hold phase, intervening troops must deliver security and essential services, gain the local population's trust and support, and begin the long transition to the Build phase to provide sustainable infrastructures for governance. Successful counterinsurgency requires occupying armies to reduce the number and effectiveness of insurgents while increasing the number and efficiency of government troops.

The contours of this debate are not new. Analyzing force-on-force strength in the First World War, Frederick Lanchester discovered that fighting strength is a function of unit effectiveness (measured by killing rate) and troop numbers. But troop numbers are the key. Drawing on Lanchester's "square law," an army fielding twice the number of enemy troops quadruples its field strength while tripling its forces increases strength ninefold. In contrast, improving a soldier's effectiveness by offering superior technology (e.g., better weapons, armor, or biomedical enhancement) has but a linear effect on troop strength. In state-on-state conflict, therefore, numbers count while "a small performance advantage (via enhancement) in force-on-force, should generally result in a *small* change in the outcome" (Williams 2008: 15).

In asymmetric war, the diminished role of enhancement is striking. Most often, small numbers of insurgents can successfully hold off far higher numbers of conventional troops because guerrillas shed their uniforms, blend in with the civilian population, and conduct rearguard actions (Gross 2015). Guerrillas remain hidden while state troops stand out, thereby allowing guerrilla troops to identify and locate their enemy quickly and mount ambushes or remote improvised explosive device (IED) attacks with concentrated power and deadly precision. State forces, on the other hand, cannot clearly distinguish guerrillas from insurgents, while concerns for noncombatant casualties frustrate attempts to use air power or long-range artillery effectively. At the same time, states must defeat guerrillas decisively, while guerrillas need only persevere by attrition. This narrow strategic goal allows guerrillas to use their small numbers effectively, even when poorly equipped. States can prevail in combat. But without alternative avenues to reduce enemy forces, they require large numbers of troops, sometimes estimated as high as 10 times the number of insurgents they face (Deitchman 1962: 820; also Bellany 2002; MacKay 2015).

States, however, are not always willing to respond with the requisite personnel. US defense officials went to war in Iraq with approximately 130,000 troops (Belasco 2009) only to discover they needed double the number once the war settled into an insurgency in late 2003 (Schmitt 2003). Budgetary and political constraints led the United States government to refuse additional deployments. To cover the shortfall, advocates of enhancement hope to increase soldiers' performance capabilities (Beard, Galliott, and Lynch 2016). But performance enhancement is the wrong target because it does not address the root causes of inefficiency. Ironically, nonstate armies would benefit from enhancement far more than state armies would because their numbers are so small that sophisticated warfighting skills are a premium.

Table 9.2 highlights the effective strategies of counterinsurgency. Enhancement is missing from most counterinsurgency strategies, just as it is absent from force protection strategies. Targeted killing and Special Operations Forces (SOF) reduce insurgent numbers directly. At the same time, population-centered policies that deliver health care, effective policing, education, employment, and other essential services can decrease the motivation to join guerrillas and increase the motivation of insiders to defect (Kilcullen 2010; Paul, Clarke, and Grill 2010; Vizzard and Capron 2010). Public diplomacy and campaigns to win hearts and minds (Chapter 10) similarly aim to stem recruitment and encourage defection. Degrading insurgents' combat effectiveness depends upon intelligence and

Table 9.2. Goals and Strategies of Successful Counterinsurgency (COIN)

Goal	Strategy
Reduce Insurgent Numbers	
Disable combatants	Drones/Ground forces
Decrease recruitment	Population-centered COIN
	Essential services and human security
	Public and medical diplomacy
Degrade Insurgent Combat Effectiveness	Jamming and surveillance
	Cyber and financial warfare
Increase Coalition Numbers	Boots on the ground
	Improve survivability
	Decrease fatigue
Improve Coalition Combat Effectiveness	Leadership training
	Advanced weaponry
	Medical enhancement

surveillance, electronic jamming, cyberattacks on information systems, and economic warfare to diminish financial resources by blocking bank accounts or imposing sanctions. Gladiatorial enhancement has a place here. It may improve Special Operations Forces who hunt guerrillas or boost the stamina and acuity of drone operators. It also may improve troop effectiveness. Nevertheless, improving the killing rate is only a small part of the counterinsurgency (COIN) puzzle, and physical enhancement is only a small part of improving the killing rate.

On the government side, higher troop deployments (surges) will increase the number of boots on the ground, while better medical management and armor will augment numbers by improving survivability. Decreasing sleep requirements also effectively increases troop numbers (Williams 2008). Reducing a person's need for sleep by 20%, for example, is an enhancement. Still, it works not by making the individual soldier a more effective warfighter but by effectively increasing soldiers' numbers by 20%. Finally, consider that medical enhancement is not the only way to improve combat effectiveness. Leadership training and advanced weapons systems are the time-honored methods that drew Lanchester's attention.

Nevertheless, it is crucial to understand what enhancement can do. At one level, neuroscience, for example, can improve military training and learning through neuroplasticity and memory exercises. Neuropsychological testing, neuroimaging, and screening for genetic and other biomarkers of successful performance can optimize recruitment and selection (DARPA 2019b; Flower et al. 2012; JASON 2010). As they do so, these technologies enhance *organizational* effectiveness. At the operational level, the National Research Council (NRC 2009: 75) takes notice of "mission enabling neuroscience technology opportunities" to "contend with an ever-increasing river of information . . . avoid information overload and successfully synthesize information that selectively highlights the mission-critical features from multiple sources." Applicable technologies include noninvasive, human-computer interfaces, remote physiological monitoring for stress, neural signals to control external systems, and virtual reality training (NRC 2009: 75–76). These training and information processing capabilities eschew the unrealizable "bionic soldier" (NRC 2009: 8) and draw attention to mission success in asymmetric war. Nevertheless, Special Operations Forces suggest a case where performance enhancements have their place.

Special Operations Forces and Military
Medical Enhancement

Special Operations Forces (SOF) are small, cohesive, independent units that spend long periods in the field to conduct search and rescue, strategic reconnaissance, unconventional warfare, and counterterrorism while often engaging guerilla forces in close combat. These tasks make speed, agility, alertness, strength, and quick decision-making particularly important. Looking to future conflict, the US military increased the numbers of SOF from 33,000 in 2001 to 70,000 in 2018 (Feickert 2018: 7). Strengthening SOF offsets conventional troop reduction with smaller, more flexible, and better-trained units while avoiding the political repercussions of placing greater numbers of personnel in the field (Hennigan 2017). As they assume the brunt of counterinsurgency warfare, however, SOF turn increasingly to population-centered strategies including internal defense, civil affairs, humanitarian assistance, and information operations. Internal defense trains host-nation forces to provide local security. Civil affairs and humanitarian assistance help local governments build medical, educational, judicial, and other service infrastructures by partnering with local stakeholders, international nongovernmental organizations (NGOs), and military forces (Kilcullen 2006; FM 3-24 2006: Chap. 2). Information operations offer the means to communicate with domestic and international audiences through print, news, and social media.

These strategies seek to decrease the number of insurgents and degrade their effectiveness without fighting. For this purpose, administrative capabilities, language proficiency, cultural understanding, and negotiation skills supersede physical strength and endurance, and assume greater importance as SOF take on civilian-related tasks. The requisite enhancement technologies are not exoskeletons or blood doping, but specialized neuro-training techniques such as TNT and memory enhancement, information processing technologies, and the appropriate neuroscientific tools to optimize the selection and recruitment of SOF team members.

In the final analysis, enhancing state fighters or Special Operations Forces may not appreciably affect the outcomes of asymmetric war any more than it affects conventional war. On the contrary, the most critical determinants of success in asymmetric war are the size of state forces, the rate of guerrilla recruitment, and the effectiveness of guerrilla fire. A state increases its numbers by recruiting more soldiers, bringing them to the field, and ensuring their survival as best it can. Dedication to force protection accounts for the substantial investments in armored vehicles, technologies to defeat IEDs, and medical care to return the injured to duty.

Degrading insurgent capabilities further depends on tactics to deplete their financial resources and defeat insurgent propaganda. Decreasing insurgent numbers is a continuous challenge. It is not about body counts but about diminishing support for guerrillas by offering young men and their families incentives to work and live peacefully rather than join the ranks of insurgents. This strategy requires investment in infrastructures to provide security, employment, health, and education as well as a horizon for transitioning to local autonomy and control. As nations prosecute an asymmetric war, therefore, they often will find organizational enhancements more valuable than gladiatorial enhancements, and the proper target of researchers and funding agencies. Pursuing organizational enhancement, researchers confront distinct ethical challenges.

Moral Dilemmas of Medical Enhancement Research

Central to medical research are dilemmas of distributive justice. How large a research budget does enhancement development merit, and who gets it? Answering this question compels policymakers to compare the costs and benefits of developing enhancement technologies to those of other assets required to wage war, whether weapons systems, therapies to treat the sick and wounded, or employment opportunities for young men. Although addressing the complex political and ethical issues surrounding funding for war is beyond the scope of this book, funding for enhancement research merits a closer look.

Having apportioned funds for new enhancement technologies, policymakers must then decide among them. Despite its engaging public profile, DARPA enjoyed a modest 3.6-billion-dollar budget in 2020. Of this, DARPA (2019a: Vol 1-47, 53ff, 121) allocates just over $250 million for biomedical technology, biologically based materials and devices, and basic operational biomedicine. Consistent with priorities to fund combat casualty care research (GAO 2013), much of DARPA's budget goes to therapeutic and preventive biomedicine, not performance-enhancing research. DARPA-approved enhancement-related projects appear in Table 9.3.

Ideally, ethics should drive budget allocations. Nevertheless, ethics can learn much from policy decisions. First, emphasizing utility and warfighter

Table 9.3. DARPA-Approved Enhancement Research Projects for 2020

Project (page citation, DARPA 2019a, Volume 1)	Budget (USD)
1. Genetic screening for "improved personnel placement" (1-57)	17M
2. Genetic protection technologies to defend against "the effects of accidental or malicious misuse of gene editing technologies" (1-130)	17M
3. Transient and reversible gene modulator therapies to "bolster intrinsic host defenses" (1-132)	16M
4. Neural Signal Interfaces and Applications (NSIA), "non-invasive neurotechnologies to interface with the nervous system with high resolution and precision without surgery" (1-54)	19M
5. Noninvasive devices to "promote plasticity for improved learning paradigms" (1-129)	15M
6. Wearable force protection (1-100)	26M
7. The Analysis and Adaptation of Human Resilience to "explore new methods to maintain and optimize warfighter health in response to environmental insults such as new and emerging infectious diseases" (1-51) [This program ended in 2019 and was superseded by Improved Intervention (Item 8).]	4M
8. Improved Interventions: "Novel pharmacological interventions to optimize the performance of the healthy warfighter ... [and] capable of modulating multiple targets within biological systems of the body, which will reduce side effects and promote safety ... [and] augment physical fitness training and maintenance for military populations" (1-50)	14M

healthcare rights, DARPA's overall budget highlights research that serves warfighting, force protection, and curative medical science, in roughly that order. Second, enhancement research emphasizes noninvasive, transient, and reversible technologies. Finally, the budget entirely ignores civilian needs. Looking past warfighters, policymakers cannot neglect research to fortify civilian resilience if they hope to wage a successful humanitarian war. The first is a question of distributive justice, the second and third speak to medical rights and vulnerable populations.

Medical Enhancement Research and Distributive Justice

Most of DARPA's budget has little to do with biomedicine. Its funding goes mainly to basic and applied research to serve warfighting needs: information, communication, electronic, material, and tactical technology; space and aerospace systems; network-centric warfare; and sensor technology. Setting these aside and turning to biomedicine, the first fault line appears between therapeutic and enhancement research. Each consumes about half of the resources devoted to biomedical research. Therapeutic research addresses both curative and rehabilitative treatments for ill or disabled warfighters (e.g., prosthetic devices), as well as preventive care to protect forces and conserve fighting strength. However, DARPA (2019a) funds little of the curative research described in the previous chapter. Their few clinical studies address the prevention of infectious disease among troops (2019a: Vol. 1-48.49), the development of noninvasive neuro-technologies (Table 9.3: 4), and treatments for traumatic injuries (2019a: Vol 1-58, 59, 135). DARPA's budget does, however, shed light on the competing claims of preventive care and enhancement research.

Preventive care does not enhance warfighters' capabilities but maintains their normal range of health. Preventive care supports unit readiness by identifying bio-threats, preventing infectious disease, boosting immunity, and slowing damage from traumatic injury. In this sense, some enhancement research projects spill into prevention as genetic protection, human resilience, and "Improved Interventions" programs demonstrate (Table 9.3: Items 2, 7, and 8). These projects pursue pharmacological or genetic agents to forestall disease and malicious intervention, and improve resilience and fitness. Gene modulation, technologies that alter a gene's expression of particular proteins (Table 9.3: Item 3), are mostly preventive but skirt enhancement when no longer transient or reversible. The remaining enhancement technologies address such institutional needs as screening and training (Table 9.3: Items 1 and 5) or improve warfighter performance with wearable or other noninvasive human-computer interfaces that facilitate information processing (Table 9.3: Items 4 and 6).

To guide allocations for therapeutic and enhancement research, pertinent criteria invoke rights and utility. Curative and rehabilitative research satisfy healthcare claim rights for those in need, and benefit military medicine by conserving human resources and providing force protection. Rights and utility may conflict. Many curative therapies improve return-to-duty rates, but others do not. Narrow beneficence and associative duties of care, however, generate claim rights for exceptional care independent of military utility. These rights compel state military organizations to allocate sufficient sums to attend to wounded warfighters and veterans, whether they can return to duty or not (Chapter 12).

Unlike curative therapies, enhancement is not rights driven. Utility understood as force protection or mission success is their only metric. When rights are absent, efficiency prevails. Therefore, if the cost of developing and implementing gladiatorial enhancements overshadows their limited role in counterinsurgency warfare, then research and development are difficult to justify. Rights, however, do not disappear entirely. Were performance enhancements militarily useful, warfighters could claim a right to obtain them, just as they might demand effective weaponry. However, it is important to note that the claim right only follows once enhancement is proven militarily necessary. This caveat is not true of curative or rehabilitative technologies. They need only be medically efficacious before triggering a prima facie claim right. This conclusion brings us full circle: The primary justification for enhancement research is military necessity. If so, why then is there a distinct preference for noninvasive technologies? The answer appears to be twofold. First, invasive enhancement research is ethically problematic, and second, its fruits offer no benefit over noninvasive enhancement.

Invasive Enhancement Research

Medical invasiveness highlights a bright line in military medical enhancement research that few are willing to breach. Commenting on surgically implanted neuro-technologies to improve control of prosthetic limbs, treat depression, or restore memory, a recent DARPA memo adds:

> Due to the inherent risks of surgery, these technologies have so far been limited to use by volunteers with clinical need. For the military's primarily able-bodied population to benefit from neurotechnology, *nonsurgical interfaces are required* . . . Teams are pursuing a range of approaches that use optics, acoustics, and electromagnetics to record neural activity and/ or send signals back to the brain at high speed and resolution. The research is split between two tracks. Teams are pursuing either completely non-invasive interfaces that are entirely external to the body or minutely invasive interface systems that include nanotransducers that can be temporarily and nonsurgically delivered to the brain to improve signal resolution. (DARPA 2019c, emphasis added)

Here, DARPA raises the conundrum of nontherapeutic research and suggests that enhancement studies cannot utilize invasive interventions to benefit able-bodied service members. But why not? There is no obvious reason that enhancement research or its utilization requires only nonsurgical interfaces. Perhaps DARPA believes that investigators need to be exceptionally careful with soldiers and avoid undue risk. If so, such caution reflects the same self-imposed restraint that hampered the experimental clinical trials described in the previous chapter and is equally unfounded. DARPA follows the same US Department of Defense (DoD) and Food and Drug Administration (FDA) rules that guide all military medical research. These rules protect service personnel from undue coercion. There are, however, no legal or ethical reasons to prevent fully informed, healthy, and competent test subjects from consenting to invasive enhancement research. Nevertheless, noninvasive research is prudent for two reasons. First, invasive research is riskier than noninvasive enhancement research. Second, its risk is far harder to quantify, making it difficult for research subjects to give fully informed consent.

Unlike noninvasive research, invasive and irreversible enhancement studies may bring undesirable and harmful physiological, cognitive, and psychological side effects that impair personal health, warfighter performance, and postdeployment integration into civilian life. Assessing plans to develop an invasive enhancement technology demands answers to two questions: (1) Does the invasive enhancement improve upon noninvasive technologies for successfully waging modern war? (2) If yes, is the invasive technology as cost-effective as noninvasive alternatives considering the costs of obtaining informed consent, health risks, and the smooth integration of biologically or genetically modified soldiers into military and, later, civilian life?

Consider, for example, neural interfaces. Commenting on HAND (human-assisted neural device), Nick Evans (2011: 108) explains how it might improve upon wearables by offering "all the advantages of URVs (unmanned robotic vehicle) in allowing an individual to control a robot in the field but without the problems of interface management, lack of proprioception and tactile senses and so on." In a constant state of development, HAND must address its relative advantages. And, for the reasons that Evans enumerates, HAND may be far more beneficial than URVs. Addressing the second question, however, is more complicated than comparing technical specifications and asks: Is technological superiority offset by the myriad of medical, ethical, and military obstacles its research and utilization pose?

Among the obstacles, researchers will consider how a permanently enhanced warfighter may weaken unit cohesion when performance-enhancing measures create significant disparities between normal and "super" personnel (Mehlman 2013: 39). Although challenging, the costs of these sorts of inequalities would not necessarily concern individual research subjects. Instead, they will want to know about the personal costs of experimentation as they weigh their consent. These costs may be unbearably high.

Apart from significant health risks, affronts to dignity and cognitive liberty are one cost enhancement research subjects may face. Beta-blockers, for example, may blunt PTSD or moral injury by hindering the consolidation of traumatic memories. Here, Jessica Wolfendale (2008) raises compelling concerns about how these agents may diminish moral responsibility or undermine personal integrity if they deprive warfighters of memories or remorse (also Robbins 2013). Moral injury is a particularly vexing challenge for military medicine. Moral injury speaks to the psychologically debilitating effects of *permissibly* killing enemies in war. Unlike PTSD, moral injury follows a deadly act of commission that brings overwhelming guilt and shame. PTSD, on the other hand, follows from a traumatic attack on one's person that brings incapacitating fear and insecurity (Litz and Kerig 2019, for review). PTSD is a psychological wound medical science should always cure. Moral injury is not. Killing in war should not be free of the moral distress inherent in what W. H. Auden (1937) once called, "the conscious acceptance of guilt in the necessary murder." Otherwise, war will rage rampant. But killing in war should not be so damnable as to debilitate soldiers and make just war impossible. On this subject, at least, medical science walks a fine line between defeating an enervating injury through enhancement and preserving basic human emotions.

Another personal and social cost looks to the future as research subjects think about civilian life following military service. Adam Henschke (2019) describes genetic modifications that suppress the trust-building hormone oxytocin. As a result, soldiers are appropriately wary when fighting in urban environments. Upon discharge, however, the same warfighters may be incapable of the trust necessary to sustain civilian relationships, a risk difficult for research subjects to evaluate in the early stages of experimental trials.

The preceding discussion exemplifies some of the medical, personal, and social costs difficult for research subjects to assess. Uncertainty about the short- and long-term effects of invasive enhancement research complicates researchers' cost-benefit calculations and make it difficult for test subjects to evaluate risk and provide fully informed consent. Nevertheless, these reservations should not suggest the futility of offering research subjects reliable data. The quality of information will undoubtedly improve, but more exact knowledge about a technology's many medical and social costs and benefits does not preclude a thorough assessment of its military necessity. Ethicists can provide cogent answers to many complex questions about enhancements, but not until they know that pending research is (1) necessary for modern war and (2) technologically superior to any alternative. The result is to narrow the footprint of research protocols that merit ethical scrutiny. Unlike the growing need for clinical therapeutic studies, the draw of invasive enhancement research is weaker. Therapeutic needs and force protection dictate urgency as casualty rates rise; enhancement needs do not. They remain speculative, and research, by necessity, proceeds at a slower, more deliberate pace to protect experimental subjects.

Still, it is reasonable to think that invasive enhancement will engage serious attention. Electric nerve stimulation improves neuroplasticity in rats and is the next logical step for humans (Waltz 2017). Similarly, neural implants may replace wearables as technology facilitates a move from human-computer interfaces to a brain-computer interface. Nor is it the end of the strategic debate. Critics of population-centered COIN describe it as little more than colonial warfare that degrades, inflames, and endangers the civilian population while trying to vanquish insurgents with brutal campaigns of counterterrorism. "Historically," concludes Douglas Porch (2013: 338), "COIN succeeds, at least temporarily, by disrupting and fragmenting communities rather than by knitting them together, which rather defeats the proclaimed state-building purpose of modern intervention." Scientific advances, coupled with revisionist assessments of counterinsurgency doctrine, may transform thinking about future warfighting. One consideration should be enhancements for civilians.

Enhancement for Civilians

Enhancement for civilians is on nobody's drawing board, yet begs attention. When casus belli for just war appeals to humanitarian relief, intervening states incur an obligation to enhance the welfare of those they take up arms to save. Otherwise, there is no just cause for intervention. Humanitarian war restores host-nation welfare through armed regime change, human security, and the reconstruction of essential infrastructures. These are the fundamentals of a "Clear, Hold, and Build" strategy that enhancement technologies, perhaps more than other tactics, can serve. Medical diplomacy, for example, often falls short because it lacks any long-term or systematic commitment to the local population. Medical care to win hearts and minds is usually transient, uneven, and inadequate (Chapter 10). If, on the other hand, human security and political reconstruction are the keys to successful counterinsurgency and subsequent state-building, then it behooves intervening states to see how enhancements might improve their military and political efforts. Research to enhance civilian resilience to the stressors of war—hunger, disease, danger, displacement, or family loss—can offer them the same endurance, stamina, and judgment that cognitive and physical enhancement affords warfighters. The question, then, is not how to transition wartime enhancements to peacetime, but how to *simultaneously* apply wartime warfighter enhancement to wartime civilian enhancement.

In humanitarian war, such enhancement is mainly preventive. Consider the following programs drawn from DARPA's 2020 budget proposal (DARPA 2019a):

- *The Expanding Human Resiliency Program* will "develop new technologies to control and manipulate the microbiome to enable peak human performance . . . to facilitate human functions (e.g., immunity to disease, metabolic performance, tolerance to chemical exposure, etc.) and behaviors (e.g., mood, decision making, ability to work as a cohesive team, etc.) using specific microbial consortia living in the gastrointestinal tract, respiratory tract, skin or mouth" (Vol. 1-133,134).
- *The Analysis and Adaptation of Human Resilience* program will explore "new methods to slow and limit damage caused by acute trauma, infection . . . and infectious diseases" (Vol. 1-49, 51).
- *Biological Complexity*: Fiscal Year 2020 plans to "demonstrate counter pathogens and antibiotic resistance, regulate inflammation from Traumatic Brain Injury (TBI), and maintain a healthy gut" (Vol.1-40).

These enhancements might mitigate wartime and postwar health threats that endanger civilians. Additionally, there is no reason why civilians would not benefit from institutional enhancements that optimize recruitment and training. Intervening nations have not always devoted the resources necessary for reconstruction, human security, and political stability. If emerging individual and institutional technologies can effectively enhance postwar well-being and improve governance, then they are an essential part of the reconstruction process that humanitarian forces must implement.

The duty to provide civilians with effective means of enhancement also requires humanitarian forces to develop and test the same technologies. This obligation would require research organizations such as DARPA to flag dual-use technologies and build their research protocols to meet military *and* civilian needs. Research subjects for enhancements currently draw from young, healthy service personnel. Whether this is sufficient to develop and test enhancements suitable for indigenous civilians is unknown. Given the urgency of wartime distress, however, local public health officials may adapt noninvasive enhancement technologies just as they will adapt successful, evidence-based medical products from high-income countries to the needs of lower-income countries during postwar reconstruction (WHO 2007: 21).

Initially, evidence of efficacy can only come from clinical studies in high-income nations. Any need to draw on civilian populations in combat zones to conduct even noninvasive medical research raises many ethical concerns. Victims of war are vulnerable populations in the extreme. Most are traumatized and many are injured, ill, displaced, and bereaved. There are no research protocols suitable for this population that would not run afoul of charges of uninformed consent, coercion, manipulation, or exploitation. Nevertheless, WHO officials often ascertain a medical product's effectiveness under local conditions and weigh its cost and benefits across the entire population (Newbrander et al. 2014). To test new medical products in a developing nation, civilian researchers will undoubtedly conduct postwar retrospective and prospective observational studies consistent with appropriate research guidelines. Concern for local civilians in the context of humanitarian intervention expands the scope of military medical enhancement research to offer its benefits to civilians during war and after.

Enhancement research for civilians bears many of the hallmarks of curative, rehabilitative, and preventive therapeutic research that invoke healthcare and political rights rather than military necessity alone. Civilian populations threatened by brutal regimes call upon the international community to exercise its responsibility to protect and rebuild. Many enhancement technologies serve this purpose. And although choosing human subjects for research poses ethical challenges, there are few reservations about clinicians who undertake research to enhance civilian health. However, one cannot be so sanguine about their contribution to protocols designed to improve warfighter efficiency.

Should Doctors Help Build Bombs?

Commenting on American and British efforts to recruit physicians to develop chemical and biological weapons, I asked two questions: "Is medicine a pacifist profession or should doctors help build bombs?" (Gross 2008b). The short answer to the first question is, "No"; medicine is not a pacifist profession, despite physicians' prominent role in antiwar movements. The answer to the second question is, "Yes"; physicians should build bombs when their expertise is required for national defense. The medical community does not exist in a superior moral universe where its members may benefit from others who take on warfighting or building the weapons warfighters need to kill. I will not review this argument here but only ask whether and how it might apply to enhanced soldiers.

If enhancement is not therapeutic, then it must offer either better protection akin to a ceramic vest or vaccination, or afford a warfighting advantage akin to a cutting-edge rifle or fighter jet. Enhancement often does both, and thus poses the very problem that confronted medical personnel employed to build weapons. One difficulty facing anyone asked to design chemical or biological weapons is the ethics of the weapons themselves. Serious concerns about chemical or biological weapons arose early on, but none were unlawful until 30 years after World War II. Even today, chemical weapons are only restricted, not banned entirely. Still, enhancement does not raise any obvious concerns about building weapons of mass destruction, so that many existing or proposed technologies are useful and permissible.

A second impediment facing weapons designers is the inability to distinguish between offensive and defensive research. Following World War II, it was common to direct PhDs, microbiologists, or chemists, for example, into offensive weapons development, and medical doctors into defensive research. If offensive research experimented with pathogens, its defensive counterpart worked on vaccines. This dichotomy, however, made no more sense than trying to distinguish between a tank's armor and its cannon. Both are necessary to battle. Early vaccines were part of a program to tailor antidotes, pathogens, and chemical weapons so that an army could wage chemical or biological warfare with abandon knowing they monopolized the disease and its cure. This picture changed once nations closed their chemical and biological weapons programs and developed antidotes solely for self-defense. Until then, offensive and defensive research were two sides of the same coin.

Enhancement technologies pose similar challenges. The enhanced warfighter is a weapon who hopes to monopolize the battlefield with superior technology. If the technology is a critical determinant of military success and does not violate the warfighters' rights, then there is no prima facie reason for medical practitioners to refuse their expertise. When they do comply, however, military physicians endanger their immunity from attack under international law. International law subjects loss of immunity to two tests: the commission of acts that (1) are harmful and (2) fall outside the humanitarian duties of tending the sick and wounded. Prescribing medical enhancements for warfighters on the battlefield meets both (Liivoja 2017: 440; 443). If nontherapeutic enhancements do not restore health but push it beyond the normal baseline, they are a medical weapon, and their purveyors cannot lay claim to special protection under current law. As medical enhancements gain greater attention, Rain Liivoja suggests transferring the personnel responsible for battlefield enhancement to nonmedical units where they serve as ordinary combatants.

One might be skeptical of this advice. First, it would invite abuse. A medical facility that housed a hospital and "enhancement wing" might lose its immunity entirely, just as it might if it housed armed fighters. As armed attacks on hospitals increase, there is no reason to give states such as Russia any further excuse to shell protected facilities. Second, shifting some medical personnel to combatant positions prevents them from performing their regular medical duties and wastes prized assets. Assuming that many state armies will think likewise, it is worth remembering that medical immunity is a convention born of mutual self-interest among belligerents (Chapter 2). The plainest solution, therefore, is for the contracting parties to amend international humanitarian law to protect all medical personnel, including those who administer or supervise enhancement protocols.

Immunity for civilian researchers poses a different problem. As a general rule, civilian industries that deliver *war-sustaining* aid, whether they make uniforms or canned rations, retain immunity from attack. Those that provide *warfighting* assets, for example, tanks or guns, do not. Law and practice, however, often distinguish between facilities and personnel (Melzer 2009: 53 n.135, 56). A weapons factory is fair game, but its staff is not necessarily liable to attack at all times. Off duty, civilian workers retain noncombatant immunity. This is not necessarily true, however, if particular workers own significant, portable expertise that they can transfer at will as needed. The targeted killing of nuclear scientists is a recent and controversial example. Tamar Meisels (2014) explains how these and other senior weapons developers are liable to assassination. Assassination, however, should be cause for pause, and reserved for the rare cases when the target poses an extreme threat, and when attempts at arrest and incarceration fail.

The current state of the art, however, gives these questions some context. As Liivoja argues, attributing liability to battlefield medical staff administering enhancing agents like Modafinil poses a pressing issue that international law must address. Concerns about researchers' liability, however, are less urgent. Many technologies, particularly gladiatorial enhancements, do not yet afford necessary or cost-effective means to wage modern war. Of those that do, the most promising improve institutional performance but fall short of a threat on par with nuclear bombs. This situation may change, and as answers about the cost and benefits of performance-enhancing research emerge, medical professionals may reconsider their collaborative roles. Alternatively, they may double down. As they do, researchers may face the same risk of defensive killing as other developers of deadly weapons.

The Ethics of Military Medical Research

This chapter and the previous one link three distinct aspects of military medical research: investigational drugs, therapeutic clinical studies, and non-therapeutic enhancement. The ethical challenge of developing all three turns on satisfying military necessity, respecting patient self-determination, and protecting vulnerable populations. Since the outrages perpetrated by the Germans and Japanese during World War II, medical research has striven to safeguard patients' interests and autonomy. The result has been to tighten research protocols to prevent abuse. At the same time, however, tighter protocols hampered the research necessary for military medicine. Unlike civilian medicine, military medicine turns on mission success and the conservation of fighting capabilities. These are public rather than private goods that nations strive to attain during war.

Attention to public, collective goods will sometimes demand exceptions and impose high risks on service personnel without necessarily obtaining their consent. This occurs when military planners require investigational drugs to meet potentially catastrophic medical threats in war. Chemical or biological threats short circuit standard medical research when they offer grounds to administer incompletely tested but promising pharmaceuticals. Controlled clinical studies, by contrast, typically fall back on standard research protocols but impose additional constraints when recruiting vulnerable populations. One result is to confine military medical research to retrospective or observational studies and severely limit valuable prehospital and battlefield research necessary to ensure warfighter health and mission success. Restoring controlled clinical studies to military medicine does not infringe on the rights of service personnel. Instead, it requires close attention to existing regulations that permit waivers of informed consent, consideration of British models that allow for a nonfamily legal representative and retrospective consent, and the recruitment of civilians to aid military medical research.

Enhancement research raises these and additional demands. Enhancement challenges military physicians, commanders, and philosophers as they consider the physical, emotional, and cognitive risks to warfighters, respect for their autonomy and dignity, and the effects of enhancement on unit cohesion and civilian-military relations. Nevertheless, and as thorough as they are, these discussions fail to weigh the relative military value of various enhancement technologies. To sharpen the debate, I raise logically prior but ever neglected questions. Foremost, an ethical inquiry must reach into strategic planning to determine the military necessity of individual and institutional enhancements. The result is to place a premium on technologies that enhance institutional performance by improving information processing, training, and recruitment. Technology, moreover, is not the only tool for optimizing performance. To improve and sustain total force fitness, Deuster, O'Connor, and Lunasco (2017) underscore the essential place of social (family and unit cohesion), spiritual (ethics, meaning, and purpose), and environmental (air and water quality) health alongside physical and psychological well-being.

Once past the necessity threshold, enhancement research balks at invasive technologies and requires pause. Nontherapeutic research is particularly problematic because it holds no potential benefit for the test subject. True, subjects on the placebo arm of a clinical study will also not benefit from research, but they might benefit should they fall into the experimental arm. But no arm of enhancement research offers the subject a clear benefit. As a result, only competent research subjects can consent, leaving no place for waivers of informed consent or surrogate decision-making.

Of course, many potential enhancement technologies began their lives as therapeutic interventions to treat brain injury, trauma, PTSD, memory impairment, and limb loss. Here, clinical trials such as those outlined in the previous chapter are acceptable protocols. When research subjects are not competent, surrogate decision-makers or legal representatives can provide consent. Once tested, these therapies may gain sufficient scientific weight to transition from experimental to investigative or standard interventions. At this point, the ethical questions turn from research to utilization and echo those surrounding anthrax, PT, and BT vaccines (Chapter 4). Benefits and risks are the primary criteria. An investigative drug or enhancement must afford military benefits, but the attendant risk may be permissibly high when military benefits are substantial.

This chapter offers a corrective to the many enhancement ethicists who neglect to question the strategic and tactical value of gladiatorial enhancement. Answering these questions before asking about rights and utility will provide funding guidelines and frame the appropriate ethical debate about utilizing enhancements. At present, the ethical challenges are not insurmountable. As new projects come online, they will raise diverse and challenging ethical questions. Among the first is a careful assessment of how prospective technologies contribute to the mutable atmosphere of contemporary warfare.

Enhanced soldiers are weapons of war. Pushing past battlefield therapy to return warfighters to duty, medical science works to create a better fighting machine. Some of the technology is awe-inspiring. Sometimes, however, all it takes to weaponize medicine is an attentive ear. Playing on the promise of routine but life-saving care, medical diplomacy sets out to defeat an insurgency by winning hearts and minds.

10

Medical Diplomacy and the Battle
for Hearts and Minds

I will put my laws in their minds and write them on their hearts. I will be their God, and they will be my people. Jeremiah 31:33

Politicos and their gods have been after hearts and minds for a long time. Methods have changed. Today we see how military medicine is inextricably linked with "winning hearts and minds" through medical diplomacy: the judicious and strategic use of medical care to influence the local population to support a government at war. But "medical diplomacy" is an incongruous construction. Medicine is about repairing hearts and minds, not winning them. Nor does medicine have anything obvious to say about diplomacy. Although warring sides sometimes enlist physicians as mediators or are willing to accept medical facilities as neutral conflict-free zones for negotiations (Iacopino and Waldman 1999; MacQueen and Santa Barbara 2000), this says nothing about *medical* diplomacy. Physicians may be acceptable mediators because they are neutral and impartial but not because of any medical service they provide in the name of diplomacy. Diplomacy, for its part, has little obvious connection to medicine. Diplomats assuage hurt feelings, mobilize coalitions to protect national interests, and defuse (or ignite) international crises.

Winning the backing of the local and international community, however, is a central goal of modern war and counterinsurgency. Widespread support is particularly crucial if nations wage war to rescue a foreign people from a rights-violating regime. Given that one would reasonably expect gratitude from rescuees, the goal of ongoing diplomacy is not so much winning hearts and minds, but not losing them as the unpredictable course of armed conflict may soon leave local nationals wondering, "with friends like this, who needs enemies?"

During the wars in Iraq and Afghanistan, three providers attended to medical relief. Military forces dominate during the invasion period; nongovernmental organizations (NGOs) assume growing responsibility during the post-invasion and transition period, and local government agencies are poised to take over during reconstruction. At no time, however, does a single provider take exclusive control. Instead, each keeps a constant presence that is a source of both support and friction. Nevertheless, military forces dominate. They supply the lion's share of relief funding and assume direct responsibility for the security without which NGOs and local government facilities cannot operate. Multinational forces, particularly the United States, dictate operational strategies that employ medical care to defeat an insurgency, provide long-term humanitarian relief, and restore governance.

As military medicine turns from its narrow therapeutic goal of saving lives and alleviating suffering, to the political and military aims of medical diplomacy, questions about medical neutrality and impartiality loom again. In Chapter 2, I explained why military medicine is neither neutral nor impartial concerning the belligerents it aids. Military medicine takes sides and distributes care to conserve force capabilities and prevail in just war. Medical diplomacy serves the same goals, and there is no compelling prima facie reason to reject medicine's diplomatic role in war. But, again, the devil is in the details. The following sections investigate three interrelated topics: (1) the aims and efficacy of medical diplomacy, (2) the ethics of utilizing medicine to enhance a counterinsurgency by encouraging patients to rally behind the local government, and (3) the challenges of conscripting humanitarian NGOs to the war effort.

The efficacy of medical diplomacy is still unsubstantiated. Medical diplomacy hovers between relief efforts to alleviate present suffering and longer-term objectives to stabilize fledgling regimes. Neither may be particularly effective as each falls prey to corruption, mistrust, hostile cultural norms, competition among stakeholders, and conflicting interests. Nevertheless, medicine may sometimes motivate patients to supply strategically important aid. The effect is to weaponize medicine and erode its commitment to patient rights. Similarly, state military organizations may co-opt impartial, neutral, and independent NGOs when recruiting humanitarian agencies to their side of a war. Military medicine may reject impartiality and neutrality, but humanitarian NGOs do not. They take pains to preserve their humanitarian space and independence as they deliver medical services. The dilemma for humanitarian organizations is whether and how to accept aid from military forces. The dilemma for military forces, which concerns us here, is how far to compromise humanitarian NGOs to pursue military aims.

Medical Humanitarianism in the Field

In contrast to medical *relief*, the opportunistic and ad hoc care of a civilian population suffering the ravages of war, medical *humanitarianism* is a strategic goal of armed conflict. Through short-term relief projects and long-term reconstruction, medical humanitarianism serves the military mission by ameliorating suffering, undermining support for insurgents, and solidifying cooperation among civilians, international forces, and the new regime. Medical humanitarianism is not an afterthought but a central component of human security. It is not subordinate to the military mission but defines it. It is, therefore, no accident that military forces are the first purveyors of civilian medical care. Facilities include front-line combat support hospitals, Medical Civic Action Programs (MEDCAPs), and Provincial Reconstruction Teams (PRTs).

Front-Line Medical Humanitarianism

The medical rules of eligibility afford no room to regularly treat local civilians except when military operations threaten their lives, limbs, or eyesight and when bed space is available. When the fighting dies down, however, Coalition hospitals would sometimes admit local nationals who would not otherwise qualify for care. Apart from emergency trauma cases, burns, and fractures (Bonnet et al. 2012; Woll and Brisson 2013), specialized care might include neurosurgery (Schulz, Kunz, and Mauer 2012), craniofacial repair (Neff et al. 2017), and pediatric care (Burnett et al. 2008). Between 2001 and 2011, in-theater multinational medical facilities treated over 7,500 children and 25,000 adults (including local security forces) in Iraq and Afghanistan (Borgman et al. 2012).

Although combat medical units did not formally pursue medical diplomacy, surveys and anecdotal reports reveal significant enthusiasm for using medicine to win hearts and minds and to reinforce support for multinational forces. In a 2014 survey of 266 deployed surgeons in Iraq and Afghanistan, a majority believed that surgical care for local nationals generated goodwill

(68%), significantly aided the US counterinsurgency (54%), benefited the local population (64%), and maintained/improved surgical skills (50%) (Porta et al. 2014). Humanitarian surgery and other medical interventions aid counterinsurgency efforts and protect forces by building "trust and comradery to establish deep relationships between two very different cultures" (Porta, 2018; also Willy et al. 2011). Pediatric care, of no medical value to military forces, was lauded. "The fastest and most effective way to win the hearts and minds of the local population is to care for their children" (Neff et al. 2017: 555), provide children with "humanitarian care" (Bolt and Schoneboom 2010: 133), or perform eye surgery on children (Enzenauer, Vavra, and Butler 2006).

Despite the enthusiasm, a minority of the combat surgeons worried that attending civilians "was not part of the mission (15%)," "interfered with trauma care (16%)," "misused personnel/supplies (13%)," and "compromised unit security (6%)" (Porta et al. 2014: 769). Other concerns included ineffective care despite occasional life-saving surgery (Beitler, Junnila, and Meyer 2006) or worries that the extraordinarily high level of Coalition medical care would erode the status of local doctors, hospitals, pharmacists, and healthcare officials who could not compete on anything approaching a level playing field. The early years of the fighting brushed aside these concerns, but they would recur as MEDCAPs and PRTs institutionalized medical diplomacy.

Medical Civic Action Programs

Medical Civic Action Programs (MEDCAPs) employ the medical staff of combat units to build clinics and train local doctors and nurses to tend the local population. Their history is checkered. In the Vietnam War, MEDCAPs drew charges of providing poor and erratic care, jeopardizing the neutrality of medical doctors, and using medicine to browbeat the local population (Gross 2006: 198–210; Wilensky 2004). Following the invasions of Afghanistan and Iraq, military units established MEDCAPs to provide "on-off non-emergency aid within a security envelope provided by Coalition forces" (Bricknell and Cameron 2011: 476). MEDCAPs built clinics and training facilities for doctors and nurses, conducted vaccination campaigns, and afforded sporadic care. Early in the fighting, MEDCAPs rushed to win hearts and minds with reconstruction projects and assistance to local surgeons (Richardson 2008; Rush et al. 2005). In Afghanistan, a typical weeklong MEDCAP mission employed 29 staff members and treated 4,179 patients and 456 animals in a village known as a "hot spot for anti-coalition militia activity." "The goal was to provide acute and preventative medical, dental and veterinary services to enhance the standing of the government of Afghanistan (GOA) and foster a positive relationship between the Coalition, the Provincial Government, and the local population" (Malsby and Territo 2007: 40).

Short time frames were the norm for MEDCAPS. Projects included vaccination campaigns, deworming, emergency dentistry, and mobile clinics that periodically stopped in remote villages. Their mission included health *and* stability operations. Health operations deliver medical attention to civilians until NGOs and public healthcare facilities assume this responsibility. Stability operations utilize medical services to control territory and maintain order by building host-nation capacity that strengthens the local government and weakens support for insurgents (Malish, Scott, and Rasheed 2006; Olsthoorn, Bollen, and Beeres 2013). In this way, MEDCAPs can be integral for stabilizing or pacifying newly controlled territory during the Clear and Hold stages of counterinsurgency. But MEDCAPS only delivered transient care with little follow-up or evaluation (Kauvar and Drury 2013). In time, they gave way to the more systematically organized Provincial Reconstruction Teams.

Provincial Reconstruction Teams

More comprehensive and better funded than MEDCAPS, Provincial Reconstruction Teams (PRTs) initiated long-term and sustainable public works projects to provide essential services (sewage treatment, roads, bridges, medical clinics, courthouses), economic development (job training, microlending), and governance (professional training, oversight, election monitoring) (FM3-24 2006: §3–68; §5–11). PRTs moved beyond MEDCAPs to establish and fund larger-scale cooperative ventures with governmental, nongovernmental, and international agencies to jumpstart development and reconstruction.

First established in Afghanistan in late 2002, PRTs came to Iraq in 2005. Their numbers, staff, and budgets were not large. Some 31 multinational PRTs operated in Iraq and 26 in Afghanistan. The staff numbers ranged from 75 members in American facilities to over 100 civilian and military personnel on British and German teams (ISAF 2009: 105–111; SIGIR 2013: 44). In Afghanistan, for example, 1,021 military personnel and 49 civilians staffed US-run PRTs (GAO 2008). In Iraq, Economic Support Fund (ESF) funding for *all* PRT projects—water, sanitation, education, electricity, microlending, and health—reached about $1 billion through September 2012 when PRTs wound down (SIGIR 2013: 64, 109, 152). To provide healthcare services, PRTs partnered with NGOs to build or refurbish health clinics, train health-care workers, and conduct public health campaigns that included preventive medicine, waste management, and health education. Successful military medical programs trained Iraqi medical personnel to evacuate and treat Iraqi battlefield casualties in local facilities (Yarvis 2011). Major civilian projects included the Missan Surgical Hospital ($16 million) and the Erbil Emergency Hospital ($13 million) (SIGIR 2013: 109–111).

Given such modest means, the stated mission of PRTs was exceptionally ambitious:

The PRT program is a priority joint Department of State/Department of Defense initiative to bolster moderates, support US counterinsurgency strategy, promote reconciliation, shape the political environment, support economic development, and build the capacity of Iraqi provincial governments to hasten the transition to Iraqi self-sufficiency (CALL 2010: 17).

These are enormous demands but consistent with medical diplomacy. Without much elaboration or appropriate metrics of success, PRT projects hoped to influence the local population and instill loyalty to the local government by trumpeting enhanced security, employment opportunities, and upgraded services, including health care.

Given the divergent aims of medical diplomacy and medical relief, there was considerable friction between military-run PRTs and civilian NGOs. Non-governmental agencies accused PRTs of subordinating humanitarian needs to military interests, ignoring local power structures, and partnering with powerful but corrupt contractors (Olson 2006). Circumstance and necessity, however, brought multinational forces and humanitarian aid organizations together from the beginning. NGOs delivered organization, contacts, and expertise, while military forces supplied funding, security, and technical support. As the wars progressed, USAID (US Agency for International Development) would team up with PRTs and NGOs to rebuild local infrastructures to ensure human security. In Afghanistan, some 80 NGOs worked in the health sector and managed over 80% of the healthcare projects, while a similar number managed 317 projects in Iraq in 2003 (Jones et al. 2006: 198, 241). Funneled through the Development Assistance Committee, American aid to Iraq and Afghanistan totaled $7 billion and $1 billion respectively in 2005, and $2.5 billion in each nation in 2009. The largest benefactor was USAID, followed by the Departments of Defense, Treasury, and Agriculture (OECD 2006, 2011). Only a small part of these funds went to humanitarian aid and health care. In Iraq, foreign donor nations contributed $453 million toward humanitarian assistance through 2005, before dropping to $95 million in 2006 (NCII and Oxfam 2007).

Medical Humanitarianism in Iraq and Afghanistan: Success or Failure?

The empirical and moral questions are closely related. Empirically, we can first ask (1) "Does diplomacy-motivated medicine offer good medical care?" and (2) "Did medical care win hearts and minds and enhance counterinsurgency capabilities?" The short answer to both is, "No." The ethical questions, therefore, take a hypothetical turn: Were medicine to win hearts and minds successfully, should multinational forces deliver medical care to encourage patients or their families to aid counterinsurgency efforts? At the same time, should foreign or local military forces recruit humanitarian NGOs for the same purpose?

Does Diplomacy-Motivated Medicine Offer Good Medical Care?

The answer to this question varies with the provider. Combat support hospitals provided a high standard of acute care consistent with American and European standards but were not a designated vehicle for medical diplomacy. MEDCAPs and, to a lesser extent, PRTs, on the other hand, afforded relatively meager treatment while actively seeking hearts and minds. There is widespread agreement that MEDCAPs did not work. Evaluating its MEDCAPs in Afghanistan, NATO (2010: B7–8) criticism was blistering:

Lessons gained in ISAF Regional Command South concluded that MEDCAPs were neither providing lasting healthcare benefits to the local population nor supporting the MoPH [Ministry of Public Health] in creating a sustainable healthcare system. Furthermore, MEDCAP has the potential to compete with the indigenous healthcare providers, with the impact to disrupt rather than enhance local healthcare capabilities.

This report and others describe how mobile clinics or other "tailgate" facilities carry inadequate diagnostic equipment, fail to keep medical records or follow patient progress, undermine the status of local physicians, bankrupt local pharmacies by distributing free drugs, elicit charges of favoritism, and seed resentment (Bulstrode 2009; Chamberlin 2013; Lesho et al. 2011; McInnes and Rushton 2014). Nevertheless, MEDCAPs doggedly retain their appeal. "Medical care in Afghanistan is often poor at best," ISAF medical staff at a MEDCAP facility in Kabul told researchers. "If we can help people while showing them that we really do care, it becomes a win-win situation. This is a 'hearts and minds' type of scenario" (Shafran 2007: 9).

PRT medical projects—building and staffing clinics and medical training programs—hoped to correct some of the glaring deficiencies of MEDCAPs by implementing long-term, sustainable, and capacity-building projects through close cooperation with local stakeholders and NGOs. Medicine was, however, only one of many PRT projects, so that healthcare benefits were diffuse. The 2010 *Handbook of the Iraq Provincial Reconstruction Team*, for example, acknowledges its health-related aims of medical training, mentorship, and refurbishment of healthcare facilities. Nevertheless, no health-related project makes its list of the 10 major PRT achievements in Iraq (CALL 2010: 52–57). Instead, top projects included microlending, government training, vocational education, and construction. Nor was medical management a top priority in Afghanistan. Although initial projects concentrated on security infrastructure, only later-phase programs addressed "the softer end" that included support for schools and clinics (Gordon 2010). Despite their attention to reconstruction, PRTs devoted significant resources to training security forces, confiscating illegal weapons, and clearing mines. The result, writes Frederic Labarre (2011: 25), was "a militarized PRT that violated COIN tenets that urged intervention with a civilian face" (also Perito 2005). Without their civilian face, PRTs found it increasingly difficult to cooperate with NGOs wary of overt ties to the military. Co-opting some NGOs and driving others, such as MSF (Doctors Without Borders), from the country, PRTs were often ineffective in the development sphere.

Does Good Medical Care Enhance a Counterinsurgency?

As Iraqis begin to trust and embrace their national and provincial governments and rely on essential government services such as medical care, they will reject the insurgency. (Baker 2007: 73)

Baker's description draws directly on American counterinsurgency (COIN) doctrine that relies on security, essential services, governance, and economic development to degrade support for insurgents, increase trust in the government, and "advance US interests and values" (DoDD 2005: §4.2; also FM 3–24 2006: §5.7–§5.18).[1] To accomplish these aims, security projects train local military and police forces or initiate programs to integrate insurgent forces into the national army. Public works projects also incentivize civilian-military cooperation. By backing the government and rejecting insurgent overtures, local stakeholders and gainfully employed young men work with the local government to protect their investments, jobs, and income.

Conceptually, COIN and US Department of Defense (DoD) policies draw on the logic of soft power, public diplomacy, and global health diplomacy. Soft power and public diplomacy eschew coercive force in favor of persuasive tactics, such as public works or economic development, to garner crucial support from domestic and foreign publics (Nye 2008). Turning to global health diplomacy, nations endeavor to win hearts and minds, project power and influence, and enhance security by exporting medical expertise and personnel (Fauci 2007; Feldbaum and Michaud 2010). Nations as diverse as Cuba, Great Britain, and China reaped diplomatic and economic dividends from their healthcare initiatives in South America, Africa, and East Asia (Feinsilver 2010; Kevany 2014; Swerdlow 2016; Zajtchuk 2003).

The causal mechanism to translate medical attention into political support is amorphous. Drilling into the emotive effects of soft power, Vuving (2009) suggests that a successful campaign to win hearts and minds instills gratitude, admiration, and reverence in the target audience. Life-saving medical care is a potent source of all three. When local civilians believe they can benefit from "superior medication, skill or knowledge, or that Americans will cure their children of incurable diseases" (Rice and Jones 2010: 53), there is every expectation that they will enthusiastically back their government and foreign troops. Ordinarily, healthcare diplomacy utilizes health care as a *substitute* for armed force. During armed conflict, however, medical diplomacy serves as an *adjunct* to armed intervention and an instrument of stability operations. Is it effective?

Evidence of successful military medical diplomacy is sparse. Following several years of PRT operations in Afghanistan, support for the US military grew from 67% in 2004 to nearly 80% in 2005 before showing signs of strain as violence increased and reconstruction efforts faltered (Jones 2008). One account from Iraq (2007–2008) is telling:

> We successfully achieved our [PRT] mission, if you're tracking incidents of significant violence against the brigade . . . The record shows that there was a significant reduction in violence. What was the chain of causality? I don't know, but I think we were successful. (Naland 2011: 6–7)

Indeed, assessing the chain of causality to determine whether and how PRT projects contributed to COIN objectives is a major bugbear. Medical metrics of success include epidemiological and public health outcomes, and the number of patient visits, additional clinics, and newly trained personnel (Lougee 2007). More generally, counterinsurgency endeavors aim to restore essential services, support economic development, and improve security to strengthen pro-government attitudes (FM 3-24.2 2009: §6.119–§6.123). Despite concerted efforts, firm consistent evidence to confirm these outcomes is unavailable. Recounting the capture of Tal Afar, Iraq, in 2005, for example, Jay Baker (2010: 15) describes how "US forces seized the hospital from enemy control, denied refuge to enemy combatants, and extended the reach of essential services to the local populace. These actions were subsequently used in successful information operations to build legitimacy for the Iraqi government." And, while the operation improved security and services, there is little indication of enhanced legitimacy. In Afghanistan, for example, public opinion vacillated. By 2008, and in contrast to the opinion polls from 2005, there was "little concrete evidence in any of the five provinces that aid projects were having more strategic level stabilization or security benefits such as winning populations away from insurgents, legitimizing the government, or reducing levels of violent conflict" (Fishstein and Wilder 2012: 3; Langer 2005). Despite some anecdotal support for PRTs and MEDCAPs, they could not offer sustained quality health care and had little influence on local attitudes.

Military medical diplomacy failed for many reasons. Poor planning, endemic corruption, insecurity, lack of long-term commitments, and inattention to local stakeholders are the usual suspects. To enhance performance, oversight and review boards called on PRTs to increase data collection to avoid waste; improve communication with United Nations officials and local leaders; vet contractors to diminish corruption; focus on small, short-term projects; push operations into remote areas; and address frequent staff rotation (CALL 2011: 174–211; also Thompson 2008; Wilton Park Conference 2010). Recommendations to reduce friction between military and humanitarian organizations turn to civilian agencies and private contractors to provide relief groups with financial, logistic, and technological services so they need not rely upon the armed forces (Carpenter and Kent 2016; Oliker et al. 2004: 106–109). By putting some distance between NGOs and the armed forces, civilian and private contractors can leave multinational troops to attend to security and thereby preserve the humanitarian space that relief agencies require to operate effectively.

Military medical diplomacy confronts acute security challenges, political instability, and fragile local government partners. In this austere environment, it may be impossible to implement medical diplomacy successfully. Alternatively, reforms may indeed better performance. PRTs, however, wound down by 2012 (Iraq) and 2014 (Afghanistan), leaving many suggestions for improvement untested. Therefore, the ethical discussion must turn on the hypothetical: Could MEDCAPs and PRTs successfully motivate local civilians to support the military and political goals of a counterinsurgency? Are military-run civilian medical services a permissible weapon of war? Here I consider two separate questions. First, taking an extreme case, is it permissible to use medical services to gather intelligence to degrade insurgent capabilities? Second, may intervening forces recruit humanitarian NGOs to attain military objectives?

The Ethics of Medical Diplomacy (I):
Intelligence Gathering

Consider four anecdotes:

1. "The care provided to just one child can affect an entire village's perception of the Coalition (to the extent that civilians provided information

that led directly to the capture of numerous insurgents)" (Burnett et al. 2008: 264).

2. "[Medical personnel] care, but they care in order to obtain information, which they refer to as 'force protection'" (Lundberg et al. 2014: 822).

3. "Surgery can be a useful commodity to gain positive influence with or to trade for intelligence from key local, national leaders" (Becker & Link 2011: 12).

4. "Civil-military operations can be an excellent way to gather intelligence . . . Locals were often so thankful for receiving healthcare from US military forces that on numerous occasions, patients in health clinics and host-nation personnel volunteered combat information to US forces concerning IEDs and weapon caches, as well as enemy activity in the region" (Jones 2008: 100; also Fishstein and Wilder 2012; Bryan 2009).

Intelligence gathering can be a significant side benefit of civilian medical attention. Unlike nebulous support for insurgents or government forces, intelligence is a concrete, immediate, and actionable metric that lends itself directly to "capturing and killing insurgents" (FM 3-24 2006 §5-111). As a test case for the ethics of medical diplomacy, intelligence gathering offers greater benefits than other deliverables. It is also intensely problematic. The Geneva Conventions caution medical personnel, "never to act in conflict with the wounded person's interests . . . and never to abuse his sense of dependence on the person administering care, particularly not with a view to gaining an advantage from him" (ICRC 1987: Art 16, §658). Abusing a vulnerable patient's sense of dependence violates human dignity egregiously and can occur whenever military authorities trade medicine for collaboration.

The Ethical Challenges of Intelligence Gathering

Moral objections to using medicine to gather intelligence emphasize mistrust of physicians, patient exploitation, and violations of medical neutrality (Cameron 2011; Chamberlin 2015; NATO 2010: 27). As the preceding chapters demonstrate, military medical providers are not neutral. They instead place medical science in the service of war. Charges of patient exploitation, on the other hand, raise serious concerns.

To address these concerns, Eugene Boneventre and Valérie Denux (2013: 205) turn to the doctrine of double effect (DDE):

> If the military delivers health care according to needs and if beneficiaries share information as a result, such passive collection of information may be acceptable as a secondary benefit under the ethical principle of "double effect," but it should not be the primary reason that the military delivers care.

Boneventre and Denux portray intelligence gathering as an unintended side effect of medical attention. As such, the medical staff does not condition specific treatment, say a course of antibiotics, on their patient delivering intelligence. Nor do anecdotal accounts depict a coercive atmosphere. Still, as some of the citations above suggest, it is difficult to ignore a more proactive, strategic interpretation of utilizing military-provided civilian health care to curry favor. For this reason, recourse to the DDE is unconvincing. As outlined in Chapter 1, the DDE generates an intended and unintended effect or outcome. If intelligence is a condition of medical attention, it cannot be the second, unintended effect. Instead, intelligence gathering is the intended effect. But by violating respect for patient autonomy and self-determination, it is impermissible. If information is a byproduct of medical attention, then it fails the DDE because the second effect must be incidental, that is, of no benefit to the agent of the first effect. Intelligence, however, is exceptionally valuable.

If the DDE fails, might a lesser-evil argument offer a more compelling defense of some forms of intelligence gathering? Intelligence gathering contends with two evils. One evil invokes the harm befalling multinational forces when intelligence sources go unmined. The second evil speaks to two costs: inferior medical care for refusing to provide intelligence, and the affront to dignity that comes with exploitation or manipulation. Is anything in this trade-off permissible?

Answering this question depends upon actual practice. One practice is ad hoc and describes how villagers provide intelligence following medical care for themselves or their families (Cases 1 and 4 above). Or, before or during treatment, medical staffers raise questions about insurgent forces in the area (Cases 2 and 3 above). Each case suggests an implicit or explicit quid pro quo. A quid pro quo, however, is not necessarily objectionable. As Cécile Fabre argues, much depends on one's ability to refuse (2021: 164-158). In one instance, medical officials might condition care on information and say: "Give us information or we won't care for you or your family." Alternatively, a patient may manipulate medical officials and say: "Treat me, and I will give you information." In each case, one party exploits the other, but only the first case is impermissibly coercive. In the second case, officials may choose to refuse or accept the offer of aid.

The distinction between exploitation and coercion helps us navigate the ethics of medical diplomacy. A medical quid pro quo is coercive in ways that other services are not. While a person has no choice but to accept life-saving care, one may reasonably refuse household electrification or paved roads. The sick and injured do not freely consent to collaboration, but comply because they have no choice. If they refuse, moreover, medical providers deny them or their family their rightful care. Rights to road or home improvements are less compelling than the fundamental right to health care. Medical diplomacy differs from public diplomacy in these crucial ways. As a result, the lesser evil argument provides no defense. Regardless of any significant military advantage intelligence may afford, the lesser evil—indignity and coercion—falls beneath minimum human rights requirements. Although military medicine sometimes subordinates a person's best interest to broad beneficence in wartime, the lesser evil cannot deprive individuals of their fundamental rights regardless of the greater good.

A Limited Role for Medical Diplomacy

Intelligence and other forms of political and material support will undoubtedly accrue as local civilians enjoy life-saving care. Driving global health diplomacy in peace and war, the expectation of support in return for health care is not inherently objectionable. Nations often choose aid recipients while weighing prospective benefits. With this in mind, political, logistic, or intelligence support from local civilians may guide decisions when military authorities construct clinics, hospitals, schools, or courthouses. In these allocation decisions, however, medical benefits shift from the individual to the community. One would rightly object to a physician refusing to provide medical treatment, or a judge threatening an adverse decision until the patient or supplicant delivers intelligence. But when benefactor nations or humanitarian forces condition a clinic, school, or foreign aid on cooperation and support, there is no suggestion that front-line doctors or teachers will provide health care or education on any other basis than patient or student needs. Although the decision to build a school or clinic is not impartial or strictly needs-based, conduct within the facility is.

Medical diplomacy, therefore, presents unique challenges to public diplomacy. When benefactors and recipients are caregivers and their patients, any quid pro quo is coercive, whether explicit or not. When benefactors and recipients are humanitarian forces and rescued communities or, more generally, strong and weak powers, expectations of aid and support permissibly drive decisions to build healthcare and other facilities. One must remember, however, that justice decisions are secondary to real-world feasibility and effectiveness. Failed clinics or half-built hospitals serve no military or medical purpose. At the same time, there is no systematic evidence from recent wars that medical diplomacy can effectively garner reliable intelligence or significant support from civilians.

State-implemented medical diplomacy suffers from innumerable workaday deficiencies. Although combat support hospitals sometimes deliver superior, but ad hoc, acute medical care, MEDCAPs and PRTs do not. It is no surprise that they fail to excite anyone's hearts and minds. Better-organized projects might, but that wherewithal seems rare. As such, multinational forces might do better to dispense with medical humanitarianism during armed conflict altogether and turn medical relief over to local and international NGOs. Such a division of labor, however, does not mean giving NGOs a free hand but directs NGO operations to serve the military and political interests of multinational forces. When this happens, a large swath of medical relief efforts, not just medical care in the hands of military doctors, becomes an instrument of war.

The Ethics of Medical Diplomacy (II): Recruiting NGOs to the Combat Team

In a speech before nongovernmental organizations on October 26, 2001, US Secretary of State Colin Powell stunned the attendees. "I have made it clear to my staff here and to all of our ambassadors around the world that I am serious about making sure we have the best relationship with the NGOs who are such a force multiplier for us, such an important part of our combat team" (Powell 2001). Coming not three weeks after the US-led invasion of Afghanistan, it is unlikely that Powell fully understood the impact of his words, but they sent a clear message. Moving away from the neutrality that has traditionally defined humanitarian work, Powell hoped to militarize humanitarian assistance by recruiting nongovernmental organizations to help prosecute the war on terror.

Classical and New Humanitarianism

As the fighting progressed, first in Afghanistan and later Iraq, international and local relief organizations depended heavily on the American government for funding and security. This largesse tested each agency's neutrality and independence as nongovernmental organizations coped with their sudden marriage to military forces. The result was a conflict between two humanitarian visions. Classical or "Dunantist" (after International Committee of the Red Cross (ICRC) founder Henri Dunant) humanitarianism embraces the traditional principles of humanity, neutrality, impartiality, and operational independence to provide need-based relief wherever required, regardless of national affiliation and without consideration of military or political aims (UNOCHA 2010). *New humanitarianism*, in contrast, moved closer to Powell's vision to acknowledge the political dimension of humanitarian aid and the central role it plays in armed intervention (Lischer 2007). Even before Powell appealed to NGOs to serve as force multipliers, new humanitarianism broadened its traditional mandate from the palliative role of alleviating the suffering of all comers to embrace the long-term political goals of state-building in fragile regimes (Barnett 2005). This broader outlook caused some humanitarian agencies to cooperate closely with the military forces and condition aid on respect for human rights and a commitment to good governance (Goodhand 2006: 89–91, 146–147, 187–193; Terry 2002: 20–26). Powell was not speaking in a vacuum. NATO had recognized the benefits of enlisting NGOs in support of military missions in the 1990s (Barnett and Weiss 2011: 88–93; Pugh 2001). Nevertheless, the test of the new, politicized, and "state-led" humanitarianism was yet to come as the global war on terror unfolded.

In Iraq and Afghanistan, multinational forces worked closely with humanitarian organizations by funding projects and ensuring the security necessary to maintain humanitarian space. In theory, close military–NGO cooperation dovetails with the emerging doctrine of the responsibility to protect and affords a natural partnership for states and relief agencies. In contrast to defensive or civil wars, wherein NGOs must carefully navigate the warring sides, humanitarian wars offered a shared ideal that addresses the roots of political instability to ensure long-term welfare. In practice, however, the outcomes were far from rosy. Many humanitarian NGOs blamed their close cooperation with military personnel for insurgent attacks on aid workers in Iraq and Afghanistan (Abiew 2012). NGOs chafed under the oversight they faced from DoD-run PRT projects, craved their dedicated humanitarian space, and paled when confronted with conditioning aid on gathering intelligence. At the same time, joint PRT–NGO ventures delivered few medical benefits and displayed little evidence that medical diplomacy aided counterinsurgency efforts or functioned as a force multiplier.

As friction between the military and humanitarian organizations intensified, relations frayed. In the field, the Center for Army Lessons Learned (CALL) describes how PRTs gave NGOs a wide berth to avoid harming their humanitarian activities. Rather than engaging NGOs dynamically, PRTs held back under advice to reduce their "visible military footprint" and "remain responsive to whatever communication is possible given realities on the ground." The best practical suggestion was to build a database of all PRT and NGO development projects so military personnel would not "duplicate [NGO] efforts or stumble on to them" (CALL 2011: 206, 210–11). This is hardly the paragon of well-coordinated force multiplication. Doctrinally, a growing chorus of voices repudiated the politicized new humanitarianism in favor of its classical version (Donini 2009; Duffield, Macrae, and Curtis 2001; Slim 2015; de Torrente 2004). Aiming at PRT activities, the World Health Organization (WHO) (2011: 12) "reiterates the guiding principle that health activities should be based on assessed health needs and guided by humanitarian principles, not by objectives that are either political or military in nature." "Health activities," WHO instructs, "should not be used as a component of a 'winning hearts and minds' strategy."

The debate among classical and new humanitarians remains unresolved. It is not my intent, however, to navigate NGO predicaments but to address those of military medicine. What models of cooperation might military planners consider to utilize NGO expertise while avoiding the antagonism that bankrupts joint efforts? One option is to divest the military of all medical relief and delegate those operations to NGOs entirely. As early as 2003, CARE International (2003: 5–6) admonished multinational forces to "focus their efforts on the promotion of security throughout Afghanistan [and] . . . leave the coordination of reconstruction to the Afghan government, UN and other civilian aid agencies." Dropping medical care from COIN constitutes a doctrinal shift that rejects military medical diplomacy and places all forms of medical relief in NGO hands. A revised Powell doctrine would disband PRT-like operations, as well as exempt medical NGOs from any role on the combat team, but continue to provide funding and security for relief operations.

Whether NGOs will do a better medical job than the military is a large, troubling question. As the fighting in Iraq and Afghanistan wound down, local government agencies, together with domestic and foreign NGOs, assumed the task of developing healthcare services. The results disappointed many. There was no shortage of corruption, insufficient donor funding, and turf quarrels (Chapter 11). Postwar reconstruction, however, poses different challenges than providing ongoing medical care during armed conflict where a clean break between NGOs and military organizations is not feasible until the fighting winds down. In the interim, it is worth considering steps to improve collaboration to keep humanitarian organizations near, if not on, the combat team.

Improving Military–NGO Medical Collaboration

NATO policymakers understand the dilemma of using medicine as a weapon of war.

> Specific attention is required when military medical support is used for winning hearts and minds. There is the risk of misusing medical care to achieve military objectives. In such cases, the consequence is that military healthcare loses its impartiality and potentially strays from fundamental humanitarian values bound to the Geneva Conventions and Protocols. Nevertheless, since the military is likely to be engaged at the forefront of humanitarian distress, there is a moral obligation to provide appropriate support in the humanitarian arena if aid is not provided by somebody else. (NATO 2010: iv; also Oliker et al. 2004: 103–104)

The NATO report does not repudiate medical diplomacy but warns of its risks. Nor does the report question the vital role that humanitarian agencies should play. To improve collaboration and minimize friction among military and civilian providers, the way forward calls for a clear division of duties, respect for institutional boundaries, and sustained funding. Just as important, however, is a clear understanding of each organization's mission, constraints, and obligations. Humanitarian forces and humanitarian agencies share key operational goals. Although many commissions address NGO ambivalence or their frustration with military forces, they neglect each institution's responsibility to explain its respective rights, duties, and demands. This is the functional role of moral discourse and addresses such topics as the justice of humanitarian intervention, shared (and antagonistic) security interests, and military medical ethics' unique principles.

The Justice of Humanitarian Intervention

Justice is not the sole concern of NGOs, but of every actor present. Aid organizations, however, face a particular dilemma. To collaborate with military operations, NGOs must know that humanitarian forces prosecute war only after exhausting less violent alternatives to end grave human rights abuses, have a reasonable chance of achieving significantly greater good than harm, and respect fundamental human rights as they wreak devastation. In these regards, the outcomes in Iraq, Afghanistan, Libya, and Syria are not encouraging. But if humanitarian intervention retains some appeal and NGOs are called to the combat team, aid agencies will require the knowledge to differentiate between defensive and humanitarian wars. Defensive wars aim to remove or deter an armed threat, while humanitarian wars rectify human rights abuses, vanquish an aggressor, and rebuild the target nation. These differences obligate intervening states to articulate their military and political goals clearly. In many defensive wars, NGOs will, justifiably, wish to maintain their independence, neutrality, and impartiality because there is no right side, that is, no side that shares their humanitarian interests, with which to align. They are, therefore, free to pursue medical relief to the best of their abilities. In a humanitarian war, on the other hand, NGOs can consider closer cooperation if assured of a war's humanitarian intent and prosecution. Otherwise, NGOs will resist collaboration if they fear the taint of military activities that veer too far from their humanitarian mission and embrace regimes that are little better than those they replace.

Security (1): Protecting Humanitarian Workers from Insurgents

Undoubtedly, insurgent attacks on aid workers fuel NGO averseness to close cooperation with military forces. Whether NGOs in Iraq and Afghanistan might have fared better had they refused to cooperate with multinational authorities remains speculative. Independence distances their activities from the envelope of military-provided security; dependence brings them into the fold. Back in the fold, some NGOs find that mutually beneficial relations can thrive when the military provides adequate protection, logistics, transport, training, intelligence, and liaison facilities (Bolton and Jeffrey 2008; Morton and Burham 2010). This model reinforces military–NGO cooperation that some NGOs will reject, particularly those with independent funding. Nevertheless, the many NGOs accepting belligerent funding will have little choice but to develop collaborative models of humanitarian aid that put them on the combat team. Military organizations can treat them as allies while remaining responsive to NGO sensibilities. This is not an easy task, particularly as many NGOs remain conflicted. It requires military officials to pursue successful collaboration and trust, rather than resign themselves to indifference or benign neglect as the Center for Army Lessons Learned analysis of PRT activities described (CALL 2011).

Security (2): Protecting Humanitarian Aid Workers from Themselves
Do medical aid workers compromise their immunity when they join a combat team? Although international law is emphatic that they do not, ethics equivocates when humanitarian organizations aid a grossly rights-violating state or genocidal insurgency. When anyone—soldier, civilian, doctor, or aid worker—supports rank injustice, they have no immunity and are liable to defensive measures. The ethical argument gains force when states or nonstates demonstrate unbridled brutality. As aid workers parachute into a humanitarian war, they may find that noncombatant immunity does not extend to civilians who are complicit in the target regime's abuses.

   Complicity is an abiding moral dilemma for humanitarian organizations, whether the result of omission (failing to clear refugee camps of militants who then recruit or murder compatriots) or commission (paying bribes or taxes to gain access to areas in need of aid) (Slim 2015: 183–203). In their defense, humanitarian agencies may invoke the lesser evil of doing (or permitting) harm for the greater good of attending to civilian health and welfare (Lepora and Goodin 2013: 97–129). And, their argument might be convincing. But it remains only a defense. Resort to the lesser evil might excuse complicity, but it cannot offer sweeping permission to provide medical relief aid under any circumstances. Military forces cannot be faulted for surveilling relief efforts or taking appropriate steps to impede NGO activities when necessary. Because relief workers offer nonlethal aid and support, suitable measures to thwart complicit agencies stop well short of deadly force as some observers condone (Frowe 2014: 202–207). Appropriate measures might include disabling administrative infrastructures, arresting or expelling relief workers, freezing financial assets, or conducting postwar criminal trials (Gross 2015: 68–72; Lewis, Modirzadeh, and Blum 2015: 111–142). Humanitarian agencies cannot ignore the moral hazards of complicity. The fear is, of course, that belligerents will not respect the proper boundaries. We already have seen how NGO hospitals and aid workers suffered punitive attacks by insurgents in Iraq and Afghanistan and by Russia in Syria. So while humanitarian troops are attentive to NGO complicity, their concomitant obligation requires them to safeguard civilian humanitarian workers from hostile forces.

Respect for Military Medical Ethics
Support and funding for humanitarian relief are part of a multinational military operation that works through stages of counterinsurgency to defeat a rights-violating regime, restore human security, and rebuild a devastated nation. Humanitarian intervention is an enormous undertaking that remains incomplete in Iraq, Afghanistan, and elsewhere. Although relief efforts are only part of the big picture, all operations serve the same mission. Cognizant of the imperative to use medicine to sustain a military mission (military-medical necessity) and to maximize the benefits of humanitarian war (broad beneficence), it is reasonable to direct NGOs to projects that enhance political and military goals rather than maximize the alleviation of suffering. Some new humanitarian NGOs understand this, and it remains the prerogative of the belligerents to choose their partners until the fighting ends. At that point, global health diplomacy replaces its military-medical variant as nations undertake to rebuild.

Medicine as a Weapon of War

This chapter is normative, empirical, and speculative. "Ought implies can" is a familiar ethical axiom. That medical diplomacy should win hearts and minds requires that it can. Can medical diplomacy deliver good medical care and solid military benefits? The empirical evidence is weak. Could *improved* medical diplomacy provide the medical and military benefits it seeks? That answer is speculative. Isolated success stories suggest it might. With that, the moral question returns more forcefully: Should medicine seek diplomatic gains?

Here, I offer a tentative answer. Writing about medical humanitarianism post-Vietnam, I explained how MEDCAP projects could enhance state-building in Cambodia or Thailand by strengthening the existing healthcare system and training medical workers. In a nonconflict setting divorced from the morass of Vietnam, the idea of using medicine to ensure the health of a political community and its members is eminently sensible and, indeed, a moral imperative (Gross 2006: 206). During armed conflict, however, the challenge is considerably more complex because the immediate goal is not nation-building through health, but violent regime change through health. And although neither is assured of success, the cost of placing medicine in the service of war can be far higher than when medicine serves peaceful nation-building.

Medical diplomacy, however, is ethically no different from using medical care to return soldiers to duty or enhance warfighter performance. All utilize medicine as a weapon of war. In each case, military-medical necessity, broad beneficence, and fundamental human rights govern the provision of care and the framework of cooperation with NGOs. Medical diplomacy adheres to the same criteria to demand that medical resources effectively serve a legitimate military mission, maximize utility, and respect fundamental human rights by maintaining minimal levels of care. Medical humanitarianism has struggled to perform. How well it will perform in the future remains to be seen. The next test comes when humanitarian forces must rebuild a shattered nation from the ground up. Reconstruction evokes the principles of *jus post bellum*, postwar justice, and is the subject of Part IV.

PART IV
AFTERWAR: POSTWAR JUSTICE AND THE RESPONSIBILITY TO REBUILD

11

Postwar Healthcare Reconstruction

When a nation successfully defends itself and defeats its enemy, what obligation, if any, does it owe the vanquished? The answer is often, "None": A defeated enemy has no claim to any consideration whatsoever, having forfeited its right to restitution the moment it pursued armed aggression. Taking this view, a victor might still rebuild a war-torn enemy nation if reconstruction serves broader security interests by facilitating future, peaceful alliances with former foes.

Humanitarian wars, however, are different because *jus ad bellum* and the just cause for war are linked closely to *jus post bellum*, postwar justice. When nations go to war to defend foreigners suffering from an abusive regime, defeating and deposing the government is only half the mission. Ultimately, humanitarian wars must restore and guarantee the same dignified life whose degradation justified war in the first place. Fair enough, but what level of reconstruction does postwar justice demand? A dignified life affords individuals and their communities the opportunity for intellectual, physical, emotional, and social development. Achieving a dignified life in places such as Iraq and Afghanistan pushes well past restoring the *status quo ante bellum*, because that status quo fired the war effort in the first place. Meeting claims for a dignified life by a people ravished by a brutal regime might entail far-reaching duties to rebuild.

The Responsibility to Rebuild

The International Commission on Intervention and State Sovereignty's *Responsibility to Rebuild* calls on intervening forces:

> to provide, particularly after a military intervention, full assistance with recovery, reconstruction and reconciliation, addressing the causes of the harm the intervention was designed to halt or avert . . . *as long as necessary in order to achieve self-sustained stability*. Coalitions or nations act

irresponsibly if they intervene without the will to restore peace and stability, and to sustain a post-intervention operation for as long as necessary
to do so. (ICISS 2001: xi, 64, emphasis added)

How is one to interpret this sweeping obligation, and upon whom does it
fall? Start with the second question: Who is obligated to rebuild? One answer
is the party intervening militarily. They broke it, so they need to fix it. This
recalls the "we hurt them; we fix them" explanation of medical rules of eligibility that confer priority on victims of collateral harm (Chapter 7). I rejected
it then and reject it now. Claim rights for medical attention and reconstruction do not draw from the liability of intervening forces, but from the harm
the target regime perpetrates. Rectifying this harm, argues James Pattison
(2015), falls on all those nations best situated to deliver aid. As such, humanitarian forces might say: We delivered the personnel and equipment for war;
other countries ought to shoulder reconstruction. This is a solid argument
but ignores the relative wealth of nations. Some nations, such as the United
States, enjoy pockets deep enough for military action *and* reconstruction. As
a result, the cost of intervention and postwar reconstruction falls disproportionately on able nations but relieves none of its obligations.

What is the scope of this obligation? Humanitarian forces need not build
a utopia. Obligated to provide the means to a dignified life, no intervening
or donor nation is obliged to bankrupt their citizenry into indignity. When a
people faces the threat of imminent extermination and those best placed to
beat it back lack resources for any further investment, humanitarian forces
may "dispose of cruelty" (Bass 2004: 403) without further obligation to rebuild (Bellamy 2008). Clear and present genocide, however, is not the typical
case. When it is, and an intervening force is too poor to aid postwar reconstruction, the responsibility to rebuild may fall on the international community. Elsewhere, threats emerge and morph over time. The regimes in Iraq and
Afghanistan were brutal but not genocidal. As multinational forces deposed
the Baathist and Taliban regimes, the situation deteriorated further. Forcible
regime changes and the anarchy that follows reinforce what many see as the
obligation to ensure good governance (Orend 2006: 197–202; Orend 2014),
or build a democracy (Feldman 2004: 17–19, 81; Powell 2001).

Among these obligations is the duty to rebuild shattered medical
infrastructures to deliver acute, chronic, and ambulatory care while undertaking such public health measures as immunization, health education, hygiene, and sewage treatment. As characterizes postwar justice more

generally, the obligation to provide or rebuild medical services following humanitarian wars is broader than that imposed by defensive wars. A defensive war imposes the minimal burden to rebuild consistent with the defending nation's national interests. The United States took on significant rebuilding following World War II but not out of anything it *owed* the defeated Axis nations. Had US interests dictated otherwise, the country might have walked away as easily as the Allies had in World War I. Fueled by security interests, therefore, *post-defensive-war* medical reconstruction goes as far as it must to prevent instability, the spread of terrorism, or an influx of displaced refugees. Fueled by a commitment to a dignified life and the rights-respecting institutions it requires, *post-humanitarian-war* medical reconstruction goes as far as it must to sustain the right to health care.

Did Coalition efforts meet the healthcare demands of *post-humanitarian-war* justice? Answering this question first raises another: "What is the goal of healthcare reconstruction beyond improving health outcomes?" One answer is, "None": Health care has nothing to do with anything but health. Alternatively, health care is essential for human development, a necessary condition of, or proxy for, a dignified life. Pushing the envelope further is a more expansive claim: efficient health care confers the fledgling state with authority and legitimacy and is, therefore, an essential component of state-building. In each case, the metrics of success vary. Isolated epidemiological measures of mortality underlie good health. Ethical criteria are entirely medical. Although security interests and associative duties drive the medical rules of eligibility and dominate medical care at Coalition-run medical facilities, the civilian principles of medical ethics—medical urgency, impartiality, neutrality, and independence—should guide medical management at local facilities during reconstruction. Human development and state-building push further, drawing on interrelated economic, political, and social measures of which health is only one component. Ethical demands are more complex. They shift from medical ethics to political morality. To afford a state the authority and legitimacy it needs to sustain itself, local authorities require competent institutions incorporating fair, transparent, and equitable rules of justice.

Health, human development, and state-building are normative claims about what healthcare reconstruction *should* do. What healthcare reconstruction *can* do is more modest. As a fundamental pillar of all reconstruction efforts, healthcare exemplifies the mechanics of postwar rebuilding and its limits. Rebuilding healthcare facilities highlights the costs of reconstruction efforts, the imperative of close cooperation among donor, local government, and military and civilian agencies, as well as the joint efforts required to overcome inefficiency, entrenched power structures, and corruption. Rebuilding is an intensely political process that reformulates the normative goals of reconstruction to jump-start those institutions a nation requires to build a dignified life for its people.

Rebuilding Medical Infrastructures for Health and Governance

Although some analysts locate the reconstruction period with the nominal transfer of authority in Iraq and Afghanistan soon after intervention, I take a longer view and peg the reconstruction period, as distinct from the invasion and transition periods, with the transfer of security responsibility from multinational forces to the local government. Reconstruction did indeed occupy Coalition forces, nongovernmental organizations (NGOs), and local government agencies throughout the wars. But with the transfer of security oversight to the local government in Iraq with the Status of Forces Agreement (SOFA) in 2008 and the Strategic Partnership Agreement (SPA) in Afghanistan in 2012, local governments moved to take over donor-funded reconstruction efforts. As reconstruction commenced, programs to improve health, human development, and governance took hold.

Primary Care and Healthcare Packages

Essential health packages (EHPs) are the building blocks of healthcare reconstruction and the backdrop for the Basic Packages of Health Services (BPHS) that nations such as Iraq and Afghanistan would adopt. EHPs comprise a low-income country's "limited list of public health and clinical services which will be provided at primary and/or secondary care level" (WHO 2008: 2). EHPs are a prelude to universal health coverage that includes comprehensive curative, clinical, preventive, rehabilitative, and public health services (WHO 2014). Three parameters define essential health packages: criteria, content, and cost.

Criteria for Essential Health Care
The World Health Organization (WHO) does not specify the goods and services that comprise essential health packages but leaves this to each nation to determine commensurate with its resources and preferences. WHO does,

however, supply pertinent criteria: cost-effective means to reduce the burden of disease, equitable distribution of healthcare services, equal access for all in need, poverty reduction, political empowerment, and accountability (WHO 2008). In practice, criteria directing medical treatment—cost-effectiveness and equity—dominate (Hayati et al. 2018). Sociopolitical standards—poverty reduction, empowerment, and accountability—are less conspicuous but particularly important for humanitarian forces who hope to build a rights-respecting political commonwealth. Further, United Nations (UN) criteria for healthcare require attention to the unique needs of children, women, the elderly, disabled, indigenous peoples, and workers (CESCR 2000: Art. 12, §12, 20–22).

These criteria require refinement. The metric for cost-effectiveness might be the number of lives saved (mortality) or the quality of lives saved. Many basic programs, for example, focus on infant, child, or maternal mortality because each indicator responds significantly to "simple, cost-effective and high-impact interventions" (e.g., immunization, sanitation, birth attendance, and antenatal visits) and dramatically improve overall life expectancy (UN 2015: 33). Reducing mortality is a good starting point for defining high-priority services that benefit worse off individuals. But it does not necessarily benefit *all* the worse off. The Afghan Ministry of Public Health and its donors, for example, made saving maternal and pediatric lives their priority (Dalil et al. 2014: S132). There is no parallel commitment to the elderly or indigent. Faced with limited resources, policymakers must make defensible choices. Saving the lives of mothers and children who can potentially live long and healthy lives may trump extending the lives of the elderly or indigent who suffer from chronic, debilitating, and expensive-to-treat diseases. Resolving issues like these illustrates the role of community healthcare deliberation (described later) and its legitimating function during reconstruction.

Content of Essential Health Care

Content turns on two dimensions: the minimal basket of healthcare services and essential drugs, and the "underlying determinants of health, such as access to potable water, adequate sanitation, nutrition, housing, healthy occupational and environmental conditions, and access to health-related education and information" (CESCR 2000: Art. 12, §11, §43; also Yamin and Norheim 2014). Guidelines leave each nation the flexibility to decide which among the drugs and treatments meet local healthcare needs. To contain costs, however, many EHPs do not provide all essential medicines, while others require significant copays (Chapman et al. 2017, 2018). Forced to prioritize, covered care may neglect women or other groups, fail to adopt measures to treat epidemic and endemic diseases, or forego some immunizations.

The Costs of Essential Health Care

International guidelines recognize that implementing a basic healthcare package is a gradual process, entirely dependent upon a state's funding capacity (CESCR 2000: Art. 12, §9, 30). Apart from public resources, patient fees and foreign donations underwrite healthcare costs. Each is problematic. Copays undermine fair access and equitable treatment for the poor. Financial support from foreign governments and international NGOs varies and is unpredictable. Even the largesse afforded by Western intervention is a dual-edged sword. On the one hand, Western-led humanitarian wars can expedite reconstruction. On the other, they may raise expectations unduly, fund short-term, grandiose rather than long-term sustainable projects, and exacerbate a culture of dependence. Trying to move too quickly, multinational forces sometimes lose sight of the limited capacity of the local government.

The criteria, content, and costs of health care speak to its medical and social goals. While health care's medical aims hope to reduce the burden of disease, its social goals strive to decrease poverty and enhance political empowerment. With the emphasis on medical outcomes, epidemiological measures assess life expectancy, infant mortality, or the rate of infectious disease. Although necessary, improvements in these areas are not sufficient to meet the responsibility of rebuilding. If rebuilding also means to restore a dignified life, self-governance, and a robust civil society, then good health must also contribute to development and state-building. To evaluate success in these two areas requires a broader metric than epidemiological benchmarks of relative health. These metrics include human development and state-building.

Health and Human Development

Human development evinces the material conditions a person requires to achieve a dignified life. To help states and their donors reach this goal, policymakers developed a single measure, the Human Development Index (HDI). The HDI draws on a humanist approach to well-being that emphasizes the capabilities, opportunities, and goods individuals must attain to formulate and implement a rational and flourishing life plan (Sen 2000, 2005). Requisite capabilities include agency, imagination, thought, emotional expression, sociability, and practical reason (Nussbaum 2007). None is attainable without good health, a long life, income, and education. Pushing beyond health measures alone, the HDI combines per capita gross national income (GNI), life expectancy, and educational attainment in a single, comprehensive index of well-being. (Stanton 2007). The HDI is comparative. It allows one nation (and its aid donors) to gauge its developmental level relative to another or evaluate the same nation's progress over time. The HDI designates four categories of development: very high, high, medium, and low development. These categories are descriptive quartiles, not normative or prescriptive evaluations of development. Nevertheless, the most highly developed nations are usually democracies.

Using the HDI to appraise postconflict reconstruction raises two problems. First, how high an HDI score reflects adequate human development or what Amartya Sen (2005: 159) terms, "a minimally basic quality of life"? There is no easy answer to this question. The UN Development Program explains how a 0.50 HDI score differentiates between developed and less developed nations (UNDP 2010: 49). This formulation does not get us very far. In 2017, Syria just beat that threshold (0.536) but seems light years away from affording the opportunities for a dignified life. More promising is to consider specific healthcare-related indicators of sustainable development, such as the level of poverty; infant, child, or maternal mortality; infectious disease; access to potable water; and literacy. Second, the HDI is apolitical. It does not endorse a democratic or any other kind of rights-respecting state. Saudi Arabia, for example, scores in the "high development" quartile (0.853, rank = 39) while tanking on the Freedom House (2019) Democracy Index as among the planet's worst human rights abusers. If protecting human rights is the goal of humanitarian intervention and a preeminent condition of a dignified life, then the HDI is insufficient to evaluate postconflict reconstruction. Human development, like better health, is only a necessary condition that intervening and donor states help meet by building adequate healthcare infrastructures. The sufficient conditions for a dignified life entail democratic state-building.

State-Building

State-building denotes local and international efforts to help a war-torn, impoverished, or disaster-ridden nation build the institutions necessary to ensure stability, peace, and governance. If *post bellum* obligations require humanitarian forces to construct a rights-respecting, if not democratic, polity, then healthcare reconstruction plays a central role. Apart from reducing the burden of disease and maintaining the regulatory institutions to guarantee the fair distribution of resources and equal access, healthcare systems also carry social and political duties. Socially, medical care should help reduce poverty by ensuring a healthy workforce and facilitating economic security. Politically, the World Health Organization (WHO 2008: 4) imposes "high-level" goals of political empowerment and accountability upon essential healthcare packages. Empowerment comes when communities take a role "in setting priorities, making decisions, planning, implementing, and evaluating strategies to achieve better health" (CESCR 2000: Art. 12, §54). Accountability comes with holding the state, healthcare providers, and insurers to delivering the public health services the government legislates.

In this way, a well-functioning public healthcare system can translate into trust for the government and bolster respect for its authority and legitimacy. Authority is bureaucratic, anchored in the government's capability to deliver competent health care while emphasizing its devotion to fairness, equality, and concern for citizens' welfare. Legitimacy is procedural and reflects the state's commitment to public participation and active citizenship. Ultimately, improved health care should contribute to political stability and governance by enhancing social cohesion, tolerance, resilience, fairness and equality, governing capacity, and government legitimacy (Eldon, Waddington, and Hadi 2008; Gordon 2013; Michael et al. 2013; Recchia 2009).

Measuring state-building capacity requires a metric more comprehensive than the HDI alone. Measures vary. Freedom House assesses the formal dimensions of democracy: civil liberties, political rights, participation, government functioning, associational and organizational rights, and the rule of law. The *Fragile States Index* (*FSI*) is thicker. It evaluates the relationship between security forces and citizens, communal violence, economic equality and opportunity, social services, political rights, responsive leadership, and internal displacement. Each index is useful in its way, with the *FSI* drilling into healthcare specifics: access to medical facilities, population density, orphaned children, food insecurity, clean water, mortality, and epidemics.[1]

Iraq and Afghanistan: How Do They Measure Up?

Beginning with healthcare metrics, Table 11.1 compares Iraq and Afghanistan across health outcomes. The following discussion then assesses inputs (donor funds for reconstruction) and outputs (e.g., number of clinics or trained nurses). Tables 11.2 and 11.3 examine the broader

Table 11.1. Health Care Outputs—Iraq and Afghanistan

	UN GOAL	Iraq			Afghanistan			Mideast and N. Africa[4]
	2030	2000	2008	2017	2000	2012	2017	2017
Infant Mortality[1]	12	35.5	30	23	90	59	50	20
Life Expectancy	Unspecified	69	68	70	56	62	64	73
Maternal Mortality[2]	<70	79	70[6]	79	1,450	954[6]	396–638	62
Under-5 mortality[3]	25	45	39	30	129	83	68	24
Immunization % DTP	Unspecified	80	69	85	24	67	66	89
Immunization % Measles	Eradicate	86	76	85	27	59	64	89
Universal Health Coverage (%)	Unspecified	NA	NA	63[7]	NA	NA	34[7]	65[7]
Severe multidimensional poverty (MDP)[5]	Eradicate	NA	NA	2.5%[8]	NA	NA	25%[8]	NA
Hunger % malnourished	Unspecified	29%	24%	29%	46%	23%	30%	9%
Safe and affordable drinking water[7]	Universal access	NA	NA	86%	NA	NA	63%	87%[9]
Sanitation facilities[7]	Universal access	NA	NA	86%	NA	NA	39%	81%[9]

[1] Per 1,000 live births

[2] Per 100,000 births

[3] Per 1,000 children

[4] Excluding high-income nations (except for the item "Universal Health Coverage," which includes all Mideast and N. African nations)

[5] Individuals living in severe multidimensional poverty are deprived in one half or more of the weighted indicators of multidimensional poverty; for example, health, education, housing, or standard of living (UNDP 2019)

[6] Data from 2010

[7] Data from 2015

[8] Data from 2015–2016

[9] Arab States

NA: No available data

Sources:

UNDP (United Nations Development Programme) 2018

World Bank (2018; 2020)

UNICEF (2019) Data: Iraq, Afghanistan

WHO and The World Bank 2017

Table 11.2. Human Development Index (HDI) and Indicators—Iraq, Afghanistan, and Medium Developing Countries

	Iraq				Afghanistan				Medium Developing Countries	
	2000	2008	2017	Change 2008–2017	2000	2012	2017	Change 2012–2017	2010	2017
Human Development Index *HDI/Global Ranking*	.607/126th	.646/109th	.685/120th	+11	.376/161st	.482/155th	.498/168th	–13	.592	.645
HDI indicators										
Life expectancy	69	68	70	+2	56	62	64	+2	69	69
Expected years of schooling	NA	9.7[2]	11	+1.3	NA	9.1[3]	10.4	+1.3	11.0	12
Mean years of schooling	NA	5.6[2]	6.8	+1.2	NA	3.3[3]	3.8	+0.5	6.3	6.7
Gross National Income per capita (USD)	9,590	12,360	17,785	+5,425	870[1]	1,900	2,000	+100	5,134	6,849

[1] Data from 2002
[2] Data from 2010
[3] Data from 2011
NA: No available data

Sources:
Human Development Report (UNDP 2010, 2017, 2018)
World Bank (2020)

Table 11.3. State-Building and Democracy • Fragile States Index (FSI)

	Iraq				Afghanistan			
	2006	2008	2020	Trend (%)[4] 2008–2020	2006	2012	2020	Trend[4] 2012–2020
Fragile States Index Total Score (Rank = nth worst)[1]	109 (4th)	111 (5th)	96 (17th)	+ (7%)	99.8 (10th)	106 (6th)	103 (9th)	+ (2%)
Subscores								
State Legitimacy[2]	8.5	9.4	9.1	+ (3%)	8.3	9.5	9.0	+ (5%)
Economic Equality[2]	8.2	8.5	6.4	+ (25%)	7.5	8.1	7.7	+ (5%)
Human Rights[2]	9.7	9.6	7.8	+ (19%)	8.2	8.5	7.6	+ (10%)
Public Services[2,5]	8.3	8.5	8.4	+ (1%)	8.0	8.5	9.5	– (12%)
Cohesion								
Lawlessness[3]	9.8	9.9	8.2	– (17%)	8.2	9.7	9.9	+ (2%)
Group Grievance[3]	9.8	9.8	8.5	– (13%)	9.1	9.4	7.5	– (20%)
Factionalized Elites[3]	9.7	9.8	9.6	– (2%)	8.0	9.4	8.9	– (5%)

[1] Total FSI Score: 0 (Strong) to 120 (Fragile); Ranking: 1st = most fragile; > 175th most stable

[2] Subscores: 1 = Strong; 10 = Weak

[3] Subscores: 1 = Weak; 10 = Strong

[4] Trends: growing stronger (+); growing weaker (-)

[5] Public Services = health, education, shelter, infrastructure, that is, essential services

Source:
Fund for Peace. *Fragile States Index 2006–2018, 2020.*

outcomes of post-humanitarian-war reconstruction: human development and state-building. Subject to the availability of data, each table tracks three periods: the period prior to transition (2006), the year of transition to local government authority in Iraq (2008) and Afghanistan (2012), and recent data (2020). Comparative 2020 data come from Middle Eastern and North African nations (excluding high-income countries) and medium developing countries.

Afghanistan: Healthcare Financing and Outcomes

The 2006 Afghanistan Compact set 2010 goals to improve security, governance, rule of law and human rights, and economic and social development. Healthcare goals included a Basic Package of Health Services for 90% of the population, comprehensive infant immunization, and the reduction of maternal and infant mortality by 15% and 20%, respectively, by 2010 (Afghanistan Compact 2006: 10). An essential package of hospital services, instituted in 2005, aimed to staff and equip district, provincial, and national hospitals (SIGAR 2017: 2–3). To meet these goals, the World Bank, the European Union, and the US Agency for International Development (USAID) allocated $820 million between 2003 and 2008/9 to renovate or build 763 healthcare facilities while NGOs delivered health care in 31 of 34 provinces (Frost et al. 2016: 1–2). Development assistance for health peaked in 2015 at $360 million before falling to $235 million in 2017 (Micah and Dieleman 2018: 148). Aid was, and remains, crucial. Lacking funds and plagued by high operating costs, lack of skilled staff, incomplete projects, and corruption, the national government could only fund 15% of all health care. Donor states underwrote more than two thirds of government-supplied health care while out-of-pocket payments for private medical care comprised the balance. By 2030, external donor aid is projected to drop, leaving the government to fund 50% of public health care, and the local population still dependent on private care (Micah and Dieleman 2018: 178–179, 188–189; also Rutherford and Saleh 2019).

Table 11.1 describes the state of health in Iraq and Afghanistan. Although the data draw from the WHO and the World Bank, there are discrepancies coming from charges that USAID in Afghanistan—the premier funding agency for postwar reconstruction—delivered unsubstantiated reports of improved health care based on poor data collection (SIGAR 2017).

Based on available information, indicators of life expectancy, along with infant, child, and maternal mortality, improved significantly in Afghanistan since 2000. On the other hand, not all measures achieved desirable outcomes. Falling short of broader coverage, immunization rates for diphtheria, tetanus, and pertussis (DTP) and measles reached only 66% and 64% by 2015. Universal health coverage struggled. Despite abolishing fees to encourage equitable utilization in 2008 (Steinhardt et al. 2013), coverage reached only 34% in 2017. As a result, many patients, including the poor and unemployed, sought medical attention in the private sector or abroad (Bricknell and Cameron 2011; SIGAR 2017: 12–14). Lack of access for rural residents skewed coverage across the country and imperiled equity (Acerra et al. 2009; Kim et al. 2016). In absolute terms, the numbers lagged further. Although meeting Afghan goals, mortality, and such health-related measures as poverty, hunger, pollution, and sanitation fell far behind UN goals and other developing states.

To bolster reconstruction efforts, NGOs and donor nations undertook significant measures to engage local communities. Cooperating with international forces, committees of civic leaders (*shura*) could facilitate public works projects, address grievances, and foster stability. Within communities, activists oversaw local meetings, educational outreach, resource mobilization, network building, and leadership training (Laverack 2006 for review; also WHO 2018). In health care, community-staffed hospital boards helped to maintain community-government relations by encouraging feedback and community support. Small-scale but successful community projects included immunization, first-aid training, health education, and community disaster planning (Afghan MOPH 2005: 11; Chang et al. 2010). By 2011 nearly all healthcare facilities collaborated with community groups (Newbrander 2014).

As an exercise of deliberative democracy, community health activism can strengthen social cohesion, empower the local population, and improve trust between the government and its citizens. It is a tall order for a nation embarking on reconstruction that is quickly undermined by inadequate funding and insecurity. Both these conditions plague postwar reconstruction in Afghanistan and leave its people a long way to go until the government can satisfy their rights to health care.

Iraq: Healthcare Financing and Outcomes

Comparing healthcare reconstruction in Iraq to Afghanistan, several trends stand out. First, as described in Chapter 4, Iraq's healthcare system was far more advanced than Afghanistan's when war erupted. Despite the impoverishment of Iraq following the imposition of sanctions in 1990, healthcare indicators were more robust than Afghanistan's. As a result, foreign assistance was less comprehensive. At just over $1 billion through 2012 (SIGIR 2013: 110), donor aid peaked in 2005, reaching $500 million or 15% of the estimated $3.4 billion spent on health care. Government spending and out-of-pocket costs comprised 73% and 27% of all healthcare spending, respectively, much the opposite of Afghanistan's figures. Donor aid funded one third of the public budget in Iraq rather than the two thirds it covered in Afghanistan.

Over the years, foreign assistance declined considerably to $78 million in 2010 and $15 million in 2016 or 1% of public healthcare spending. But if the goal was to wean the Iraqi government from donor aid, the brutal war with ISIS upended these plans. Facing a severe wave of internal refugees and the loss of facilities as ISIS gained control of 15% of Iraqi territory, all forms of healthcare spending increased from $3.4 billion (2005) to $6.2 billion (2016). Short of funds, however, government healthcare spending *decreased* from $2 billion (2005) to $1.6 billion (2016) after peaking at $3 billion in 2009. As a result, out-of-pocket costs for Iraqis rose from just under $1 billion (2005) to $4.6 billion in 2016 (IHME 2020). By 2016, out-of-pocket costs for private care and pharmaceuticals reached two thirds of all healthcare expenditures.

Despite its relative development, Iraq did not develop a centralized policy for essential health and hospital care as early as Afghanistan did. Lack of a comprehensive healthcare program coupled with institutional weakness in the emerging Iraqi government undercut attempts at sustained reconstruction (Jawad et al. 2010). While healthcare funding increased, plans languished, oversight was weak, and important goals remained unachieved. In 2012, some 229 poorly equipped hospitals and 2,500 primary healthcare centers delivered public health care (World Bank 2020). Many facilities were "in poor repair, inadequately staffed, and inequitably located," while pharmacies were chronically understocked (al Hilfi, Lafta, and Burnham 2013: 942–943; also Shabila et al. 2012a). The result was a thriving but mostly unregulated private sector for treatment and medicine.

Similarly, the Ministry of Health acknowledged weak accountability, regulation, and transparency, as well as "far from desired levels" of quality care in the public and private sector (Iraq MOH 2014: 5–16). A Basic Health Service Package (BHSP) aiming to "ensure the timely delivery of cost-effective, integrated and standardized health services" (WHO 2019: 1) was only first formulated in 2009 and still under development in 2014 (Iraq MOH 2009; 2014: 24) when ISIS stepped up its attacks in Iraq. That fighting ended in 2017 but not before disruptions drained funding from health care and forced hospitals and healthcare facilities to close (Webster 2016; Jaff. Leatherman & Tomaro 2019). In response, there were no increases in donor funding for health care in Iraq. In Kurdistan, an influx of Syrian refugees, coupled with disputes over central government funding, put further pressure on a fragile healthcare system (Shukor, Klazinga & Kringos 2017; RAND 2017; Shabila et al. 2012b).

Still, Iraq compares reasonably well with other developing nations and its neighbors. The trends are not linear; some indicators, such as immunization rates, deteriorated at the height of the fighting. Nevertheless, most health outcomes, including poverty, sanitation, pollution, and potable water, have improved since 2000 to put Iraq within sight of UN goals. Hunger, however, remains an acute problem in both nations. In Iraq and Afghanistan, 30% of the population remain undernourished, three times the number found in other Middle Eastern and North African nations.

Significantly, Iraq shows how the pace and prospect of successful reconstruction fluctuate subject to events beyond the control of multinational forces. Writing in 2014, Valeria Cetorelli and Nazar Shabila, for example, describe variable growth in primary care centers and hospitals across Iraq between 2003 and 2012. Although hospital growth remained static, primary care centers grew in number until the conflict with ISIS and the war in Syria intensified. Scarce funds, internally displaced persons, and refugees overwhelmed the system. These two conflicts, rather than the intervention 15 years earlier, created new and urgent demands for reconstruction. How, then, do humanitarian forces know when they have met their responsibility to rebuild? Can measures of human development and state-building tell us when this occurs?

Postwar Reconstruction: Human Development or State-Building?

Human development reflects the health, education, and material wealth required for a dignified life (Table 11.2).

Afghanistan sits well below developing nations, while Iraq reaches par. Ranked at 120 among the world's countries (medium human development), Iraq compares with India or the Philippines. Hindered by renewed fighting, however, Iraq has barely budged since 2000 after cresting in about 2010. Despite improved life expectancy, gross national income (GNI), and education, Afghanistan remains ranked 168th globally, lower than where it stood in 2010 and near the bottom of the scale.

These figures evaluate development comparatively. Raw HDI scores for Iraq and Afghanistan have improved slightly but their international rankings have not. Reconstruction has allowed each nation to keep pace and, essentially, maintain the status quo antebellum. But humanitarian intervention is supposed to do more than this. Afghanis and, to a lesser extent, Iraqis still lack the requisites to realize the full range of human capabilities. One can only look to other nations similarly situated, such as Ivory Coast or Sudan, to see how those peoples have yet to achieve a dignified life.

Albeit crucial, an individual's health, education, and income are only necessary conditions for a flourishing life. Utilizing each to attain a dignified life requires a thriving political environment to assure human security: the rule of law, essential services, fair resource distribution, and good governance. While human development measures individual well-being, human security is a political metric of collective welfare that comes with a well-governed state. In theory, then, state-building is the proper goal of humanitarian intervention. But is it effective? Does reconstruction, particularly healthcare reconstruction, foster empowerment, participation, and civilian oversight?

Various indices assess state-building in Iraq and Afghanistan. The Freedom House Democracy Index analyzes democratic institutions, political rights, and civil liberties to give countries a "Freedom Rating" of Free (1.0 to 2.5), Partly Free (3.0 to 5.0), or Not Free (5.5 to 7.0).Although Iraq and Afghanistan demonstrate considerable disparity on health indicators and human development, their state-building scores are equally poor. Following humanitarian intervention, each nation progressed from a Freedom Rating of 7.0 (not free) in 2001 to 6.0 (not free) at the start of reconstruction in 2008 (Iraq) and 2012 (Afghanistan), and to 5.5 (not free) in 2017 (Freedom House 2002; 2009; 2013; 2018). Despite the "not free" rating, each country moved slowly toward "partly free." This has to be a significant achievement that attests to the institutionalization of formal democracy in each nation. By 2019, each nation held regular elections and facilitated ethnic group representation. Nevertheless, corruption, powerful unelected factions, security threats, unfulfilled rights to freedom of assembly and movement, and the lack of an independent media and judiciary undermine the integrity of the political system. These measures barely budged despite the transfer of authority to the local government and concerted reconstruction efforts. Such uneven and slow development poses an abiding challenge to the nascent government in each nation and leaves intervening forces to wonder whether making a *Not Free* nation just a little bit freer satisfies their responsibility to rebuild.

In contrast to the Freedom Rating, the *Fragile States Index* (*FSI*) examines social, economic, and political variables that measure state legitimacy, social cohesion, human rights, and economic equality that healthcare reconstruction expects to improve directly. In Iraq and Afghanistan, the *FSI* suggests limited progress (Table 11.3).

Overall, both states remain exceptionally fragile, that is, subject to pressures that "outweigh a states' capacity to manage those pressures" (Fund for Peace 2019: 31). Although each state's overall ranking is equally poor and persistent, subscores offer a more nuanced picture. Among the expected state-building effects of a healthcare system are cohesion, a sense of shared identity, respect for human rights, economic growth, and greater state legitimacy (Kruk et al. 2010). The *FSI* measures of state legitimacy, economic equality, human rights, and cohesion do not lend ready weight to these expectations.

State legitimacy assesses public confidence, transparency, corruption, active opposition parties, and access to the political system. Economic equality drills into actual and perceived inequality, structural barriers to equality, and the opportunities to improve economic status. Human rights reflects the rule of law, respect for legal, political, and social rights, and politically inspired violence. Public services speak to health, education, welfare, water, and public security. A high *FSI* score on these measures signifies inequality, inadequate attention to human rights and public services, and weak state legitimacy. Cohesion weighs lawlessness among security service personnel, group grievances, and factionalized elites (Fund for Peace 2019: 33–40). These *FSI* scores run in the opposite direction so that social cohesion increases as lawlessness, grievances, and fictionalization decrease.

To various degrees, state legitimacy, cohesion, economic inequality, and human rights improved in each nation from the beginning of the reconstruction period to 2020. On the other hand, public services, including health, education, shelter, and infrastructures, changed little (Iraq) or deteriorated (Afghanistan). One reading suggests that relative lack of essential services, including health care, does not undermine state legitimacy or social cohesion if the state can improve security, protect human rights, and mitigate economic inequalities.

The *FSI*, however, does not isolate health care among essential services. Although Table 11.1 describes how health-related outcomes improved, this improvement may be insufficient to solidify state legitimacy when other essential services lag. Nor do these improvements tell the entire story. Enlisting health care in the cause of state-building sometimes subordinates medical goals to political goals. One result is to favor immediate high-impact projects over long-term sustainability (Philips and Derderian 2015). Another is to avoid risky projects whose failure only excites animosity toward government agencies (Jones et al. 2006: 187–275).

Alternatively, state-building indicators are so poor across the board that the causal chain is still indiscernible. Poorly developed public services coupled with slowly improving but still inadequate attention to human rights, economic inequality, and group grievances may be simply insufficient to build the trust necessary to boost state legitimacy and sustain social cohesion. Each state also suffered political shocks that undermined its legitimacy. In 2014, ISIS brought Iraq to the brink of civil war. Renewed intervention and the growing numbers of refugees who swamped the local healthcare system did nothing to fortify state legitimacy. Iraqi numbers are only just returning to pre-2014 levels. In Afghanistan, on the other hand, state legitimacy and public services went south with the departure of NATO troops and remained stubbornly weak as intense fighting with the Taliban continued into 2019. Social cohesion, economic equality, and respect for human rights improved modestly. Support for state legitimacy would strengthen by 2019 but remain below 2006 levels. Despite modest health-related improvements, essential public services have yet to catch up.

Mission Accomplished?

The preceding discussion raises one question and hints at another. First, when does the responsibility to rebuild end? Second, is the postwar responsibility to rebuild any more compelling than the responsibility to build a country unaffected by war but similarly distressed? These two questions are intimately connected. Military ethics imposes the obligation of postwar reconstruction following armed intervention. Severe prewar distress and imminent harm justify military engagement when other avenues of relief fail. Armed intervention, however, cannot privilege the rescued nation over similarly deprived peoples whose rescue does not require war.

Resources are limited, so nations capable of rendering aid must expend personnel and materiel judiciously. Judiciously rescuing the many deserving nations or peoples resembles wartime triage. Rescue may demand attention to the most urgent cases first, that is, those communities facing immediate extermination. Or, rescue may require attention to a much broader class of less immediate threats short of genocide that endanger a people's right to a dignified life. Intervening states, therefore, consider two criteria when declaring, "mission accomplished" and moving on. One is internal: The job ends when they meet their designated outcomes. The second is external: The job has not yet ended, but the call of other victims supersedes the current relief operation. Having secured some measure of betterment relative to a reasonable baseline, intervening states turn their attention to the new worse off. The questions remain, however. Where is the baseline, and does it matter that other nations are in the rescue queue?

Internal Criteria: Where is the Rescue Baseline?

The preceding sections suggest criteria for a baseline that satisfies the responsibility to rebuild. This chapter does not attempt to survey the many dimensions of reconstruction but uses medicine and health care as an important proxy for operationalizing its goals. Like security, health care is essential for any dignified life. Unlike security building, which is forever tricky to quantify and measure, healthcare building enjoys widespread consensus about many of its goals—diminished mortality and greater life expectancy, for example—that are relatively easy to measure and compare. There is no limit to healthcare building. Nevertheless, a basic healthcare package can achieve a level of viable health so that rescued people can take over state-building and deliver healthcare services. As they developed in Afghanistan and, to a lesser extent in Iraq, basic healthcare packages offered an effective means for improving key health indicators. At one point, then, it may be time to look at the plight of others in distress.

"At one point," can mean that things are approaching United Nations healthcare goals. By that standard, Iraqi health care is reasonably well along despite its many shortcomings. Afghan health care is not. Alternatively, policymakers might set reconstruction goals relative to developing nations or neighboring states. Each comparison is arbitrary. "Developing state" is a self-defined label, often affixed for political reasons. Nor is there any apparent reason to compare Iraq or Afghanistan with its neighbors as an early RAND Corporation study does (Jones et al. 2006). One option, perhaps, is to pick a reasonably peaceful and stable emerging nation in the "partly free" category of Freedom House to emulate. By this index, 75% of all nations are free or partly free, surely a reasonable goal.

As a thought exercise, this generates some intriguing examples. Both Nepal and Papua New Guinea, for example, are partly free but developing states (Freedom House 2019). Each falls between Iraq and Afghanistan on indicators of life expectancy; infant, maternal, and under age 5 mortalities; and universal coverage (World Bank 2020). Politically, each hovers at the top quartile of fragile states but ahead of Iraq and Afghanistan (Fund for Peace 2019). Perhaps, then, humanitarian forces can aim no higher than to reach the level of a state such as Nepal or Papua New Guinea. But as the Iraqi case demonstrates, superior health care alone cannot accomplish this. Reconstruction must address a great many other economic, political, and social matters. The question for multinational forces is to determine when target states can function competently to take the wheel, not when they have successfully reached their destination. This goal requires a minimally functioning state whose people are at least partly free and who have moved beyond the most fragile states. In this context, health care is not an end in itself but a necessary condition without which state-building cannot commence.

Nevertheless, there are many things humanitarian forces cannot do. They can build schools or medical facilities, and train teachers and healthcare workers, but they cannot compel patients to seek treatment or parents to send their children to school. Multinational troops can help establish the institutions of democracy but cannot democratize, cement social cohesion, or enhance state legitimacy. Only the local population can complete these processes. At best, the responsibility to rebuild coalesces around the minimal facilitating conditions for human security. These efforts reflect inputs, that is, the funding and resources to train security forces and build schools, hospitals, and courts. Outputs, that is, completed and functioning infrastructures, offer an additional metric of successful rebuilding but are far more capricious than inputs due to circumstances donor nations cannot control.

Healthcare building is an excellent example of the challenges that face reconstruction. On the one hand, health care lends itself to clear goals, costs, and responsibilities. Immunization campaigns and neo/antenatal, maternal, and pediatric care draw on well-established goals and programs. As such, they enjoy universal appeal and precedents of success that allow humanitarian troops to calculate and allocate the cost of rebuilding. On the other hand, factors beyond donors' control can stymie their efforts. Healthcare workers lose their lives trying to implement immunization programs. Many healthcare projects fell prey to endemic corruption, delays, conflicts of interest, interference, and incompetence. In this environment, intervening states and NGOs jump-start state-building and provide the rudiments of human security so a traumatized people can build a dignified life. For health care, this means to develop a basic package of primary hospital care and health care, fund immediate infrastructure needs, implement training programs, and underwrite publicly provided services until the government gains its legs. After that, it is time to wind down. Still vastly expensive, these steps coalesce around inputs, resources, and funding. They are only the "means to the means" of a dignified life, but the most the responsibility to rebuild can impose.

Of course, this is what multinational forces try to do. The trick is not to look directly at the broader goals of human development and state-building but to do basic reconstruction better. The lessons are there, buried in mountains of reports from governmental, nongovernmental, and international organizations. Beginning with the 2006 RAND Corporation report, *Securing Health: Lessons from Nation-Building Missions* (Jones et al. 2006), numerous studies by USAID, the World Bank, UK Department for International Development, and the Special Inspectors General for Afghanistan and Iraq Reconstruction (SIGAR and SIGIR), carefully explain how humanitarian and donor states can encourage stakeholder and community cooperation and avoid paternalism while they nurture independence, ensure security, promote transparency, monitor the public and private sector, and fight corruption (Rutherford and Saleh 2019 for partial review). Unfortunately, institutional memories rapidly fade once military and civilian experts leave their posts and move on afterwar.

In this context, it is critical to recognize how setting the bar for reconstruction affects the bar for intervention. If the responsibility to rebuild entails democracy building, then any nondemocratic state is a candidate for intervention. If the responsibility to rebuild demands the means for a dignified life—health, security, education, and income—then only near dispossession of any feature of human security justifies armed involvement. Under these circumstances, only grave injustice, severe deprivation, and extreme desperation warrant armed intervention.

External Constraints: Whom to Rescue, and for How Long?

The previous section asked: What is the rescue baseline? The answer is: the means for a dignified life, including primary health care. Those nations or peoples falling below that baseline enjoy the right of rescue, an obligation falling on those best situated to help. "Best situated" means to command the necessary military and/or financial resources and the national will to use them. But resources and will are limited, leaving each potential rescuing nation to decide whom to rescue and for how long.

The responsibility to rebuild is not limited to humanitarian intervention. Rather, military force is a last resort "should peaceful [i.e., diplomatic or humanitarian] means be inadequate . . . " (World Summit 2005: §139). It is a common misconception to link the duty to rebuild to the harm multinational troops bring when they employ armed force. Short of acting negligently or criminally, however, a country at just war incurs no responsibility to rebuild. Instead, the duty to rebuild draws on the harm a people suffers at the hands of its government *before* intervention. Foreign military intervention does not trigger that duty. Armed intervention may create unique or special needs (e.g., reconciliation, economic recovery, or resettlement; ICISS 2001: §5.6) but not special rights. Nowhere does the responsibility to protect or rebuild suggest that the beneficiaries of an armed humanitarian mission have an exclusive claim to world resources. Post-*war* rebuilding, therefore, has no superior status to post-*disaster* rebuilding. In response to either, the world community may choose armed force or material aid to strengthen human security in some of the most fragile states. The fact that one engaged military force and the other did not does not alter the responsibility to rebuild.

A plethora of threats to life and dignity leaves the best-situated nations with the duty to choose their operations wisely. The many candidates for rescue compel intervening nations to husband their resources and aid as many distressed nations as possible rather than undertake a colossally expensive war to aid one or two. Returning then to countries populating the lower rungs of the *Fragile States Index*. All face a different threat. Syria's savage war against its people garners the most attention. Genocide, war crimes, and crimes against humanity characterize a desperate situation that no Western military operation seems able to address. Civil war embroils some of the others. In Yemen, the most fragile of all states, Western intervention via Saudi Arabia is feasible but has, to date, only exacerbated the conflict. Elsewhere, Chad, Zimbabwe, or Sudan owe their fragility less to civil war and more to the political instability that comes from hostile external forces or authoritarian and kleptocratic leaders. They do not yet require military assistance but could undoubtedly benefit from human security as their people attempt to build a dignified life.

The many peoples deserving protection raises the triage question: whom to choose and how much to give them? The previous section answered the second part: a suffering people deserves more than being pulled from the flames; they also need the means to soldier on and rebuild their lives. Triage demands we attend the worse off first, assuming we can help at all. Syria may be the worse off of all, but most of the world community stepped back. Either military operations were infeasible (we lack the resources to pull it off) or ineffective (military intervention will not unseat Assad and improve things).

Turning from war-racked Syria leaves one to choose among other candidates. The obvious criterion is: Where is the biggest bang for the buck? Where is an intervention, military or otherwise, likely to be effective and leave the target nation with sufficient capacity to build a dignified life? The subclause, "military or otherwise," is vital because military intervention is neither necessary nor sufficient to trigger the responsibility to rebuild. On the contrary, the responsibility to protect demands alternative avenues of engagement before military action. Stripped of military force, the responsibility to protect is nearly synonymous with the responsibility to rebuild. It is also less expensive. Nonmilitary intercession may rescue far more peoples than armed force and avoids the tremendous costs of veteran care.

If a relatively simple cost-benefit function allows best-situated states to choose their missions, what about interventions in place? Seemingly, these end when they achieve minimal levels of human security. But what happens when new crises erupt, whether in the target nation or elsewhere? As reconstruction wound down, ISIS and the Taliban took the offensive to create chaos in Iraq and Afghanistan. Do these new events reset the clock? I think they must. Despite the enormous sunk costs that multinational forces incurred here, new threats trigger new claims for aid that compete with those of other needy nations.

Healthcare Reconstruction and the
Responsibility to Rebuild

Focusing on healthcare reconstruction affords insights into postwar justice
and the feasibility of long-term and sustainable rebuilding. The demands of
postwar justice vary with the cause of war. When wars are defensive, postwar
justice affords occupying forces the right to undertake reconstruction when
necessary to meet narrow security interests. In contrast, wars of aggression
impose stringent obligations on invaders to restore the status quo ante and
make reparations to a violated nation as Iraq was required to do following the
invasion and occupation of Kuwait in 1990. The obligations of humanitarian
forces fall somewhere in-between. The substance of "in-between" depends
upon the material conditions that justify humanitarian military intervention. Usually, these conditions are so dire that restoring the status quo ante
does not get us very far. But neither do intervening forces have any obligation
to refashion host-nations into liberal democracies.

The experience of rebuilding a shattered healthcare infrastructure in Iraq
and Afghanistan shows how modest gains are feasible when pursued as a
basic healthcare package that provides the foundation, and only the foundation, for the health care necessary to build a dignified life. Focusing on
feasible accomplishments requires humanitarian forces to look far ahead
and husband their resources for modest rather than grandiose projects. Such
foresight and restraint often present a difficult challenge. Operating rooms
are far more glamorous, and far more attractive to donors, than chemical
toilets. Nevertheless, throttling back at the beginning is the only reasonable
way to preserve the resources to rebuild as the war winds down and interest
wanes. This is the proper interpretation of the International Commission on
Intervention and State Sovereignty (ICISS 2001: 64) instruction "to provide,
full assistance . . . as long as necessary in order to achieve self-sustained stability." "Full assistance" means broad-based but modest infrastructures consistent with the rudiments of a dignified life. "Self-sustained stability" is the
political goal of rebuilding. It occurs as all the necessary infrastructures—
health, education, banking, security, and so on—gain modest traction.

Given the disparate obligations of defenders, aggressors, and
humanitarians to rebuild, one might reasonably ask: Were Coalition armies
defensive, occupying, or humanitarian forces? I will not try to settle this question but only suggest that the wars in Iraq and Afghanistan were not pure
types. Each began with a declaration of security interests, namely to destroy

weapons of mass destruction (Iraq) or decapitate al Qaeda (Afghanistan). Whether one justifies the wars or not, occupation and regime change quickly followed each country's invasion. What may have begun as a defensive war morphed into a humanitarian war, or to some, a war of aggression and conquest. The responsibility to rebuild evolved accordingly. Had the United States found weapons of mass destruction and removed bin Laden without regime change, its obligation to rebuild goes only as far as its national interests dictate. Alternatively, had the United States stayed on to subjugate these forlorn countries, then its responsibility to rebuild is far-reaching. Doing neither, but remaining to ameliorate people's lives puts multinational forces on course to pursue the middle ground of humanitarian intervention.

Postwar justice starts and ends with the obligation to rebuild. Sometimes, rebuilding embraces national reconciliation. Often reserved for war-torn nations, national reconciliation speaks to criminal trials for agents of the deposed regime and compensation for its victims. In contrast, we often fail to address postwar reconciliation within nations who deploy humanitarian forces. As their troops return home, postwar justice demands significant resources to attend soldiers' physical and psychological injuries. Medical care for veterans is the subject of the final chapter.

12

Veteran Health Care

There were thirty million English who talked of England's might,
There were twenty broken troopers who lacked a bed for the night.
They had neither food nor money, they had neither service nor trade;
They were only shiftless soldiers, the last of the Light Brigade.

They felt that life was fleeting; they knew not that art was long,
That though they were dying of famine, they lived in deathless song.
They asked for a little money to keep the wolf from the door;
And the thirty million English sent twenty pounds and four! . . .

O thirty million English that babble of England's might,
Behold there are twenty heroes who lack their food to-night;
Our children's children are lisping to "honour the charge they made –"
And we leave to the streets and the workhouse the charge of the
     Light Brigade!
                    (Rudyard Kipling, *The Last of the Light Brigade*, 1890)

[In 2011, the US Department of Housing and Urban Development
(HUD 2019) estimated that 65,455 American veterans were homeless on any given night.]

Stirred by the carnage of the Italian war of independence and the abandonment of the wounded on the field, Henry Dunant established the
International Committee of the Red Cross in 1863. Grossly neglected for
most of the 19th century, the severely injured enjoyed but rudimentary
care that did little to return them to duty or leave them capable of leading a
healthy life. Dunant would labor tirelessly to convince military and public
officials of their duty to evacuate and treat the wounded. But as Kipling caus-
tically reminds us 30 years later, medical attention and support for veterans

were not foregone. Today the obligation a state owes its warfighters and veterans seems self-evident. It is not.

Historically poor care for sick or wounded veterans, and the periodic scandals that wrack veteran health care in the United States and elsewhere, rightly directs our attention to the duty the state owes its disabled warfighters. When Dunant (1862: 126–127) wrote that "the soldier who receives a bullet in defense of his country deserves all that country's solicitude," or, a century and a half later, when President Obama (2014) spoke of a *sacred* obligation to "make sure all our veterans get the benefits they've earned," several related questions arise. First, why do military veterans *deserve* special medical attention? Why must one *earn* the right to decent health care as Obama suggests? I will argue that there are no reasonable grounds for desert; soldiers' right to health care is no more, or less, compelling than that of their compatriots. As a result, they do not deserve *all* their country's solicitude because this unfairly disadvantages others. Instead, warfighters deserve their fair share of medical resources based solely on the gravity of their injuries or illness. Should this be less than they deserve, veterans have the same right to demand redress as anyone else. Veterans own no exclusive rights or entitlements upon which to base their claim to health care.

To address the complexity of postwar military medicine, this chapter first describes veteran health care in the United States and United Kingdom. American and British forces suffered the lion's share of casualties in Iraq and Afghanistan, including tens of thousands of physically wounded and many more who require mental health care (Chapter 4). To care for veterans, each nation employs radically different healthcare systems. In the United States, the Department of Veterans Affairs (VA) provides veterans with an exclusive, dedicated healthcare system. In the United Kingdom, veteran care is embedded in the National Health System (NHS), which, nevertheless, carves out a unique niche for veterans.

With national pictures in mind, I ask: Do these schemes satisfy veteran healthcare rights? But first: To what medical care are veterans entitled? Do the rights of veterans differ from those of civilian compatriots? Understanding the entitlements of each group raises questions of allocation. How should healthcare systems allocate resources among citizens? Answering this question leads to the next: When a state goes to war, how much of its military resources should it reserve for postwar medical management?

Veteran Health Care in the United States

Representing the last vestige of military hospitals that have largely disappeared with the advent of national health care, military health care in the United States is unique. While various branches of the armed forces provide ambulatory and hospital care for active service personnel and their families, the Veterans Health Administration, as part of the Department of Veterans Affairs, treats some, but not all veterans. Established in 1930 to deliver medical services in the absence of any institutionalized healthcare system for veterans, the VA operates 170 medical centers, 1,074 outpatient clinics, and serves 9 million veterans (VA 2019a). This number includes close to 800,000 veterans who served in Iraq and Afghanistan (Geiling, Rosen, and Edwards 2012: 1235). The most common injuries are amputations, traumatic brain injury (TBI), post-traumatic stress disorder (PTSD), moral injury, and mental illness. Recognizing the VA's limited resources, recent legislative initiatives, such as the 2018 VA Mission Act, allow the VA to fund outside providers to treat eligible veterans that the VA cannot attend to on a timely basis. The VA's budget request for FY 2019 was $98 billion (up from $25 billion in 2003; Perlin, Kolodner, and Roswell 2004) or $14,000 per veteran per year (compare $11,000 per US Medicare patient in 2014; Fulton and Brooks 2018). Of this, disability costs for veterans of the war in Iraq and Afghanistan reached $35 billion through 2013 (Bilmes 2013). The total expenditures for veteran health care and disability payments over their lifetimes are likely to exceed $700 billion (Bilmes and Stiglitz 2011).

Not every US veteran is eligible for government health care. Instead, eligibility turns on four criteria in roughly the following order of priority: military merit, service-related medical injuries, nonservice catastrophic disabilities, and financial need. Military merit includes Medal of Honor recipients, and over 50,000 service personnel awarded the Purple Heart for battle injuries (CRS 2020). Eligible battle injuries do not include PTSD. PTSD and other mental health injuries may fall into the second priority category, where eligible service-related injuries comprise any injury causing greater than 10% disability. Lower priority categories are not service-related and reflect social rather than military criteria of eligibility. These include catastrophically disabled or impoverished veterans (VA 2019b). A qualifying catastrophic disability is any that "permanently compromises the ability to carry out activities of daily living" and "requires personal or mechanical assistance to leave home or bed." Financial need must also be extreme, but not as extreme as Medicaid (the

US healthcare insurance for the poor and disabled) demands of impoverished nonveterans. In 2019, the maximum allowable income for VA eligibility was $34,171 (single veteran) and $45,707 (three dependents, VA 2020a) compared to $17,236 and $35,535 for many Medicaid recipients (HHS 2019).

Assessments of VA health care vary. In 2014, VA scandals erupted when some administrators manipulated waitlists to improve performance measures (Hayward 2017). Allegations of poor nursing care also rocked the VA in 2018 (Slack and Estes 2018). Scholarly reviews show a mixed picture of VA care that compares favorably with other US government healthcare programs. Surveying 69 studies from 2005 to 2015, O'Hanlon and colleagues (2017) conclude, "the VA often (but not always) performs better than or similar to other systems of care concerning the safety and effectiveness of care" (2017: 105; also Blay et al. 2017; Penn et al. 2019; Price et al. 2018). Nevertheless, the mounting costs of caring for an aging population of veterans, and efforts to improve access and delivery, have prompted proposals to phase out the VA entirely in favor of private insurance or Medicare/Medicaid (Hynes et al. 2007).

Veteran Health Care in the United Kingdom

The last military hospital in the United Kingdom closed in 2007, allowing the country to consolidate the medical management of soldiers and veterans under NHS auspices. To serve critically injured service personnel, the Royal Centre for Defence Medicine (RCDM) operated a dedicated military medical unit in the University Hospitals Birmingham NHS Foundation Trust from 2001. Veteran care, however, largely remains the purview of the NHS and mirrors health care for nonveterans with two exceptions: priority treatment and bespoke care.

Priority Treatment

The Armed Forces Covenant of the United Kingdom declares:

> The Veterans receive their healthcare from the NHS, and should receive priority treatment where it relates to a condition which results from their service in the Armed Forces, subject to clinical need. Those injured in Service, whether physically or mentally, should be cared for in a way which reflects

the Nation's moral obligation to them whilst respecting the individual's wishes. (UK MoD 2011: 10)

The NHS (2020) adds a caveat:

> [P]riority access to NHS care . . . is always subject to clinical need and does not entitle you to jump the queue ahead of someone with a higher clinical need.

Veterans may, however, jump the queue ahead of someone with *comparable* clinical needs. As such, military service functions as a tiebreaker, which raises the compelling question: Why is military service a justifiable criterion for the distribution of health care, all things being equal? One can certainly think of other reasons for preferential treatment. If military service confers special rights, what about others who perform public services, such as police officers, firefighters, or teachers? Alternatively, perhaps, one may attend to indispensable figures first, such as the head of a household with many dependents. The possibilities are endless and perplexing.

Moral qualms about offering veterans priority medical attention have not gone unnoticed. Commenting on a question to square the principle of priority care with the principle of equal access, UK Minister Jackie Doyle-Price responded:

> There is a tension there, because the military covenant clearly says that we should prioritise delivering services for veterans, which is absolutely true. But it is also a fundamental principle of the NHS that no one is given favour over anyone else. We have chosen to deal with our obligation to veterans through specialist commissioning, so we are giving access to bespoke services for veterans. (House of Commons Defence Committee 2018: 19–20)

No one has repudiated the principle of equal access, but affording special services solely for veterans is the emerging policy in practice.

Bespoke Healthcare Services

"Bespoke" can refer to either tailored or additional care for veterans. For example, the Veterans Trauma Network establishes a personalized treatment program that matches patients with NHS experts. It does not bestow priority access or any additional care that similarly injured civilians would not receive but functions to streamline treatment. Several programs, however, offer veterans *additional* care. One is prosthetics. In 2013, the government announced an £11 million program for "injured war heroes to receive *improved* care from the NHS." The program earmarked £6.7 million for designated centers to "access the latest technology and provide the highest quality of prosthetic care for veteran amputees" while noting "other services will benefit too—with a £1 million fund to ensure that all prosthetics services across England improve" (UK MoD 2013). Here, funding designates two classes of amputees: service members and civilians, and provides significantly different sums for each.

Bespoke care offers grounds for pause. On the one hand, some benefits are relatively meager. An extra £11 million may benefit veterans more than civilians, but it is a paltry sum in an NHS budget of over £125 billion. On the other hand, bespoke care speaks to a unique obligation to attend to veterans. Tailored bespoke care utilizes existing resources more efficiently for the benefit of veterans than other protocols do. In contrast, additional bespoke care attempts to meet this obligation by recognizing unique healthcare entitlements.

The preceding discussion of veteran health care in the United States and United Kingdom highlights disparate ethical issues. The dedicated US system is unique; the UK system is not. Many other nations, Canada and Australia, for example, attend to veterans through their national health care networks. There, veterans enjoy additional healthcare benefits that allow some Canadian veterans prior access to beds in long-term health care facilities or offer Australian veterans prescription drugs unavailable to others (Office of the Veterans Ombudsman 2013; ADVA 2019). The US and UK cases raise different but related ethical questions. For the United States, the initial question is very broad: Does the state owe continued health care to its veterans in a political environment wherein the universal right to health care is tenuous? Their emerging answer was, "Yes," and policymakers translated this obligation into a comprehensive healthcare system whose eligibility criteria gave disabled veterans greater access to health care than many others had. Within the VA, the same commitment gave weight to military merit when establishing eligibility criteria.

In contrast, post-World War II national healthcare systems afforded primary health care to everyone and thereby allowed the United Kingdom and other nations to sidestep the broader question plaguing the United States. Nevertheless, the United Kingdom recognized a singular obligation to veterans and embraced the principle of priority access and bespoke services. Although the reach of US and UK policy is different, both raise the same question: What special healthcare obligations does the state owe veterans? In contrast to the prevailing sentiment, the correct answer is, "None."

The Obligation to Care for Veterans

- "This country has a moral obligation to provide our servicemen and women with the best possible care and treatment," President George W. Bush (2007).
- "Taking care of our veterans and their families is a sacred obligation. And now that we've ended the war in Iraq, and as our war in Afghanistan ends as well, we have to work even harder as a nation to make sure all our veterans get the benefits and opportunities they've earned. They've done their duty, and they ask nothing more than that this country does ours— now and for decades to come," President Barack Obama (2014).
- "The (UK) Armed Forces Covenant is the expression of the moral obligation the Government and the Nation owe to those who serve or have served in our Armed Forces and to their families . . . They deserve not only our respect and gratitude, but also our constant attention to how they are treated and the impact that Service life has on them and on their families" (UK MoD 2011).

Many share these sentiments that echo obligation, duty, and desert. Evoking Dunant, modern political leaders recognize a special responsibility toward those who risk their lives in their country's defense. In the United States, this recognition built an entire healthcare system for a relatively small segment of the population. In the United Kingdom and elsewhere, it generated special privileges. What is the nature of this right, and does it offer justifiable privileges?

Several factors may affect healthcare entitlements. Social criteria weigh utility and determine healthcare privileges based on an individual's present or future contribution to the war effort (military necessity) or society more generally (social utility). Behavioral criteria weigh actions and intentions. Meritorious or virtuous behavior affords grounds for enhancing healthcare rights when some individuals, such as veterans, act heroically or risk their lives to aid others. Negligent conduct, on the other hand, offers reasons for restricting healthcare rights when individuals behave irresponsibly and recklessly risk their health. These are not new questions, but dogged modern bioethics from its inception. They have yet, however, to engage military medical ethics. The following sections explore this context more closely.

Allocating Scarce Medical Resources: The Early Debates

Until the invention of dialysis, kidney failure was a quick and fatal disease. With dialysis, a process to mechanically clean the blood of toxins, patients gain the time to recuperate from kidney disease or obtain a transplant. Hemodialysis is not cheap and costs $90,000 per patient annually in the United States (UCSF 2019). First commercially available in the 1960s, there were few dialysis machines. This shortage confronted providers with an acute allocation dilemma: Who should get lifesaving access to dialysis machines? Should it be those who had curable renal disease or those who required dialysis their entire lives? Should it be the young or the old?

To select among the many candidates for treatment, the first dialysis center in Seattle, Washington, established medical and social criteria. To ensure successful treatment, medical criteria required patients no older than 45 years, without a history of hypertension or vascular disease, and sufficiently mature to comply with strict dietary guidelines (Blagg 2007). To select among those who fulfill the medical criteria, social measures weighed such factors as marital status, educational background, occupation, and past and potential contributions to society (Jonsen 1998: 212). Social criteria mask two contrasting principles. *Future* contributions to the community or one's family speak to the benefits that will come following successful treatment. *Past* contributions speak to merit, to virtuous (or villainous) behavior for which one deserves something more (or less) than others. Social criteria sparked enormous controversy, and although unaddressed in military medical ethics, they mirror preferential treatment for veterans.

Social Utility and a Dignified Life

In the early years of the dialysis debate, a minority view held that access to scarce, publicly financed healthcare resources should weigh social utility.

When public funds finance a good such as medical care or research, then the public (represented by a lay committee) has the right, indeed, the duty to see that it gets the best return on its investment. What might this return be? Outputs are the most straightforward: save those who, once cured, offer society significant material, intellectual, or creative goods (Rescher 1969). One person may care for aged parents, while another enriches cultural events with fine art or music. Neither contribution is easy to measure or compare, and all are value-laden. Comparing the social worth of families with dependents to those without hinges on social judgments about the value of various lifestyles as well as the ability to weigh the significance of each person's contribution accurately, whether material, artistic, or scientific.

Looking at the value of a particular contribution or life plan, however, is the wrong way to look at social utility because it deprives individuals of their equal worth as human beings. To grant overriding weight to some rational life plans over others, and reward their agents accordingly, is to disadvantage equally potent life plans that might fulfill another person's ambitions and aspirations. Social utility, therefore, is not a measure of the value of one person's particular plan or contribution, be she a married professional with children or a single, childless bohemian (or some combination thereof). Instead, social utility maximizes life plans that develop each person's capabilities as a human being, while disregarding an individual's substantive contribution to society. In this way, social utility endorses an equal chance for each person to flourish. Social utility is sensitive to need, not contribution. Among these needs, good health is paramount.

The idea of measuring social utility as future contributions, therefore, is deficient. It cannot justify prior access to any scarce medical resource, whether for those suffering from kidney failure or the ravages of combat. But perhaps, understanding utility in terms of military necessity might offer a better way to substantiate unique healthcare entitlements for veterans. By this reasoning, veteran health care is a necessary component of military success. There is some appeal to this approach. After all, military necessity is an important criterion for providing military medical health care.

Social Utility and Military Necessity

Military necessity allocates medicine to conserve force capabilities and return the highest number of wounded to duty (Chapter 1). Noting its mission to care for warfighters, soldiers for life, and their families, the revised Army Medicine Vision (US Army 2016: 10) concludes: "We are focused on being a well-integrated part of one team with one purpose—*conserving the fighting strength.*" Conserving this fighting strength, not saving lives per se, is the principal function of battlefield medicine. Force conservation is a criterion of medical care unique to military medicine. It reflects an objective measure of a soldier's ability to do his or her job. To keep soldiers fit to fight, military medicine devotes enormous resources to maintain or restore their health so they may continue to serve vital national interests. This argument sounds very much like the view of social utility just debunked; it justifies privileged health care for soldiers because their present and future contributions serve the national interest. In this way, it echoes justifications for priority medical care for first responders during a natural disaster or national emergency. Here, the idea is to attend first to those who treat or protect others. In this case, then, why not first offer dialysis to a researcher on the cusp of an important scientific discovery that will benefit humankind?

Answering this question suggests the need to balance the right to determine a rational life plan with two primary goods necessary to achieve any life plan, namely, security and health care. During national emergencies, medical care might be required to ensure the health of those charged with maintaining security. Temporary, priority care for first responders during a disaster or for warfighters during a war helps ensure the background conditions—security, law, and order—necessary for any life plan to succeed. War, earthquakes, epidemics, or floods are transient conditions that temporarily restructure allocation schemes. Once the threat subsides, preferential allocation schemes lose force. Priority treatment for a scientist may also qualify if one can successfully identify an impending, significant breakthrough without which the background conditions necessary for self-determination fail. The idea is to prevent deficits rather than encourage specific gains. Human society requires refuge from war and pestilence, lest it descend into chaos. Society does not need a cure for cancer to survive. To reward scientists in the absence of dire threats affords special entitlements to an entire class at the expense of others pursuing alternative rational life plans. Such a policy very quickly impoverishes the public good.

Veterans, however, are no longer first responders so that social utility and military necessity no longer justify any unique medical entitlement. It may be, however, that this interpretation construes military necessity too tightly. Perhaps health care for veterans is a necessary condition of morale, without which soldiers will be reluctant to fight. In this view, future care for veterans affects the way soldiers fight today. This is undoubtedly true in cases where warfighters went to war with no prospect of decent medical attention whatsoever. It is no surprise, therefore, that the abandonment of the wounded and substandard medical treatment substantially debilitated morale and sapped fighting strength throughout history (Gross 2006). This is not true, however, of state armies today. Where nations have a national healthcare system, veterans have no worries, and it is unlikely that the modest bespoke benefits the United Kingdom offers its veterans significantly affect morale on the battlefield.

The situation in the United States is more complicated than Britain's. American warfighters enjoy superlative medicine. The US Army (2016: 13) further acknowledges that care for a warfighter's family "allows the Warfighter to remain focused on the task at hand," a concern unintelligible in any nation with national health care. While present-day care might keep warfighters focused, what of future care? Does the prospect of future care, or lack thereof, also affect the morale of American soldiers? It is difficult to say. Although the updated US Army Medicine mission statement emphasizes care of the soldier *for life*, this is not the case. Apart from the war-wounded, disabled, and indigent, the American warfighter has no assurance that he will receive future medical attention. Mental health care, for example, is only available for most veterans if they served in a combat zone (Hester 2017; Burnam et al. 2009; VA 2019c). Access for others is difficult, just as it is for those living far from VA facilities.

American service members going to war know they will receive unmatched care at the point of injury and soon afterward. This is probably sufficient to allay any fears of abandonment and substandard treatment. They also know that veteran care for service-related injuries might be unavailable, inconsistent, or inferior to other options such as Medicaid or private insurance. In 2014, some 42% of the 21.6 million American veterans were enrolled in the VA, and of these, less than two thirds used VA facilities (Eibner 2016). Although impossible to discount the impact of future VA medical care on present-day morale, other factors including organizational efficiency, up-to-date weaponry, sound leadership, and a sense of comradery, are equally, if not more, determinative of military morale in the field (Chapter 5). At best, concern for morale only justifies adequate medical attention for veterans at a level every citizen should receive (or does receive in a national healthcare system). It cannot warrant preferential medical benefits. Unable, then, to anchor privileged treatment in social utility or military necessity, one might consider that military service and the readiness to risk one's life are sufficiently meritorious to warrant special medical entitlements.

Virtue or Vice as a Criterion for Medical Care

If virtue justifies preferential healthcare rights, then vice should disadvantage the same rights. Consider whether some patients might deserve *less* care because of their behavior. Should alcoholics or smokers be pushed down (or off) transplant lists? Should bikers who don't wear helmets or motorists who don't wear seat belts get the last bed in the intensive care unit (ICU), or should it be reserved for a faultless injury? These questions turn on the connection between a person's deliberate actions and his right to health care. If such virtuous behavior as risking one's life for one's nation merits special healthcare rights, then it follows that irresponsible patients forfeit these same rights. Do they?

The idea of health-care-forfeiting behavior suggests a firm distinction between those whose injury is no fault of their own and those whose injury follows from irresponsible decisions. Moral blamelessness is intuitively appealing so that a pedestrian injured by a drunk driver seems to merit prior attention and, perhaps, greater resources than the similarly injured but intoxicated driver responsible for the accident. Despite this appeal to simple justice, any such distinction is empirically and morally problematic. Empirically, it is difficult or impractical to determine the extent of an individual's responsibility for his or her medical condition (especially on a busy night in the ICU) because it may be the (partial) result of genetics, addiction, or disease. Indeterminate responsibility applies to alcoholism, smoking, overeating, and extraordinary risk-taking. In each case, write Beauchamp and Childress (1994: 359), "a denial of a person's right to healthcare would be unfair if the person could not have acted otherwise, or could have acted otherwise only with great difficulty." Theirs is a sweeping claim. It may be true of diseases that result from bad luck, but less accurate concerning such common illnesses as heart disease or diabetes, or of accidents for which one is morally blameworthy. Here, individuals bear all or some responsibility for their actions and injuries. A person may be addicted to alcohol, drugs, overeating, or nicotine, but that does not necessarily excuse their refusal to seek medical attention. Partial responsibility, then, may justify some treatment distinction.

Beauchamp and Childress hint as much when they write that denial of health care is "unfair" if a patient could not have acted otherwise. This leaves open the fair option of denying (or augmenting) health care to those who could have acted otherwise.

Further moral complications arise if we consider the difference between actions and intent. The preceding discussion emphasizes a person's actions and their outcomes. But good intentions may yield bad outcomes, just as bad intentions may yield good ones. The result is accidental heroes and villains. An accidental hero may be an officer who disobeys orders or misreads his maps but successfully outmaneuvers his enemy and saves his platoon. Accidental villains abound in war. The same platoon may take extraordinary risks and suffer massive casualties to destroy an enemy position only to discover that what they thought was a command headquarters was, in fact, a residential building. Nevertheless, and despite the practical and moral difficulties of assigning praise and blame to the sick and injured, their appeal as arbiters of scarce resource allocation remains. This appeal resonates when the sick and injured are veteran warfighters.

Virtue or Vice as a Criterion for Military Medical Care

Among veterans, too, we may ask whether some deserve greater or lesser healthcare rights. Consider first whether veterans, like smokers or reckless bikers, deserve less care than those who behave responsibly. It has been estimated, for example, that a third of the head injuries in Vietnam occurred when soldiers failed to wear helmets because they were too hot and uncomfortable (Neel 1991: 55). Similarly, in Iraq, some soldiers refused to wear goggles because they were "too ugly," and eye injuries only decreased when the "military bowed to fashion and switched to cooler-looking Wiley brand ballistic eyewear" (Gawande 2004: 2474). Are severe and incapacitating head and eye wounds resulting from what appear to be grossly irresponsible decisions somehow less worthy of attention? Conversely, should virtuous behavior, broadly defined as risking one's life for one's country, render one more deserving of medical attention?

Enhanced rights for virtuous behavior seem more compelling than restricted rights for negligent conduct. The UK Armed Forces Covenant is a statement of veterans' moral rights and the concomitant obligations of the state and government. The starting point is service members' voluntary decision to surrender their civilian freedoms and to face life-threatening dangers to defend the realm (UK MoD 2011: i). In return, service personnel "deserve [the nation's] respect, support, and fair treatment." The Covenant speaks to an implicit contract that seems fair and reasonable. "Fair," of course, is the operative word. A fair wage is one that meets minimal economic requirements for a dignified life, but whose upper limit is subject to market forces that might drive up wages to attract service personnel, particularly those with highly technical skills. Fair health care, on the other hand, is not subject to these vagaries. Neither are priority care and bespoke services that the Covenant supports.

To illustrate the complexity of using merit-based claims to allocate scarce medical resources, consider persons who lost a limb to an improvised explosive device (IED) attack, malfunctioning factory equipment, or obesity-related diabetes. In each case, the patient requires immediate reconstructive care, long-term treatment for comorbidities (weight gain, diabetes, and coronary heart disease), and sophisticated prosthetic devices. If, for example, there are 10 units of treatment ordinarily available to tend these injuries, how ought we to distribute them justly? There is little doubt that a soldier who has suffered significant physical injuries while protecting his fellow citizens has a claim that the government can only meet by allocating more medical resources than are usually available in peacetime. Following a long war, it is likely that available medical resources cannot meet everyone's medical needs. To deliver the health care necessary for a decent life, policymakers may impose a tax to pay the costs of war. Policymakers may similarly impose a tax on tobacco or sugared drinks, for example, to pay for risky lifestyles that create special medical needs. In neither case do taxes change the distribution principle that governs the allocation of health care; they only increase available medical resources. The pie is larger, but a bigger pie does not make a case for preferential treatment. Instead, additional taxes should permit a government-funded healthcare service to maintain the same high standard for everyone despite the crippling costs of war or risky patient behavior. Therefore, if an amputation requires five units of treatment, then ten available units are insufficient to attend to all three patients. Whether from increased taxes or cutbacks elsewhere, only additional funding can supply the resources to offer the three patients the same standard of care.

Fortified by additional resources, providers now have 15 units of treatment to tend the three patients just described. How should they be allocated? One option is to deliver exceptional care to the soldier (10 units) on the assumption that his contribution merits privileged treatment while the others receive inferior care (2.5 units each). But this seems unfair: The factory worker did nothing to merit less attention than he would typically receive (5 units). And the diabetic, let's assume, paid a tax on sugared beverages his whole life. Alternatively, one may distribute the resource equally and allow each patient five units of treatment. Here, no one suffers harm, but the soldier does not receive special consideration for his sacrifice. Considering the two distribution scenarios, the principle of not harming trumps one of not rewarding. That is, it is better, morally, that the faultless should not be harmed rather than the meritorious not rewarded. Equal distribution is, therefore, preferable to unequal distribution in this case. It should not go unnoticed that the first distribution scheme (10 units for the severely wounded, 2.5 units for others) occurs when a nation builds a dedicated healthcare system to tend wounded veterans and ignores vast segments of the nonmilitary population. In contrast, the second distribution scheme (equal distribution based on need) represents a national healthcare system.

Fair Access to Medical Care

For the reasons just described, *access* to health care also should be blind to merit, responsibility, and past contributions. The US Veterans Administration employs tests for eligibility to access the VA system that evaluate merit, military service, disability, and income. Assuming that a dedicated healthcare system is only justified in the absence of a national healthcare system, one may ask: Are these criteria morally defensible? Specifically, are there any grounds for using criteria other than medical urgency to determine access to care? Merit is entirely contingent on random events, while courage under fire is the product of a particular personality. Forced to choose between a relatively healthy Medal of Honor recipient (Priority category 1) and a 40% disabled veteran (Priority category 2), there is no compelling medical reason for the VA to offer the medal recipient priority care. Morally, the disparate priority categories force a choice between denying one an honor and harming the other. Each is denied a right. Nevertheless, the right not to suffer severe preventable harm (and the concomitant duty to cure severe preventable harm) overwhelms the loss of military honors, which is a right of limited substance and subject to transient social norms. The outcome of honoring or rejecting each right is equally determinative. Denied access to the VA, the healthy medal recipient suffers no medical harm and retains the honorific and attendant approbation. The disabled veteran, on the other hand, experiences pain and suffering if denied access.

Nonservice-related catastrophic disabilities and impoverishment raise similar questions. A veteran suffering a 10% service-connected disability (Priority category 3) enjoys access ahead of those suffering nonservice-related disabilities or penury. Impoverishment and catastrophic disabilities are related. Absent a national healthcare system, individuals must turn to private insurance schemes. Impoverished individuals, and those with exceptional medical needs who cannot afford or obtain sufficient insurance, turn to the state. Government-supported insurance fulfills the state's obligation to ensure the right of primary health care for all. Such coverage is the purpose of Medicaid in the United States. There is no reason that the VA cannot take on the same obligation for the catastrophically ill or impoverished, assuming it is sufficiently funded and utilizes eligibility criteria *identical* to other insurance schemes such as Medicaid. Military service affords no grounds for preferred access. Instead, the pertinent criteria—medical and financial need—should be uniform for all citizens irrespective of the source of one's disability. Ideally, a well-conceived national healthcare system would have no reason to utilize any merit-based criteria to access care. However, this is not entirely true of Britain.

In the United Kingdom, access to health care is always subject to clinical need. Veterans, therefore, cannot move ahead of patients whose medical needs are greater. The idea seems innocuous: Veterans get priority access to medical care, *all other things being equal,* that is, when there are no others with more pressing medical needs. Conceptually, though, this is an impossible condition: There are always those with more significant medical needs somewhere. As such, the NHS must mean there is no patient with greater need when and where the veteran seeks medical attention. This qualification does not improve matters much. Consider first non-urgent care. The maximum wait time for non-urgent surgery in the United Kingdom is 18 weeks (NHS 2019). Assuming that many cases are equally non-urgent, a veteran with the same non-urgent condition as another patient has the right to jump the queue. Non-urgent, however, does not mean non-harmful. Non-urgent illnesses or injuries may bring anxiety, inconvenience, or moderate discomfort. These are nontrivial harms that priority access allows a veteran to avoid.

Harm becomes significant when cases are urgent. Consider two equally critical transplant patients, a veteran waiting a week and a nonveteran waiting six months. Alternatively, consider two accident victims vying for a single ICU bed. Phrased in this way, priority access is no different from preferential attention. In non-urgent cases, disease-free time is the resource, and the veteran collects a greater-than-equal portion. In the urgent case, life or quality of life is the resource, and, here too, the veteran enjoys a larger share, while others, through no fault of their own, receive less. If merit cannot morally justify preferential treatment, then it cannot justify priority access. Instead, when all things are equal, one turns to "first come, first served" or a lottery when medical need among patients is identical. In this context, it is essential to see that military service cannot function as a tiebreaker in the same way associative duties do when choosing to attend to compatriots before host-nation soldiers on the battlefield (Chapter 5). The two are not analogous. Associative duties are special obligations of care that supplement and, sometimes, supplant other obligations. Merit for public service, on the other hand, occasions public recognition, not the duty of care.

Health Care as a Primary Good and Fundamental Human Right

Utilitarian and merit-based justice arguments fail to justify special care for veterans because they ignore the special status of health care as a primary good due to all persons equally. Human rights and primary goods are necessary conditions for, and not contingent upon, virtuous behavior. The right to health care, therefore, cannot draw from such fortuitous events as financial success or social contributions or turn on future potential that often requires luck, education, social status, and *good health*. Likewise, military service cannot add to or detract from an individual's right to health care. Conditioning scarce medical care on factors that require good health damns many to ill-health and creates an impregnable fortress of health care for those already advantaged.

In summary, there are good reasons to reject anything but urgency and clinical-medical necessity as the sole criterion of veteran care. Military necessity regulates the provision of health care on the battlefield but has nothing to say about treating those who no longer contribute to the war effort. Associative duties cannot affect healthcare decisions among members of the same moral community. Resource allocation based on past or future contributions ignores how primary resources such as health care are prior and necessary components of anyone's ability to contribute to society. No life plan is feasible without good health, education, moderate resources, and political liberties. The allocation of the primary goods necessary for a decent life cannot depend on how that life performed without restricting a dignified life to those fortunate to have the right parents, community, and nation, or, in the case of veterans, the right war. None of this means, however, that one may not compensate veterans for the risks they incur by offering them financial remuneration.

Taxes and Compensation: Money for Meritorious Behavior

Military service and heroism are virtuous behaviors that undoubtedly merit recognition. Dunant is correct; those willing to risk their lives for their country's defense *deserve* its solicitude and its gratitude. Desert, however, is not the same as military necessity or utility. Tasked with deciding between treating an injured first responder (police, fire, or medical personnel) or an injured civilian during a terror attack, one may legitimately attend to the former first, assuming that he or she can return to the field and save more people. Desert is not a factor here. The first responder does not deserve attention because he behaves heroically but receives priority care to enable the conditions necessary for everyone else to lead a dignified life. If social utility is forward-looking, desert looks to past actions. Desert creates a select category of entitlements based entirely on one's efforts where success depends crucially on good mental and physical health. Like merit, desert cannot be a condition for good health. Desert can, however, be grounds for rewards, compensation, or honors.

How do we recognize virtuous and other forms of exceptional behavior? One way, of course, is with public honors and rewards. Medals are common for military service; cash awards are not. Nevertheless, educational benefits for American veterans, for example, can be substantial (VA 2020b). Such payments are a form of compensation for taking on a dangerous and risky job, and familiar to many professions. Police officers, firefighters, and warfighters *require* higher compensation to draw them to the profession and *deserve* higher compensation for their willingness to risk their lives for the common good. If the public wants these services, this is the price it must pay. The UK Covenant is explicit in this regard: In return for defending the realm and risking their lives, service personnel *deserve* support and fair treatment. Desert translates to educational, tax, consumer, housing, and other financial benefits.

Compensation also may reflect payments for loss. Insurance companies pay for the loss of a stolen car. Alternatively, a manufacturer may compensate consumers for injuries caused by product failure. In these cases, a contractual obligation with the insurance company or the manufacturer's liability gives the insured or consumer the right to receive payment. Public servants often have contractual arrangements with the government to disburse lump sum or periodic payments as compensation in the event of death or injury. In these circumstances, compensation is a welfare right to guarantee the financial means necessary to maintain a decent life. Funding for the former comes from government-mandated employer contributions, while the latter draws on the same tax revenues that support the military. Compensation benefits vary. The United Kingdom, Canada, and Australia allot various combinations of disability pensions and lump-sum compensation, while the United States grants monthly disability payments for service-related injuries or illness (VAC 2019; ADVA 2020; UK MoD 2020b; VA 2020c). Unlike preferential medical attention or priority access, veterans' compensation benefits do not adversely affect others' rights. At the same time, however, compensation is no substitute for dignified care.

Dignified Health Care for Veterans

To the question: What do veterans deserve? The answer is: the same as everyone else. Public officials, therefore, must allocate sufficient resources during and afterwars to attend to veterans at the same level as all other citizens. The question: "What does everyone else deserve?" is not one for military medical ethics but one for distributive justice. The answer is: sufficient resources, medical and otherwise, to lead a dignified life, and all this entails. The narrower question is how to pay for this level of health care when wartime injuries require costly acute and long-term care. It is hard to see how the United States, for example, will meet these needs without securing additional revenues for veteran care through higher taxation or reallocation of resources. Reallocation only goes so far before it impinges on what everyone else requires for a decent life. Governments, therefore, must explain to their public how they plan to pay for the direct cost of war, mostly personnel and materiel, and the long-term "hidden" costs of expensive medical management for the high numbers of wounded that modern war generates.

Once a government delivers universal health care at the level required for a dignified life, concern about priority access or bespoke services should dissipate. In contrast to compensation, no state has a solid moral basis to establish exclusive healthcare entitlements for military veterans. There is no military necessity or medical need for special privileges, while merit or social contribution is an indefensible criterion to distribute medical assets. As the dialysis case demonstrates, medical care should remain unaffected by a person's virtues or vices.

Coming home, severely wounded veterans should find a level of health care that meets their basic medical needs as well as it meets the needs of their compatriots. Sick and injured defense contractors, whom Riley and Gambone (2020) call "the new veterans," can make the same claim. Given that wounded soldiers have not often received medical care on par with compatriots, this alone is a significant step forward. Echoing Kipling, the NHS updated its Covenant in 2015 to ensure that "those in the armed forces, reservists, their families, and veterans are *not disadvantaged* in accessing health services in the area they reside" (DHSC 2015). "Disadvantaged" is often the reality of veteran health care, a condition the British sought to alleviate by apportioning additional resources and recruiting charitable organizations to provide added services to veterans (Herman and Yarwood 2015; Mumford 2012).

The claim for preferential treatment or exclusive entitlements for veterans only gains significant ground in those nations, such as the United States, where historically there is no minimally mandated level of health care for all citizens. In such a hostile environment, it is indeed unfair if critically wounded soldiers returning from war must fend for themselves or endure substandard care. Against the backdrop of no medical care whatsoever, it made sense to ask about the kind of health care that disabled veterans deserve (because, like anyone else, they certainly deserve something). As the years went by, the same question addressed various ad hoc segments of the American population—the elderly (Medicare), the poor (Medicaid), children, and so on—but only recently the populace at large.

Focusing on the rights of discrete groups, rather than on the universal right to health care distorts the debate in the United States and gives way to the peculiar language of special entitlement. But it is a vestige of an earlier time, and with the advent of universal-like health care in the United States, any grounds for preferred veteran care should disappear. There are already calls to disband the VA due to high cost and inefficiency, and to integrate veteran health care into Medicare (Fulton and Brooks 2018). But apart from the economic arguments, there are also sound moral grounds to subsume health care for veterans under the healthcare programs the state provides for all.

On the battlefield, military medicine remains committed to force conservation where the rules of triage and limited patient rights hold sway. During war, military medicine is subordinate to the dictates of military necessity, and this demands the allocation of resources necessary to wage war effectively and protect national interests. Despite inefficiencies, few complain if the emergency redistribution of resources during war reduces care available to civilians when medicines, machines, and personnel rush to the front. Off the battlefield, however, a different paradigm takes hold: military and civilian health care merge, guided by the criterion of medical urgency. A merger is not only true in practice—as the steady closure of military hospitals attests—but an ethical imperative as well. Once seriously wounded and unable to return to war, veterans join the rank of citizens and compete equally for medical resources.

Given the debt that we often believe a nation owes its defenders, many will find this view disconcerting. Wounded veterans, it seems, should enjoy privileged health care. If beds, medicines, and medical personnel are scarce, then those seriously wounded in war should receive the very best care possible. As nations think about distributing health care to all their citizens, the moral justifications for privileged care are difficult to articulate. These concerns gain traction when scandals erupt, and veterans are abused. By 2019, some 37,085 veterans remained homeless (HUD 2019), an improvement since 2011 but a travesty for any country, whether the dispossessed are veterans or not. The answer, then, is to restore veteran health care to the national baseline and maintain the national baseline so all can enjoy a dignified life.

Conclusion

Military Medical Ethics and Just War:
The 21st Century and Beyond

Conclusions can be as dangerous as introductions, lulling readers into a false sense of competence after they have read both. To avoid this pitfall, this concluding chapter only offers a parsimonious synopsis to remind readers how the key points tie together, as well as some thoughts on military medical ethics in future war.

A Parsimonious Synopsis

After kindly reading most of this book all the way through, George Lucas offers a crisp takeaway: *proper, ethically informed, and legal medical practice during wartime cannot be separated from the transformative background of just war theory.* "Cannot be separated" is to understand that military medicine is a practice of war, not of medicine alone. Military medicine saves lives and heals bodies to maintain a fighting force whose members must kill, injure, or cajole others in the violent continuation of politics. There are no two ways about it. To gain moral purchase, military medicine must serve just war. As it does, medical ethics adapts to war.

But here, military medical ethics has stumbled. It did not falter because of Abu Ghraib. Abu Ghraib was a reprehensible act of brutality, the proper purview of criminal justice. Military medical ethics faltered because it never reconciled, or thought to reconcile, state sovereignty, human rights, and the fundamental entitlement to health care during war. As a result, practice diverges from theory across the board. Failing to fully grasp theory, military medicine did not always do what it should. Failing to fully understand its practice, military medicine sometimes did what it should but couldn't explain why. When practice wanders from the theory, we must adjust one or the other, or both.

Opening the discussion in Part I, we take our cue from military ethics, the theory of just war, and the law of armed conflict. The Geneva Conventions codify international humanitarian law. The Conventions are just that, agreements among states to adopt principles that protect their material and moral interests. This is not a realist view of the international order, but one which understands how compliance with ethical norms are as crucial to reason of state as power, status, and security. Each impacts the practice of war. The principles of noncombatant immunity and proportionality are one result. One saves lives, the other sets rules for taking them. A cogent theory and practice of military medical ethics must navigate similar straits.

The Geneva Conventions do not assist us much. They say nothing about veteran health care or postwar reconstruction. Their view of civilian care is haphazard; only vague references address some minimal level of health care that all deserve. Fleeting references acknowledge associative duties but do not attempt to integrate them into a broader theory. Military medicine struggles with its weaponization with little help. Nor does civilian medical ethics offer much guidance. In fact, it cannot. Committed to impartiality and narrow beneficence, civilian medical ethics is unsuited to war. Wrapped by military ethics, however, military medical ethics takes a different tack. As it does, medical impartiality and neutrality fall to the rear, while the necessities of war and collective well-being step to the fore. This inversion underscores the transformative effects of just war theory.

The two aims of just war bind the permissible practices that populate this book: self-defense and humanitarian intervention. Throughout this book, I draw data from nearly two decades of warfare in Iraq and Afghanistan. Prosecuted by multinational forces, these conflicts toggle between defensive and humanitarian war accompanied by no small doses of aggression, occupation, and futility. There are no pure types, but these conflicts illustrate pockmarked exemplars of just war or, to hedge even further, of wars that skirt the pit of manifest injustice without tumbling in.

To wage a just war, however flawed, one can think of a set of distilling principles. Utility and military necessity are the first. They only offer a coarse test: the reasonable expectation that a tactic, operation, or practice will improve an army's capability to prevail in just war. In terms of straight-up medical care, bald utilitarian calculations direct military medicine to return the wounded to duty. With this singular goal in mind, military medicine freezes out anyone whose contribution to the war effort is marginal, including critically wounded soldiers and most injured or sick civilians.

Nevertheless, it would be misleading and, indeed, cavalier to think that military necessity and utility do all the work of military medical ethics. Additional principles intercede to refine theory and practice further. One is associative duties, those special obligations that reach beyond utility to obligate friends, family, and comrades-in-arms to care for one another. Military necessity and associative duties, however, focus on specific groups of beneficiaries. Therefore, they miss the big picture. Still needed is the more expansive norm that coalesces around the human right to a dignified life. Among its necessary conditions is the universal right to adequate health care, that neither military necessity nor associative duties can supersede.

The tension among these principles is palpable. Military necessity serves a collective good and the health of the political commonwealth. Human rights, on the other hand, are acutely individualistic. Associative duties span both boundaries. Military necessity sacrifices vast numbers of lives, while human rights protect them. There is no easy way for military ethics or military medical ethics to ever get this exactly right. But taken together, we can understand how utility, associative duties, and human rights propel the many practices of military medicine.

Part II of this book describes how these principles align to drive the duty to tend compatriot and allied warfighters, detainees, and civilians. Everyone clamors for life-saving care. The medical rules of eligibility get some of it right. Priority care goes to those who can return to duty and to any wounded compatriot. But instead of carving out a special place for detainees and collateral casualties, the rules of eligibility would better serve justice by treating all local nationals without distinction. The cost of universal, primary health care would be considerable. Much may have to wait until the fighting dies down and reconstruction begins. Nevertheless, modest health care for the local population counts among the prevailing duties of intervening forces.

Part III drills deeper into medicine's warfighting role as it pursues medical diplomacy, experimental research, and warfighter enhancement. Beyond battlefield care, medical research and medical diplomacy are adjuncts to war. Stymied by close attention to patient rights, in-theater research suffered during the war years. "Stymied" is a strong word. How can one ever pay too much attention to patient rights? To be clear: medical research is experimentation. Experimentation requires safeguards, and military personnel are as vulnerable as any other patient. That said, we have seen how life-saving clinical studies could not always meet strict standards of consent. So we modify those standards to facilitate wartime research. Still, the transformation is modest insofar as emerging protocols attend the aims of just war and still protect service members' rights.

Medical enhancement and diplomacy take us far from routine medical practice. Enhancement raises all kinds of fascinating challenges for medical ethics. But I don't get that far because most enhancement technologies fail the first test of military ethics: utility. Apart from very modest, noninvasive enhancements that raise few ethical concerns, technologies to create super soldiers offer few, if any, benefits to nations fending off insurgents. Medical diplomacy, on the other hand, might be enormously useful. "Might be" is an important caveat because evidence of success is partial at best. Using or, perhaps, exploiting medicine to win hearts and minds, providers are in a unique position to build trust, gain support, and, yes, gather intelligence from needy civilians. The exigencies of war do not necessarily prohibit conditional medical care. Nevertheless, the details are knotted and require constant attention to avoid undermining the basic medical attention that all enjoy by right.

Part IV seeks closure. Killing in war is for naught without a feasible program to rebuild shattered states and care for those who fought. With what might come as a relief to some readers, military necessity falls back, and medical impartiality steps forward as military medicine attends to postwar reconstruction and veteran care. In each case, medicine slowly emerges from the all-embracing grip of the military. Still, vestiges of military and political necessity remain. Western armies did not come halfway around the world, spend trillions of dollars, and suffer the casualties of war merely to restore the dismal status quo ante bellum. Sunk costs such as these sometimes ignite ambitious goals, nothing less than erecting stable and vigorous democratic states. Sunk costs such as these also throw good money after bad. Eventually, and with good reason, humanitarian forces and international nongovernmental organizations (NGOs) seek more modest goals so they can pack up and go home.

At home, the sick and injured of war await. Veteran care, too, speaks to a dignified life in the shadow of war. More than an appeal to a fundamental human right, veteran health care evokes gratitude and guilt; gratitude to those who put their lives on the line, and guilt when the grateful nation fails to deliver decent medical attention. Neither emotion is appropriate. As compelling as they are, warfighters' heroism and sacrifice find no place in postwar medicine. Instead, we are better left to lean on every person's right to health care. Equality of care attuned solely to medical need is not a fixture of wartime military medicine but dominates postwar. It is, therefore, enough to provide veterans with the same decent level of care that each person deserves. National health care systems understand this implicitly, but the patchwork healthcare system of the world's wealthiest nation does not quite get it.

Military medical ethics gains its rigor by consistently applying military necessity, associative duties, and the fundamental right to a dignified life to the practice of wartime medicine. The first two principles are foreign to civilian medical ethics but central to military medical ethics. What, at first, appears to be a blanket of incongruous practices fall into place in the context of just war. Theory and practice slowly reconcile in preparation for what awaits.

Future War

If the future is now, we can look back two decades to see how considerably military medical ethics has evolved since the end of the previous century. The enthusiasm for humanitarian intervention and democratic state-building put medical care for civilians squarely on the agenda of military medicine. This is why pediatricians went to war. And why, for the first time, an occupying army paid compensation to civilian victims of collateral harm. And why postwar reconstruction loomed so large. Civilian demands, coupled with claims for medical treatment by host-nation allies, besieged an infrastructure solely designed to tend the wounds of compatriot warfighters and marked for dissolution with the war's end. The immediate answer to such unfulfillable demands was to formulate medical rules of eligibility. By invoking military necessity and associative duties, these operative rules relegated many patients' medical needs to second place. Controversy brews here. The longer-term solution for adequate civilian health care was to pour huge but inadequate funds into postwar reconstruction. More controversy and pinched budgets beset the efforts of humanitarian forces.

Some of the lessons learned were not. Detainees suffered abuse. Spurred by Vietnam era "medical stability operations," purveyors of medical diplomacy continued to hope medical care would sway hearts and minds. They did not deliver any better now than then. Medical research during war faltered; veteran care during and afterwar lagged. As many more soldiers from the Iraq and Afghan theater survived with severe physical and psychological wounds than in previous wars, financial obligations pile up with no solution yet in sight. Some lessons just need to be relearned.

All along, science galloped ahead. The relationship between physicians and military technology was always testy. During and after World War II, physicians were summoned to build chemical and biological weapons. Some refused; others sought refuge in defensive research. Today, human enhancement to improve cognitive and physical performance, and instill the resilience needed to fight and kill, sets off similar alarms. The specter of medical scientists building warfighting machines introduces new meaning to "care," "treatment," and "therapy" entirely unanticipated by the debate surrounding chemical and biological weapons. Surprises await.

Back to Future War

Looking forward, the old adage warns about generals preparing to fight the last war. One must, therefore, resist preparing military medicine to fight the last war, too. Nevertheless, a variety of potential scenarios come to mind. Consider conventional war first. By conventional, I mean a war fought by bombs, bullets, and missiles. In this regard, conflict in the Middle East still percolates. From this vantage point, my own, things are not going to change very quickly. Future wars will look a lot like past and present wars. Without trying to invite any more controversy at this point, I will assume for a moment that some of these neighborhood feuds bear the mark of defensive war. In this context, military medicine attends to the military and political interests of state. When wars are defensive, defending nations have less compelling obligations to tend enemy civilians killed or injured in battle. When these wars are also asymmetric and the motivation for reciprocity is weak, the stronger party may forget its medical obligations toward detainees.

When war is very close to home, state of the art medicine is 15 minutes away. Scarcity, therefore, is not the same problem it is when wars are far from home. But we can expand the scope and also think about faraway wars. Confrontation with North Korea, for example, might be conventional or nuclear. Far from home means limited medical resources and demands for prioritizing care for compatriot or multinational forces. Nuclear confrontation, however limited, means pressing needs for battlefield research and enormous resources for postwar veteran care. Confronting an authoritarian state raises the prospect of rescue together with obligations of care and reconstruction for the formerly subjugated population. In this case, the principles and practices described throughout this book provide useful templates.

In-between asymmetric war in the Middle East and apocalyptic war in East Asia, lie myriad civil wars, proxy wars, despotic regimes, and failed states that invite intervention by multinational forces. Countries such as Ukraine, Venezuela, or Yemen might tempt Western powers to join the fray, as might regret over the half-done job in Libya and Syria. There, the world witnessed massive casualties, chemical warfare, bombings of hospitals, atrocities, and mass displacement. The impulse for regime change may emerge again to mimic the wars in Iraq and Afghanistan if our collective historical memory fails. In which case, the lessons military medical ethics gleans from the past two decades are pertinent. Unless, of course, we forget these, too.

Speculation about conventional confrontations puts a tentative name to the belligerents, but pondering unconventional warfare does not. Future war scenarios about cyber operations, information warfare, or killer robots are abstract and anonymous. What challenges might these raise for military medical ethics? One foray takes us back to enhancement. Hardcore neural enhancement to build cyborgs finds little place in a conventional war but may occupy our attention in future conflicts. One can imagine all kinds of novel questions that would confront medical scientists who build human/machine warfighters. Still, the principles of military necessity and human rights set the stage for the discussion. Is enhancement necessary for the future battle-field or just something we'd like to have before anyone else does? Does enhancement violate or infringe on fundamental human rights? Answering this question draws in lesser-evil arguments. I discussed and dismissed many of these philosophical exercises because enhancement fails the test of necessity in war as we know it. But in the future, it may not.

Cyber warfare, the latest twist in the art of war, raises issues of its own. Like drone operators, cyber warriors operate far from physical danger but skate on thin psychological ice. The effects of sustained cyber warfare remain unexamined, but one might expect fatigue, stress, burnout, PTSD, and moral injury. At this writing, cyber operations have yet to kill or seriously injure anyone. Nevertheless, the potential for deadly harm is ever-present, while theft or destruction of property is common. Such outcomes combine to excite mental suffering, anxiety, and distrust in ways that track conventional war and terrorism (Gross, Canetti, and Vashdi 2017). As soldiers and civilians suffer injury, the same demands of appropriate research, medical care, and compensation surface as in conventional war. Economic sanctions, campaigns of disinformation, and psychological operations can be equally pernicious. While nonkinetic warfare might avoid many of war's physical harms, it exacerbates its psychological wounds. In response, the loci of military medical ethics in future wars may shift, but the ethical dilemmas of medical care remain the same.

Far-Future War

In a 1967 episode of *Star Trek,* "A Taste of Armageddon," the USS *Enterprise* comes between two planets perpetually at war. The planets war by computer, but the casualties are real. Following a virtual attack appearing only on a computer screen, the residents of a "bombed" city are declared "dead" and must report to a disintegration center for elimination. Cities and civilizations endure whole, but millions lose their lives. In an alternate scenario, there are also virtual "wounded" whom doctors and nurses must "tend" by amputating their limbs or by breaking their bones. Kirk is appalled, but Spock senses a certain logic to all this. Controlled conflict is an effective way to fulfill the destructive inclinations of the planets' inhabitants without risking obliteration. Undeterred by efficiency, Kirk refuses to let them play their game. Destroying each planet's ability to curb the intensity of its attacks, he leaves them only two options: peace or mutually assured destruction. The warring sides step back.

In this far-future war, doctors and nurses euthanize the "dead" and mutilate the "injured," while in contemporary wars, they enable others to kill and injure. The difference may not be so striking. Realizing this, doctors and nurses may think about pulling their support for war. Some do, but most do not. Like any reflective person, they know that self-defense and the defense of others may necessitate armed force. Medical care and research are crucial tools of defense that cannot ignore the demands that just war places on the practice of medicine. The war Kirk will defuse is unnecessary and, therefore, manifestly unjust. Others are not. The challenge for military medical ethics, like all ethics, is to tell them apart and guide us to act accordingly.

Notes

Chapter 2

1. This case was discussed under Chatham House rules. For information, please contact the author.

Chapter 5

1. I thank Major Jacob F. Collen, M.D., for providing this case for discussion. See also Collen et al. 2013.
2. I am grateful to Yitzhak Benbaji for clarifying the contractarian aspects of associative duties.

Chapter 6

1. Citing its confidentiality policy in response to the author's request to confirm this classified summary, the ICRC wrote: "This report was leaked from the US cables, and appears to resemble ICRC's report, however we can't confirm its veracity" (ICRC personal communication, 24 March, 2020).

Chapter 7

1. Defining emergency care to save life, limb, and eyesight reflects the exigencies of modern asymmetric war. Before the wars in Iraq and Afghanistan, US military field manuals emphasized the urgency of life and limb-saving care alone. IEDs, however, raised special concerns about eye injuries. Only prompt and sophisticated treatment kept the rate of eye removal at a relatively low 13% of eye injuries in the early years of the Iraq War (Thach et al. 2008). As a result, rapid treatment for eye trauma was a dominant feature of battlefield care.

Chapter 8

1. My thanks to Therese A. West, Civilian Deputy Director of the Combat Casualty Care Research Program, for providing the program's research data.

Chapter 10

1. The phrase "advance US interests and values" does not appear in the 2009 revised directive (DoDI 2009).

Chapter 11

1. Additional indices include the Economist Democracy Index (2019) and the Organisation for Economic Co-operation and Development (OECD) States of Fragility Index (2019). Each offers some but not all of the variables the *FSI* and Freedom House provide to evaluate the hypothesized benefits of state-building and healthcare reconstruction.

References

21st Century Cures Act. (2016). Public Law 114–255—Dec. 13, 2016 130 Stat. 1033, 21st Century Cures Act, 12/2016, Section 3024.

ABA. (2010). *Standards on treatment of prisoners*. American Bar Association. https://www.americanbar.org/groups/criminal_justice/publications/criminal_justice_section_archive/crimjust_standards_treatmentprisoners/

Abiew, F. K. (2012). Humanitarian action under fire: Reflections on the role of NGOs in conflict and post-conflict situations. *International Peacekeeping*, 19(2), 203–216.

Acerra, J. R., Iskyan, K., Qureshi, Z. A., and Sharma, R. K. (2009). Rebuilding the health care system in Afghanistan: An overview of primary care and emergency services. *International Journal of Emergency Medicine*, 2(2), 77–82.

Adams, D. P. (1991). *The greatest good to the greatest number: Penicillin rationing on the American home front, 1940–1945*. New York: P. Lang.

Afghanistan Compact. 2006. The London Conference on Afghanistan, January 31–1 February 1, 2006. https://www.nato.int/isaf/docu/epub/pdf/afghanistan_compact.pdf

Al Hilfi, T. K., Lafta, R., and Burnham, G. (2013). Health services in Iraq. *The Lancet*, 381(9870), 939–948.

Alkire, S. (2002). Dimensions of human development. *World Development*, 30(2), 181–205.

Allhoff, F. (2008). Physician Involvement in Hostile Interrogations. In F. Allhoff (Ed.), *Physicians at war: The dual-loyalties challenge* (pp. 91–104). Dordrecht: Springer.

Allhoff, F. (2012). *Terrorism, ticking time-bombs, and torture: A philosophical analysis*. Chicago: University of Chicago Press.

American College of Surgeons. (2014, 3 January). Statement on advance directives by patients: "Do not resuscitate" in the operating room. American College of Surgeons. Retrieved from https://www.facs.org/about-acs/statements/19-advance-directives.

American Forces Press Service (AFPS) (2008). "Running a city" in southern Iraq. *DoD News*, March 18. https://www.nationalguard.mil/News/Article-View/Article/573192/running-a-city-in-southern-iraq/

American Medical Association (AMA). (2006). *Physician participation in interrogation*. Council on Ethical and Judicial Affair. Opinion of Council on Ethical and Judicial Affairs (Resolution 1, 1-05), In F. Allhoff (Ed.), *Physicians at war* (pp. 261–270). Dordrecht: Springer.

American Psychological Association (APA). (2002). *Ethical principles of psychologists and code of conduct, Section 1.02: Conflicts between ethics and law, regulations, or other governing legal authority*. https://psycnet-apa-org.ezproxy.haifa.ac.il/fulltext/2002-11464-006.pdf

American Psychological Association (APA) (2010). Amending the ethics code. *APA Monitor* 2010, Vol 41, No. 4 https://www.apa.org/monitor/2010/04/ethics.aspx

Annas, C. L., and Annas, G. J. (2009). Enhancing the fighting force: Medical research on American soldiers. *Journal of Contemporary Health and Policy*, 25(2), 283–308.

Annas, G. J. (1998). Protecting soldiers from friendly fire: The consent requirement for using investigational drugs and vaccines in combat. *American Journal of Law and Medicine*, 24(2,3), 245–260.

Annas, G. J. (2005). Unspeakably cruel—Torture, medical ethics, and the law. *New England Journal of Medicine*, 352(20), 2127–2132.

Annas, G. J., and Crosby, S. (2019). US military medical ethics in the war on terror. *Journal of the Royal Army Medical Corps*, 165(4), 303–306.

AR 220-1. (2007). *Field organizations: Unit status reporting*. Army Regulation 220-1. Washington, DC: Department of the Army. https://www.ssi.army.mil/ncoa/AGS_SLC_ALC_REGS/AR%20220-1.pdf.

AR 40-66. (2008). *Medical Services: Medical record administration and healthcare documentation*. Army Regulation 40-66. Washington, DC: Department of the Army. https://armypubs.army.mil/epubs/DR_pubs/DR_a/pdf/web/r40_66.pdf

AR 40-3. (2013). *Medical services: Medical, dental, and veterinary care*. Army Regulation 40–3. Washington, DC: Department of the Army. https://armypubs.army.mil/epubs/DR_pubs/DR_a/pdf/web/r40_3.pdf.

AR 600-20. (2014). *Personnel-general: Army command policy*. Army Regulation 600-20. Washington, DC: Department of the Army https://armypubs.army.mil/epubs/DR_pubs/DR_a/pdf/web/r600_20.pdf

AR 25-22. (2016). *Office management: The army privacy program*. Army Regulation 25–22. Washington, DC: Department of the Army. https://www.cadetcommand.army.mil/res/files/AR%2025%E2%80%9322%20The%20Army%20Privacy%20Program%20(22DEC16).pdf

Army Technology. (2013). Brain computer interfacing: A big step towards military mind-control. *Army Technology*, July 16. https://www.army-technology.com/features/featurebrain-computer-interfacing-military-mind-control/

Associated Press. (2003). Court-martial for refusing anthrax shot. April 5.

Auden, W. H. (1937). Spain. Cited in Galvan, R. (2018). *News of war: Civilian poetry 1936–1945*. Oxford: Oxford University Press.

Australia Department of Veteran Affairs (ADVA). (2019). Factsheet HSV92—Repatriation pharmaceutical benefits scheme. https://www.dva.gov.au/factsheet-hsv92-repatriation-pharmaceutical-benefits-scheme

Australia Department of Veterans Affairs. (2020). Compensation. https://www.dva.gov.au/financial-support/compensation-claims

Avery, G. H., and Boetig, B. J. (2010). Medical and public health civic action programs: Using health engagement as a tool of foreign policy. *World Medical & Health Policy*, 2(1), 59–81.

Bacevich, A. J. (2016). *America's war for the greater Middle East: A military history*. New York: Random House.

Baker, J. B. (2007). Medical diplomacy in full-spectrum operations. *Military Review*, 87(5), 67–73.

Baker, J. B. (2010). The doctrinal basis for medical stability operations. *Military Medicine*, 175(1), 14–20.

Baker, M. S. (2014). Casualties of the global war on terror and their future impact on health care and society: A looming public health crisis. *Military Medicine*, 179(4), 348–355.

Baker, R., and Strosberg, M. (1992). Triage and equality: An historical reassessment of utilitarian analyses of triage. *Kennedy Institute of Ethics Journal*, 2(2), 103–123.

Balazs, R. (2019). NATO trauma registry—evidence based military medical care for the alliance. *Worldwide Military Medicine*, January 21. https://www.military-medicine.com/article/3618-nato-trauma-registry-evidence-based-military-medical-care-for-the-alliance.html

Barfield, T. (2010). *Afghanistan: A cultural and political history*. Princeton, New Jersey: Princeton University Press.

Barilan, Y. M. (2017). The role of doctors in hunger strikes. *Kennedy Institute of Ethics Journal*, 27(3), 341–369.

Barilan, Y. M., and Zuckerman, S. (2013). Revisiting medical neutrality as a moral value and as a doctrine in international law. In M. L. Gross and D. Carrick (Eds.), *Military medical ethics in the 21st century* (pp. 97–110). Farnham, UK: Ashgate Publishing.

Barnett, M. (2005). Humanitarianism transformed. *Perspectives on Politics*, 3(4), 723–740.

Barnett, M., and Weiss, T. G. (2011). *Humanitarianism contested: Where angels fear to tread*. London: Routledge.

Bass, G. J. (2004). Jus post bellum. *Philosophy & Public Affairs*, 32(4), 384–412.

Bassiouni, M. C. (2010). SOFA status and occupation: Legal status of US forces in Iraq from 2003–2008. *Chicago Journal of International Law*, 11(1), 1–38.

Bazargan-Forward, S. (2019). The identity-enactment account of associative duties. *Philosophical Studies*, 176(9), 2351–2370.

Beam, T. E., and Howe, E. G. (2003). A proposed ethic for military medicine. In T. E. Beam and L. R. Sparacino (Eds.), *Military medical ethics* (pp. 851–865). Falls Church VA: Office of The Surgeon General.

Beard, M., Galliott, J., and Lynch, S. (2016). Soldier enhancement: Ethical risks and opportunities. *Australian Army Journal*, 13(1), 5–20.

Beauchamp, T. L., and Childress, J. F. (2009; 1994). *The principles of biomedical ethics (6th ed; 4th ed)*. Oxford: Oxford University Press.

Becker, T., and Link, M. (2011). Medical rules of engagement negative patients: The dilemma of forward surgical teams in counterinsurgency operations. *Journal of Special Operations Medicine: A Peer Reviewed Journal for SOF Medical Professionals*, 11(2), 12–15.

Bedau, H. A. (ed.). (1969). *Civil disobedience: Theory and practice*. Indianapolis, IN: Bobbs Merrill.

Beekley, A. C., Bohman, H., and Schindler, D. (2012). Modern warfare. In E. Savitsky and B. Eastridge (Eds.), *Combat casualty care, Lessons learned from OEF and OIF* (pp. 1–38). Washington, DC: Office of the Surgeon General, Department of the Army.

Beitler, A. L., Junnila, J. L., and Meyer, J. H. (2006). Humanitarian assistance in Afghanistan: A prospective evaluation of clinical effectiveness. *Military Medicine*, 171(9), 889–893.

Beitler, A. L., Wortmann, G. W., Hofmann, L. J., and Goff, J. M. (2006). Operation Enduring Freedom: The 48th combat support hospital in Afghanistan. *Military Medicine*, 171(3), 189–193.

Belasco, A. (2009). Troop levels in the Afghan and Iraq wars FY2001–FY2012: Cost and other potential issues. Congressional Research Service, Report No. R40682. https://fas.org/sgp/crs/natsec/R40682.pdf

Bellamy, A. J. (2008). The responsibilities of victory: Jus post bellum and the just war. *Review of International Studies*, 34(4), 601–625.

Bellany, I. (2002). Fighting asymmetric wars: An application of Lanchester's square-law to modern warfare. *The RUSI Journal*, 147(5), 72–76.

Belmont Report. (1979). Ethical principles and guidelines for the protection of human subjects of research. The national commission for the protection of human subjects of biomedical and behavioral research. Department of Health, Education, and Welfare. https://www.hhs.gov/ohrp/sites/default/files/the-belmont-report-508c_FINAL.pdf

Benard, C., Edward O., Cathryn Quantic Thurston, Villamizar, A., Loredo, E. N., Sullivan, T., and Goulka, J. (2011). *The battle behind the wire: U.S. prisoner and detainee operations from world war II to Iraq.* Santa Monica, CA: RAND Corporation.

Benatar, S. R., and Upshur, R. E. (2008). Dual loyalty of physicians in the military and in civilian life. *American Journal of Public Health*, 98(12), 2161–2167.

Bennett, R. A. (2016). Ethics surrounding the medical evacuation of catastrophically injured individuals from an operational theatre of war. *British Medical Journal of Military Health*, 162(5), 321–323.

Berger, Z., Rubenstein, L. S., and DeCamp, M. (2018). Clinical care and complicity with torture. *The British Medical Journal*, 360: k449.

Bernthal, E. M., Russell, R. J., and Draper, H. J. A. (2014). A qualitative study of the use of the four quadrant approach to assist ethical decision-making during deployment. *British Medical Journal of Military Health*, 160(2), 196–202.

Berwick, D., Downey, A., and Cornett, E. (Eds.). (2016). *A national trauma care system: Integrating military and civilian trauma systems to achieve zero after injury.* Washington, DC: National Academies Press.

Bilmes, L. (2013). The financial legacy of Iraq and Afghanistan: How wartime spending decisions will constrain future national security budgets. Harvard Kennedy School. Working Paper No. RWP13-006.

Bilmes, L., and Stiglitz, J. E. (2011). The long term costs of conflict: The case of the Iraq War in the Great Recession. In D. L. Braddon and K. Hartley (Eds.), *Handbook on the economics of war* (pp. 293–307). Northampton, MA: Elgar Publishing.

Bingham, S. (2012). Refusal of treatment and decision-making capacity. *Nursing Ethics*, 19(1), 167–172.

Black, L. (2006). Defining hospitals' obligation to stabilize patients under EMTALA. *AMA Journal of Ethics*, 8(11), 752–755.

Blagg, C. R. (2007). The early history of dialysis for chronic renal failure in the United States: A view from Seattle. *American Journal of Kidney Diseases*, 49(3), 482–496.

Blay, E., DeLancey, J. O., Hewitt, D. B., Chung, J. W., and Bilimoria, K. Y. (2017). Initial public reporting of quality at veterans affairs vs non–veterans affairs hospitals. *JAMA Internal Medicine*, 177(6), 882–885.

Blitz, M. J. (2017). *Searching minds by scanning brains neuroscience technology and constitutional privacy protection.* Cham, Switzerland: Palgrave Macmillan.

Bloche, M. G. (2011). *The Hippocratic myth: Why doctors are under pressure to ration care, practice politics, and compromise their promise to heal.* New York: St Martins Press.

Bloche, M. G., and Marks, J. H. (2005). When doctors go to war. *New England Journal of Medicine*, 352(1), 3–6.

Blum, G. (2010). The laws of war and the "lesser evil." *Yale Journal of International Law*, 35(1), 1–69.

Bogue, R. (2009). Exoskeletons and robotic prosthetics: A review of recent developments. *Industrial Robot: An International Journal*, 36(5), 421–427.

Bohannon, J. (2011). War as a laboratory for trauma research. *Science*, 331(6022), 1261–1263.

Bok, S. (1989). *Secrets: On the ethics of concealment and revelation.* New York: Vintage.

Bolt, J. D., and Schoneboom, B. A. (2010). Operative splenectomy for treatment of homozygous thalassemia major in Afghan children at a US military hospital. *AANA journal*, 78(2), 129–133.

Bolton, M., and Jeffrey, A. (2008). The politics of NGO registration in international protectorates: The cases of Bosnia and Iraq. *Disasters*, 32(4), 586–608.

Bonnet, S., Gonzalez, F., Poichotte, A., Duverger, V., and Pons, F. (2012). Lessons learned from the experience of visceral military surgeons in the French role 3 medical treatment facility of Kabul (Afghanistan): An extended skill mix required. *Injury*, 43(8), 1301–1306.

Bonventre, E. V., and Denux, V. (2013). Military health diplomacy. In T. E. Novotny, I. Kickbusch, and M. Told (Eds.), *21st century global health diplomacy* (pp. 191–214). Hackensack, NJ: World Scientific.

Borgerson, K. (2020). What is human subjects research? In A.S. Iltis and D. MacKay (Eds.). *The Oxford Handbook of Research Ethics*. Oxford: Oxford University Press.

Borgman, M., Matos, R. I., Blackbourne, L. H., and Spinella, P. C. (2012). Ten years of military pediatric care in Afghanistan and Iraq. *Journal of Trauma and Acute Care Surgery*, 73(6), S509–S513.

Bostrom, N., and Sandberg, A. (2009). Cognitive enhancement: Methods, ethics, regulatory challenges. *Science and Engineering Ethics*, 15(3), 311–341.

Bowersox, J. C., and Al-Ainachi, S. (2006). Who will care for Iraq's wounded warriors? *World Journal of Surgery*, 30(2006), 1769–1773.

Boyle Jr, J. M. (1980). Toward understanding the principle of double effect. *Ethics*, 90(4), 527–538.

Brecher, B. (2007). *Torture and the ticking bomb*. Oxford: Blackwell.

Brevard, B. B., Champion, H., and Katz, D. (2012). Weapons effects. In E. Savitsky and B. Eastridge (Eds.), *Combat casualty care: Lessons learned from OEF and OIF* (pp. 39–84). Washington, DC: Office of the Surgeon General, Department of the Army.

Bricknell, M. C. M., and Cameron, E. (2011). International military medical engagement with the indigenous civilian health sector. *Journal of the Royal Army Medical Corps*, 157(4), S472–S476.

Bricknell, M. C. M., Jones, F. R., and Hatzfeld, J. J. (2011). Casualty estimation and medical resource planning. *Journal of the Royal Army Medical Corps*, 157(4), S439–S443.

Bricknell, M. C. M. (2014). Military medical contribution to indigenous (military and civilian) Health Sector Development (HSD) within security and stabilisation operations. In J. M. Ryan et al. (eds.), *Conflict and catastrophe medicine* (pp. 451–473). London: Springer-Verlag.

Bridges, E., and Biever, K. (2010). Advancing critical care: Joint combat casualty research team and joint theater trauma system. *AACN Advanced Critical Care*, 21(3), 260–276.

Brigham Health and Women's Faulkner Hospital. (2019). Understanding do not resuscitate (DNR) orders. Brigham and Women's Faulkner Hospital. https://www.brighamandwomensfaulkner.org/patients-and-families/advance-care-directives/dnr-orders.

Brigham, R. K. (2006). *ARVN: Life and death in the South Vietnamese army*. Lawrence: University of Kansas Press.

Brocke, A. (2017). Personal communication, Research and Clinical Innovation, Royal Centre for Defence Medicine, Birmingham, UK, September 19, 2017.

Brondex, A., Viant, E., Trendel, D., and Puidupin, M. (2014). Medical activity in the conventional hospitalization unit in Kabul NATO role 3 hospital: A 3-month-long experience. *Military Medicine*, 179(2), 197–202.

Brosch, L. R., Holcomb, J. B., Thompson, J. C., and Cordts, P. R. (2008). Establishing a human research protection program in a combatant command. *Journal of Trauma and Acute Care Surgery*, 64(2), S9–S13.

Broughton, G., Janis, J. E., and Attinger, C. E. (2006). A brief history of wound care. *Plastic and Reconstructive Surgery*, 117(7S), 6S–11S.

Brown, W. (2015). Doctors in the crosshairs: Four years of attacks on health care in Syria. *Physicians for Human Rights*, March 1. https://phr.org/our-work/resources/doctors-in-the-crosshairs-four-years-of-attacks-on-health-care-in-syria/.

Brownlie, I. (1972). Interrogation in depth: The Compton and Parker reports. *The Modern Law Review*, 35(5), 501–507.

Bryan, A. R. (2009). Field hospital support for civilians in counterinsurgency operations. *Military Review*, 89(4), 119–122.

Bulstrode, C. (2009). Medcaps—Do they work? *British Military Journal of Military Health*, 155(3), 182–184.

Burnam, M., Meredith, L., Tanielian, T., and Jaycox, L. (2009). Mental health care for Iraq and Afghanistan war veterans. *Health Affairs*, 28(3), 771–782.

Burnett, M. W., Spinella, P. C., Azarow, K. S., and Callahan, C. W. (2008). Pediatric care as part of the US Army medical mission in the global war on terrorism in Afghanistan and Iraq, December 2001 to December 2004. *Pediatrics*, 121(2), 261–265.

Bush, G. W. (2007). President's Radio Address. The White House, Office of the Press Secretary. http://www.whitehouse.gov/news/releases/2007/03/20070302-3.html.

Bush, G. W. (2010). *Decision points*. New York: Random House.

Butler, D. (2019). Kurdish MPs, prisoners end hunger strike in Turkey. *Reuters*, May 26. https://www.reuters.com/article/us-turkey-security-kurds/kurdish-mps-prisoners-end-hunger-strike-in-turkey-idUSKCN1SW08H

Butler Jr., F. K. (2017). Two decades of saving lives on the battlefield: Tactical combat casualty care turns 20. *Military Medicine*, 182(3–4), e1563–e1568.

Butler Jr., F. K., and Blackbourne, L. H. (2012). Battlefield trauma care then and now: A decade of tactical combat casualty care. *Journal of Trauma and Acute Care Surgery*, 73(6), S395–S402.

Butler Jr., F. K., Hagmann, J., and Butler, E. G. (1996). Tactical combat casualty care in special operations. *Military Medicine*, 161(suppl_1), 3–16.

Caldwell, J. A., and Caldwell, J. L. (2005). Fatigue in military aviation: An overview of US military-approved pharmacological countermeasures. *Aviation, Space, and Environmental Medicine*, 76(7), C39–C51.

Center for Army Lessons Learned (CALL). (2010). *Iraq provincial reconstruction team handbook: Observations, insights, and lessons*. No. 11–03. https://usacac.army.mil/sites/default/files/publications/11-03.pdf

Center for Army Lessons Learned (CALL). (2011). *Afghanistan provincial reconstruction team handbook: Observations, insights, and lessons*. No. 11–16. https://usacac.army.mil/sites/default/files/publications/11-16.pdf

Callahan, D., and Jennings, B. (2002). Ethics and public health: Forging a strong relationship. *American Journal of Public Health*, 92(2), 169–176.

Cameron, E. A. (2011). Do no harm—The limitations of civilian medical outreach and MEDCAP programs based in Afghanistan. *Journal of the Royal Army Medical Corps*, 157(3), 209–211.

Carpenter, S., and Kent, R. (2016). The military, the private sector and traditional humanitarian actors. In Z. Sezgin and D. Dijkaeul (Eds.), *The new humanitarians in international practice: Emerging actors and contested principles* (pp. 144–166). London: Routledge.

Casebeer, W. (2005). Torture interrogation of terrorists: A theory of exceptions (with notes, cautions, and warnings). In T. Shanhan (Ed.), *Philosophy 9/11: Thinking about the War on Terrorism* (pp. 261–272). Peru, IL: Open Court Publishing.

Convention Against Torture (CAT). (1984). *Convention against Torture and Other Cruel, Inhuman or Degrading Treatment or Punishment.* https://www.ohchr.org/en/professionalinterest/pages/cat.aspx.

Causey, M., Rush Jr., R. M., Kjorstad, R. J., and Sebesta, J. A. (2012). Factors influencing humanitarian care and the treatment of local patients within the deployed military medical system: Casualty referral limitations. *The American Journal of Surgery*, 203(5), 574–577.

Cereste, H. X. (2011). Gray matters: A deployed physician's perspective on combat medicine in Iraq. *Journal of Religion and Health*, 50(3), 527–542.

Committee on Economic, Social and Cultural Rights. (CESCR). (2000). *General Comment No. 14: The right to the highest attainable standard of health (Art. 12).* Office of the High Commissioner for Human Rights. Document E/C.12/2000/4.

Cetorelli, V., and Shabila, N. P. (2014). Expansion of health facilities in Iraq a decade after the US-led invasion, 2003–2012. *Conflict and Health*, 8(1), 16.

Chalela, J. A. (2017). Medical care of detainees in US military facilities: Unspeakable kindness. *JAMA: The Journal of the American Medical Association*, 317(11), 1119–1120.

Chamberlin, S. M. E. (2013). The complicated life of a physician-soldier: Medical readiness training exercises & the problem of dual loyalties. *Journal of Biomedical Science and Engineering*, 6(10), 8–18.

Chamberlin, S. M. E. (2015). Medicine as a non-lethal weapon: The ethics of "winning hearts and minds." *Ethics and Armed Forces*, 1, 9–16.

Chang, C. S., Bonhoure, P., Alam, S., Hansen, P., and Burnham, G. (2010). Use of the balanced scorecard to assess provincial hospital performance in Afghanistan. *World Medical & Health Policy*, 2(1), 77–100.

Chapman, A. R., Forman, L., Lamprea, E., and Khanna, K. (2018). Identifying the components of a core health services package from a human rights perspective to inform progress toward universal health coverage. *Human Rights Quarterly*, 40(2), 342–368.

Chapman, A. R., Forman, L., and Lamprea, E. (2017). Evaluating essential health packages from a human rights perspective. *Journal of Human Rights*, 16(2), 142–159.

Chenoweth, E., and Stephan, M. J. (2011). *Why civil resistance works: The strategic logic of nonviolent conflict.* New York: Columbia University Press.

Childress J. F., Faden, R. R., Gaare, R. D., Gostin, L. O., Kahn, J., Bonnie, R. J., Kass, N. E., Mastroianni, A. C., Moreno, J. D., and Nieburg, P. (2002). Public health ethics: Mapping the terrain. *The Journal of Law, Medicine and Ethics*, 30(2), 170–178.

Childress, J. F. and Bernheim, R. G. (2015). Introduction: A framework for public health ethics. In R. G., Bernheim, J. F., Childress, A., Melnick, and R. J., Bonnie (Eds.), *Essentials of public health ethics* (pp. 1–20). Burlington, MA: Jones and Bartlett Learning.

Cho, R. I., and Savitsky, E. (2012). Ocular trauma. In E. Savitsky and B. Eastridge (Eds.), *Combat casualty care: Lessons learned from OEF and OIF* (pp. 299–342). Washington, DC: The Office of the Surgeon, General Department of the Army.

CIA. (2004). OMS guidelines on medical and psychological support to detainee rendition, interrogation and detention, December 2004. https://www.thetorturedatabase.org/document/cia-memo-oms-guidelines-medical-and-psychological-support-detainee-rendition-interrogation?pdf_page=4./

CIA. (2007). Summary and reflections of chief of medical services on OMS participation in the RDI program (no dates but updated through 2007). https://www.cia.gov/library/readingroom/docs/0006541727.pdf

CIVIC. (2009). *Losing the people: The costs and consequences of civilian suffering in Afghanistan.* New York: Campaign for Innocent Victims in Conflict (CIVIC).

Coetzee, R. H., Simpson, R. G., and Sharpley, J. (2010). The doctor vs. the command: Can disagreement arise? *Journal of the Royal Army Medical Corps*, 156(3), 204–208.

Cohen, J. (1998). Democracy and liberty. In J. Elster (Ed.), *Deliberative democracy* (pp. 185–231). Cambridge: Cambridge University Press.

Cohen, R. (2015a). Understanding the U.S. military's morale "crisis." *Lawfare*, June 28. https://www.lawfareblog.com/understanding-us-militarys-morale-crisis

Cohen, R. (2015b). In the ranks: Making sense of military morale. *World Affairs*, 178(1), 59–66.

Coleman, J. L. (1976). The morality of strict liability. *William & Mary Law Review*, 18(2), 259–286.

Collen, J., O'Malley, P., Roy, M., and Sessums, L. (2013). Military medical ethics: Experience from Operation Iraqi Freedom. In M. L. Gross and D. Carrick (Eds.), *Military medical ethics in the 21st century* (pp. 17–42). Farnham, UK: Ashgate Publishing.

Cooke, M. (2006). Five arguments for deliberative democracy. In M. D'Entreves (Ed.), *Democracy as public deliberation* (pp. 53–87). London: Taylor and Francis.

Cope, V. (1941). Influence of war upon surgery. *Nature*, 148, 577–580.

Cordesman, A. H. (2017). *Afghan desertions in the U.S.: Assessing the desertion and "ghost soldier" problem in Afghan national security forces.* Washington, DC: Center for Strategic and International Studies. https://www.csis.org/analysis/afghan-desertions-us-assessing-desertion-and-ghost-soldier-problem-afghan-national-security.

Cordesman, A. H., Allison, M. and Lemieux J. (2010). *IED metrics for Afghanistan January 2004–September 2010.* Washington, DC: Center for Strategic and International Studies.

Cordesman, A. H., Loi, C., and Kocharlakota, V. (2010). *IED metrics for Iraq, June 2003–September 2010.* Washington, DC: Center for Strategic and International Studies.

Costanzo, G. and Spott, M. A. (2010). Joint Theater Trauma System (JTTS); Joint Theater Trauma Registry (JTTR), *Information Brief to DHB*. US Army Institute of Surgical Research (USAISR). file:///C:/Users/user/Downloads/71410Joint_Theater_Trauma_System.pdf

Crawford, N. C. (2013). *Accountability for killing: Moral responsibility for collateral damage in America's post-9/11 wars.* Oxford: Oxford University Press.

Crawford, N. C. (2018). Human cost of the post-9/11 wars: Lethality and the need for transparency. Watson Institute, Brown University. https://watson.brown.edu/costsofwar/files/cow/imce/papers/2018/Human%20Costs%2C%20Nov%208%20 2018%20CoW.pdf

Crosby, S. S., Apovian, C. M., and Grodin, M. A. (2007). Hunger strikes, force-feeding, and physicians' responsibilities. *JAMA: The Journal of the American Medical Association*, 298(5), 563–566.

CRS. (2020). The purple heart: Background and issues for Congress. Congressional Research Service, Report No. R42704. https://fas.org/sgp/crs/natsec/R42704.pdf

Cubano, M. A. (Ed.) (2018). *Emergency war surgery* (5th revision.). Falls Church, VA: Office of The Surgeon General.

Cummings, M. (2002). Informed consent and investigational new drug abuses in the U.S. military. *Accountability in Research: Policies and Quality Assurance,* 9(2), 93–103.

Daily Mail. (2009). Karzai's fury as NATO airstrike on fuel trucks hijacked by Taliban kills 90 in massive blast. *Daily Mail Online*, September 5.

Dalil, S., Newbrander, W., Loevinsohn, B., Naeem, A. J., Griffin, J., Salama, P., and Momand, F. M. (2014). Aid effectiveness in rebuilding the Afghan health system: A reflection. *Global Public Health*, 9(suppl_1), S124–S136.

Dao, J. and Froschdec, D. (2009). Military rules said to hinder therapy. *New York Times*. December 6.

Davies, H., Shakur, H., Padkin, A., Roberts, I., Slowther, A. M., and Perkins, G. D. (2014). Guide to the design and review of emergency research when it is proposed that consent and consultation be waived. *Emergency Medicine Journal*, 31(10), 794–795.

Defense Advanced Research Projects Agency (DARPA). (2017). TNT researchers set out to advance pace and effectiveness of cognitive skills training. *DARPA News and Events*, April 26. https://www.darpa.mil/news-events/2017-04-26.

Defense Advanced Research Projects Agency (DARPA). (2018). *Department of Defense Fiscal Year (FY) 2019 budget estimates*. https://www.darpa.mil/attachments/DARPAFY 19PresidentsBudgetRequest.pdf

Defense Advanced Research Projects Agency (DARPA). (2019a). *Department of Defense Fiscal Year (FY) 2020 budget estimates*. https://www.darpa.mil/attachments/DARPA_ FY20_Presidents_Budget_Request.pdf

Defense Advanced Research Projects Agency (DARPA). (2019b). *Understanding warfighter performance from the inside out. DARPA News and Events*. https://www.darpa. mil/news-events/2019-01-22a

Defense Advanced Research Projects Agency (DARPA). (2019c). Six paths to the nonsurgical future of brain-machine interfaces. *DARPA News and Events*. https://www.darpa. mil/news-events/2019-05-20.

Defense Advanced Research Projects Agency (DARPA). (nd). *Warrior web. DARPA Program Information*. https://www.darpa.mil/program/warrior-web

De Torrente, N. (2004). Humanitarian action under attack: Reflections on the Iraq war. *Human Rights Journal*, 17, 1–29.

Defense Health Board. (2015). *Ethical guidelines and practices for U.S. military medical professionals*. Falls Church, VA: Office of The Assistant Secretary of Defense Health Affairs.

Deitchman, S. J. (1962). A Lanchester model of guerrilla warfare. *Operations Research*, 10(6), 818–827.

Del Rosso, J. (2015). *Talking about torture: How political discourse shapes the debate*. New York: Columbia University Press.

Department of the Navy. (2002). Unreasonable refusal of medical, dental, or surgical treatment. *Navy Disability Evaluation Manual*. Instruction 1850.4E. Washington, DC: Department of the Navy.

Detainee Treatment Act. 2005. Pub. L. No. 109-148, §§ 1001–1006. https://www.govinfo. gov/content/pkg/COMPS-489/pdf/COMPS-489.pdf

Deuster, P. A., O'Connor, F. G., and Lunasco, T. K. (2017). MPH human performance optimization. In F. G. O'Connor, E. B. Schoomaker, and D. C. Smith (Eds.), *Fundamentals of military medicine* (pp. 275–283). Fort Sam Houston, TX: Army Medical Department.

Deutsche Welle. (2008). Three civilians shot dead at German checkpoint in Afghanistan. *Deutsche Welle*, August 29. http://www.dw.com/en/three-civilians-shot-dead-at-german-checkpoint-in-afghanistan/a-3602953

Dhiab v Obama. (2014). US District Court, District of Columbia, Civil Action No. 05-1457.

DHSC. 2015. *The NHS constitution for England*. Department of Health and Social Care https://www.gov.uk/government/publications/the-nhs-constitution-for-england/the-nhs-constitution-for-england

Dinstein, Y. (1985). International criminal law. *Israel Law Review*, 2(3), 206–242.

Department of Defense (DoD). (2001). *Instruction number 133.21. Code of conduct*. January 8. https://biotech.law.lsu.edu/blaw/dodd/corres/pdf/i130021_010801/i130021p.pdf

Department of Defense (DoD). (2011). *Instruction number 3216.02, November 8, 2011: Protection of human subjects and adherence to ethical standards in DoD-supported research, Enclosure 3, paragraph 9: Unique DoD Limitations on Waiver of Informed Consent*. (US) http://www.esd.whs.mil/Portals/54/Documents/DD/issuances/dodi/321602p.pdf

Department of Defense (DoD). (2015). *Ethical guidelines and practices for U.S. military medical professionals*. http://www.health.mil/Reference-Center/Reports/2015/03/03/Ethical-Guidelines-and-Practices-for-US-Military-Medical-Professionals

Department of Defense (DoD). (2018). *DoD Worldwide number for traumatic brain injury*. https://dvbic.dcoe.mil/files/tbi-numbers/worldwide-totals-2000-2018Q1-total_jun-21-2018_v1.0_2018-07-26_0.pdf

Department of Defense (DoD). (2019). *Instruction number 6025.18*. Health insurance portability and accountability act (HIPAA) privacy rule compliance in DOD health care programs. https://www.esd.whs.mil/Portals/54/Documents/DD/issuances/dodi/602518p.pdf

Department of Defense Directive (DODD). (2003). *Mental health evaluations of members of the armed forces* (Publication No. 6490.1). https://biotech.law.lsu.edu/blaw/dodd/corres/pdf2/d64901p.pdf.

Department of Defense Directive (DODD). (2005). *Military support for stability, security, transition, and reconstruction (SSTR) operations*. (Publication number 3000.05). https://policy.defense.gov/portals/11/Documents/solic/DoDD%203000.05%20SSTR%20(SIGNED)%2028NOV05.pdf

Department of Defense Instruction (DoDI). (2009). *Stability operations*. (Publication number 3000–05). https://cryptome.org/dodi/dodi-3000-05.pdf

Donaldson, R. I., Hasson, T., Aziz, S., Ansari, W., and Evans, G. (2010). The development of civilian emergency medical care during an insurgency: Current status and future outlook in Iraq. *Annals of Emergency Medicine*, 56(2), 172–177.

Donini, A. (2009). *Afghanistan: Humanitarianism under threat*. Medford, MA: Feinstein International Center, Tufts University.

Doscher, T. J. (2007). New joint theater hospital offers advanced care in Afghanistan. *DoD News*, 5 March. http://archive.defense.gov/news/newsarticle.aspx?id=3259.

Duffield, M., Macrae, J., and Curtis, D. (2001). Politics and humanitarian aid. *Disasters*, 25(4), 269–274.

Dukes, S., Tourtillott, B., Bryant, D., Carter, K., McNair, S., Maupin, G. and Tamminga, C. (2015). Finishing what was started: An analysis of theater research conducted from 2010 to 2012. *Military Medicine*, 180(suppl_3), 8–13.

Dunant, H. (1986; 1862). *A memory of Solferino*. Geneva: The International Committee of the Red Cross.

Dutton R. P., Stansbury L. G., Hemlock B., Hess J. R., and Scalea T. M. (2008). Impediments to obtaining informed consent for clinical research in trauma patients. *Journal of Trauma and Acute Care Surgery*, 64(4), 1106–1112.

Easby, D., Inwald, D. P., and McNicholas, J. J. K. (2015). Ethical challenges of deployed military critical care. In P. F. Mahoney (Ed.), *Combat anesthesia: The first 24 hours* (pp. 459–468). Falls Church, VA: Office of the Surgeon General, Department of the Army.

Eastridge, B. J., Blackbourne, L. H., Rasmussen, T., Cryer, H., and Murdock, A. (2012a). Damage control surgery. In E. Savitsky and B. Eastridge (Eds.), *Combat casualty care, Lessons learned from OEF and OIF* (pp. 165–224). Washington, DC: Office of the Surgeon General, Department of the Army.

Eastridge, B. J., Costanzo, G., Jenkins, D., Spott, M. A., Wade, C., Greydanus, D., Greydanus, D., Flaherty, S., Rappold, J., Dunne, J., Holcomb, J. B., and Blackbourne, L. H. (2009). Impact of joint theater trauma system initiatives on battlefield injury outcomes. *The American Journal of Surgery*, 198(6), 852–857.

Eastridge, B. J., Mabry, R. L., Seguin, P., Cantrell, J., Tops, T., Uribe, P., Mallett, O., Zubko, T., Oetjen-Gerdes, L., Rasmussen, T. E., Butler, F. K., Kotwal, R. S., Holcomb, J. B., Wade, C., Champion, H., Lawnick, M., Moores, L., and Blackbourne, L. (2012b). Death on the battlefield (2001–2011): Implications for the future of combat casualty care. *Journal of Trauma and Acute Care Surgery*, 73(6), S431–S437.

Economist Democracy Index. (2019). https://www.eiu.com/topic/democracy-index

Eibner C. (2016). Current and projected characteristics and unique health care needs of the patient population served by the Department of Veterans Affairs. *RAND Health Quarterly*, 5(4), 13.

Eisenstein, N., Naumann, D., Burns, D., Stapley, S., and Draper, H. (2018). Left of bang interventions in trauma: Ethical implications for military medical prophylaxis. *Journal of Medical Ethics*, 44(7), 504–508.

Eldon, J., Waddington, C., and Hadi, Y. (2008). Health system reconstruction: Can it contribute to state-building? Health and Fragile States Network. HLSP Institute. file:///C:/Users/user/Downloads/2008_Health_system_reconstruction.pdf

English, R. (2003). *Armed struggle: The history of the IRA*. Oxford: Oxford University Press.

Enzenauer, R. W., Vavra, D. E., and Butler, F. (2006). Combat ophthalmology when there isn't an assigned ophthalmologist. *Journal of Special Operations Medicine*, 6(2), 34–42.

Etzioni, A. (2002). Are particularistic obligations justified? a communitarian examination. *The Review of Politics* 64, 573–598.

Etzioni, A. (2007). Reconstruction: An agenda. *Journal of Intervention and Statebuilding*, 1(1), 27–45.

European Parliament. (2014). EU. Regulation (EU) No 536/2014 on clinical trials on medicinal products for human use, and repealing directive 2001/20/EC. https://ec.europa.eu/health/sites/health/files/files/eudralex/vol-1/reg_2014_536/reg_2014_536_en.pdf

Evans, N. (2011). Emerging military technologies: A case study in neurowarfare. In P. Tripodi and J. Wolfendale (Eds.), *New wars and new soldiers: Military ethics in a contemporary world* (pp. 105–116). Farnham, UK: Ashgate.

Even, D. (2013). Israeli doctors to give Washington tips on dealing with hunger strikers. *Ha'aretz*, July 8.

Fabre, C. (2021). *Through a glass darkly: The ethics of espionage and counter-intelligence.* Oxford: Oxford University Press.

Fang, R., Markandaya, M., DuBose, J. J., Cancio, L. C., Shackelford, S., and Blackbourne, L. H. (2015). Early in-theater management of combat-related traumatic brain injury: A prospective, observational study to identify opportunities for performance improvement. *Journal of Trauma and Acute Care Surgery*, 79(4), S181–S187.

Farley, K. M. J., and Veitch, J. A. (2003). Measuring morale, cohesion, and confidence in leadership: What are the implications for leaders. *The Canadian Journal of Police & Security Services*, 2003(1), 353–364.

Farmer, B. (2014). Help for heroes: Up to 75,000 British scarred by Iraq and Afghanistan. *The Telegraph*, October 3.

Fauci, A. S. (2007). The expanding global health agenda: A welcome development. *Nature Medicine*, 13(10), 1169–1171.

FDA Guidance. (2013). Guidance for institutional review boards, clinical investigators, and sponsors: Exception from informed consent requirements for emergency research. US Department of Health and Human Services, Food and Drug Administration. https://www.fda.gov/downloads/regulatoryinformation/guidances/ucm249673.pdf

FDA. (2018). Lasik. US Department of Health and Human Services, Food and Drug Administration. https://www.fda.gov/medical-devices/surgery-devices/lasik

Feickert, A. (2010). Mine-resistant, ambush-protected (MRAP) vehicles: Background and issues for Congress. Congressional Research Service, Report No. a502022. https://apps.dtic.mil/dtic/tr/fulltext/u2/a502022.pdf.

Feickert, A. (2018). U.S. special operations forces (SOF): Background and issues for Congress. Congressional Research Service, Report No. RS21048. https://fas.org/sgp/crs/natsec/RS21048.pdf

Feinsilver, J. M. (2010). Fifty years of Cuba's medical diplomacy: From idealism to pragmatism. *Cuban Studies*, 41(1), 85–104.

Feldbaum, H., and Michaud, J. (2010). Health diplomacy and the enduring relevance of foreign policy interests. *PLoS Medicine*, 7(4), e1000226.

Feldman, N. (2004). *What we owe Iraq.* Princeton, NJ: Princeton University Press.

Filc, D., Ziv, H., Nassar, M., and Davidovitch, N. (2014). Palestinian prisoners' hunger-strikes in Israeli prisons: Beyond the dual-loyalty dilemma in medical practice and patient care. *Public Health Ethics*, 7(3), 229–238.

Finkelstein, C., and Xenakis, S. N. (2020). Repairing the damage from illegal acts of state: The costs of failed accountability for torture. In J. B. Barela, M. Fallon, G. Gagioli, and J. D. Ohlin (Eds.), *Interrogation and torture: Integrating efficacy with law and morality* (pp. 1–18). Oxford: Oxford University Press.

Fish, P. N. (2014). *Army medical officer's guide.* Mechanicsburg, PA: Stackpole Books.

Fishstein, P., and Wilder, A. (2012). *Winning hearts and minds? Examining the relationship between aid and security in Afghanistan.* Medford, MA: Feinstein International Center.

FitzPatrick, W. J., and Zwangziger, L. L. (2003). Defending against biological warfare: Ethical issues involving the coercive use of investigational drugs and biologics in the military. *The Journal of Philosophy, Science and Law*, 3(2), 1–16.

Flower, R., Dando, M., Hay, A., Iverson, S., Robbins, T., Robinson, J. P., Rose, S., Stirling, A., Tracey, I., and Wessely, S. (2012). *Brain waves module 3: Neuroscience, conflict, and security.* London: The Royal Society.

FM 3-24. (2006). *Counterinsurgency*. Field Manual 3-24. Washington, DC: Department of the Army. https://legacy.npr.org/documents/2008/may/counterinsurgency_manual.pdf

FM 4-02.46 (2007). *Medical support to detainee operations*. Field Manual 4.02.46. Washington, DC: Department of the Army. https://info.publicintelligence.net/USArmy-DetaineeMedicalSupport.pdf

FM 3-24.2. (2009). *Tactics in counterinsurgency*. Field Manual 3-42.2. Washington DC: Department of the Army.

FM 4-02. (2013). *Army health service*. Field Manual 4-02. Washington DC: Department of the Army.

Fox, K. (2013). Ethical considerations for engineers working in cybernetic implants. In proceedings of the IEEE International Conference on Cybernetics (CYBCO) (pp. 273–277). Lausanne: IEEE.

Frame, T. (Ed.). (2015). *Moral injury: Unseen wounds in an age of barbarism*. Pontypridd, UK: University of South Wales Press.

Freedom House. (2002). *Freedom in the world. The annual survey of political and civil liberties 2001–2002*. Livingston, NJ: Transaction Publishers.

Freedom House. (2009; 2013; 2018). *Freedom in the world. The annual survey of political and civil liberties*. New York: Rowman & Littlefield Publishers, Inc.

Freedom House. (2019). Countries and territories. https://freedomhouse.org/countries/nations-transit/scores?sort=desc&order=Country

Friedl, K. E. (2015). US Army research on pharmacological enhancement of soldier performance: Stimulants, anabolic hormones, and blood doping. *The Journal of Strength & Conditioning Research*, 29(November), S71–S76.

Friedman, N. (2013). This truck saved my life: Lessons learned from the MRAP vehicle program. Joint Program Office, Mine-Resistant Ambush-Protected Vehicles. Washington, DC: Delta Resources. https://www.dau.edu/cop/pm/dau%20sponsored%20documents/mrap%20history%20final%2030june2014.pdf

Frost, A., Wilkinson, M., Boyle, P., Patel, P., and Sullivan, R. (2016). An assessment of the barriers to accessing the basic package of health services (BPHS) in Afghanistan: Was the BPHS a success? *Globalization and Health*, 12, 71.

Frowe, H. (2014). *Defensive killing*. Oxford: Oxford University Press.

Fulton, L. V., and Brooks, M. S. (2018). An evaluation of alternatives for providing care to veterans. *Healthcare*, 6(3), 92.

Fund for Peace. (2006–2018). Fragile states index (2006–2018). https://www.arcgis.com/apps/MapSeries/index.html?appid=7e7947483f8342f8a31445cebcce3754

Fund for Peace. (2019). Fragile states index annual report 2019. https://fundforpeace.org/wp-content/uploads/2019/04/9511904-fragilestatesindex.pdf

Fund for Peace. (2020). Fragile states index. https://fundforpeace.org/2019/04/10/fragile-states-index-2019/

Gabriel, R. A. (2013). *Between flesh and steel: A history of military medicine from the Middle Ages to the war in Afghanistan*. Washington, DC: Potomac Books.

Gabriel, R. A., and Metz, K. S. (1992). *A history of military medicine*. New York: Greenwood Press.

Galliott, J. and Lotz, M. (2017). Introduction. In J. Galliott and M. Lotz (Eds.), *Super soldiers: The ethical, legal and social implications* (pp. 1–8). London: Routledge.

Galuszka, D. H. (2006). *Medical logistics in a new theater of operations: An Operation Iraqi Freedom case study*. Fort Leavenworth, KS: School of Advanced Military Studies United States Army Command and General Staff College.

Government Accounting Office (GAO). (2007). *Military operations: The Department of Defense's use of solatia and condolence payments in Iraq and Afghanistan.* Washington, DC: US Government Accounting Office. https://www.gao.gov/new.items/d07699.pdf

Government Accounting Office (GAO). (2008). *Provincial reconstruction teams in Afghanistan and Iraq.* https://www.gao.gov/products/GAO-09-86R.

Government Accounting Office (GAO). (2013). Defense health: Actions needed to help ensure combat casualty care research achieves goals. https://www.gao.gov/assets/660/652139.pdf

Garasic, M. (2015). *Guantanamo and other cases of enforced medical treatment: A biopolitical analysis.* Dordrecht: Springer.

Garreau, J. (2005). Enhancing the warriors. *Fortune* 151, 11 (May 30): 101–108. Cited in McIntosh, D. (2010). The transhuman security dilemma. *Journal of Evolution and Technology,* 21(2). 32–48.

Gawande, A. (2004). Casualties of war—Military care for the wounded from Iraq and Afghanistan. *New England Journal of Medicine,* 351(24), 2471–2475.

Geiling, J., Rosen, J. M., and Edwards, R. D. (2012). Medical costs of war in 2035: Long-term care challenges for veterans of Iraq and Afghanistan. *Military Medicine,* 177(11), 1235–1244.

Gibbs, D. A., and Olmsted, K. L. Rae (2011). Preliminary examination of the confidential alcohol treatment and education program. *Military Psychology,* 23(1), 97–111.

Gilbert, P. (2013). Medical neutrality and the dilemmas of war. In M. L. Gross and D. Carrick (Eds.), *Military medical ethics for the 21st century* (pp. 85–95). London: Routledge.

Gillenwater, G. E. (2008). FDA's emergency research rule: An inch given, a yard taken. *Food and Drug Law Journal,* 63(1), 217–256.

Ginbar, Y. (2008). *Why not torture terrorists? Moral, practical and legal aspects of the "ticking bomb" justification for torture.* Oxford: Oxford University Press.

Ginn, R. V. N. (1977). *The history of the US Army Medical Service Corps.* Washington, DC: US Government Printing Office.

Giordano, J., and Wurzman, R. (2011). Neurotechnologies as weapons in national intelligence and defense–An overview. *A Journal of Science, Technology, Ethics, and Policy,* 2(1), T55–T71.

Giustino, T. F., Fitzgerald, P. J., and Maren, S. (2016). Revisiting propranolol and PTSD: Memory erasure or extinction enhancement? *Neurobiology of Learning and Memory,* 130, 26–33.

Glick, S. M. (1997). Unlimited human autonomy: A cultural bias? *New England Journal of Medicine,* 336(13), 954–956.

Global Security. (2019). Iraqi military reconstruction. https://www.globalsecurity.org/military/world/iraq/iraq-corps.htm

Goldberg, M. S. (2010). Death and injury rates of U.S. military personnel in Iraq. *Military Medicine,* 175(4), 220–226.

Goldberg, M. S. (2016). Casualty rates of US military personnel during the wars in Iraq and Afghanistan. *Defence and Peace Economics,* 29(1), 44–61.

Goldkind, S. F., Brosch, L. R., Biros, M., Sillbergleit, R. S., and Sopko, G. (2014). Centralized IRB models for emergency care research. *IRB: Ethics & Human Research,* 36(2), 1–9.

Goodhand, J. (2006). *Aiding peace? The role of NGOs in armed conflict.* Boulder, CO: Lynne Rienner.

Goodman, R., and Roseman, M. (2009). *Interrogations, force feedings, and the role of health professionals: New perspectives on international human rights, humanitarian law, and ethics.* Cambridge, MA: Harvard University Press.

Gordon, M. R., and Trainor, B. E. (2006). *Cobra II: The inside story of the invasion and occupation of Iraq.* New York: Pantheon Books.

Gordon, S. (2010). The United Kingdom's stabilisation model and Afghanistan: The impact on humanitarian actors. *Disasters,* 34(S3), S368–S387.

Gordon, S. (2013). Health, conflict, stability and statebuilding: A house built on sand? *Journal of Intervention and Statebuilding,* 7(1), 29–44.

Gordon, S. (2014). The military physician and contested medical humanitarianism: A dueling identity? *Social Science & Medicine,* 120, 421–429.

Green, L. C. (1985). Superior orders and the reasonable man. In L. C. Green. *Essays on the modern law of war* (pp. 245–283). Ardsley, NY: Transnational Publishers.

Greenawalt, K. (1984). The perplexing borders of justification and excuse. *Columbia Law Review,* 84, 1897–1927.

Greenberg, H. (2006). IDF: Malfunction possible cause of Gaza incident. *Ynet,* October 8. https://www.ynetnews.com/articles/0,7340,L-3325803,00.html.

Greenberg, K. (2006). *The torture debate in America.* Cambridge: Cambridge University Press.

Gronke, P., Rejali, D., Drenguis, D., Hicks, J., Miller, P., and Nakayama, B. (2010). US public opinion on torture, 2001–2009. *PS: Political Science & Politics,* 43(3), 437–444.

Gross, M. L. (2006). *Bioethics and armed conflict: Moral dilemmas of medicine and war.* Cambridge, MA: MIT Press.

Gross, M. L. (2008a). The second Lebanon war: The question of proportionality and the prospect of non-lethal warfare. *Journal of Military Ethics,* 7(1), 1–22.

Gross, M. L. (2008b). Is medicine a pacifist vocation or should doctors help build bombs? In F. Allhoff (Ed.), *Physicians at war* (pp. 151–166). Dordrecht: Springer.

Gross, M. L. (2010). *Moral dilemmas of modern war: Torture, assassination and blackmail in an age of asymmetric conflict.* Cambridge, UK: Cambridge University Press.

Gross, M. L. (2013). The limits of impartial medical treatment during armed conflict. In M. L. Gross and D. Carrick (Eds.), *Military medical ethics for the 21st century* (pp. 71–84). London: Routledge.

Gross, M. L. (2015). *The ethics of insurgency: A critical guide to just guerrilla warfare.* Cambridge: Cambridge University Press.

Gross, M. L., Canetti, D., and Vashdi, D. R. (2017). Cyberterrorism: Its effects on psychological well-being, public confidence and political attitudes. *Journal of Cybersecurity,* 3(1), 49–58.

Grossman, D. (2014). *On killing: The psychological cost of learning to kill in war and society.* New York: Open Road Media.

Guardian. (2019). British dead and wounded in Afghanistan, month by month. *The Guardian Datablog.* https://www.theguardian.com/news/datablog/2009/sep/17/afghanistan-casualties-dead-wounded-british-data#data.

Gutmann, A., and Thompson, D. (2009). *Why deliberative democracy?* Princeton, NJ: Princeton University Press.

Habermas, J. (1979). *Communication and the evolution of society.* Boston: Beacon Press.

Habermas, J. (1990). *Moral consciousness and communicative action.* Cambridge: MIT Press.

Habermas, J. (2006). Political communication in media society: Does democracy still enjoy an epistemic dimension? The impact of normative theory on empirical research. *Communication Theory*, 16(4), 411–426.

Hagopian, A., Flaxman, A. D., Takaro, T. K., Al Shatari, S. A. E., Rajaratnam, J., Becker, S., Levin-Rector, A., Galway, L., Al-Yasseri, B. J. H., Weiss, W. M., Murray, C. J., and Burnham, G. (2013). Mortality in Iraq associated with the 2003–2011 war and occupation: Findings from a national cluster sample survey by the university collaborative Iraq Mortality Study. *PLoS Medicine*, 10(10), 1–15.

Hague Convention. (1907). *Annex to the convention (IV) respecting the laws and customs of war on land and its annex: Regulations concerning the laws and customs of war on land.* The Hague.

Hatzfeld J. J., Childs, J. D., Dempsey, M. P., Chapman, G. D., Dalle Lucca, J. J., Brininger, T., Tamminga, C., Richardson, R. T., Alexander, S., and Chung, K. K. (2013). Evolution of biomedical research during combat operations. *Journal of Trauma and Acute Care Surgery*, 75(2), S115–S119.

Hayati, R., Bastani, P., Kabir, M. J., Kavosi, Z., and Sobhani, G. (2018). Scoping literature review on the basic health benefit package and its determinant criteria. *Globalization and Health*, 14, 26.

Hayward, R. A. (2017). Lessons from the rise-and fall? -of VA healthcare. *Journal of General Internal Medicine*, 32(1), 11–13.

Health Research Authority (UK). (2008). Medicines for human use 2004: Clinical trials regulations—Informed consent in clinical trials. Version 3. Dated 1 May 2008. National Health Service https://www.hra.nhs.uk/documents/294/informed-consent-in-ctimps.pdf

Held, V. (2006). *The ethics of care.* Oxford: Oxford University Press.

Heller, J. (1955). *Catch 22.* New York: Simon and Schuster.

Hennessy, K. (2016). *A legacy of lessons learned: Landstuhl regional medical center during wartime, 2001–2014.* Fort Sam Houston, TX: Army Medical Department.

Hennigan, W. J. (2017). The new American way of war. *Time Magazine*, November 30.

Henschke, A. (2019). Militaries and the duty of care to enhanced veterans. *Journal of The Royal Army Medical Corps*, 165(4), 220–225.

Herman, A., and Yarwood, R. (2015). From warfare to welfare: Veterans, military charities and the blurred spatiality of post-service welfare in the United Kingdom. *Environment and Planning* A, 47(12), 2628–2644.

Hester, R. (2017). Lack of access to mental health services contributing to the high suicide rates among veterans. *International Journal of Mental Health Systems*, 11(1), 47.

HHS. (2019). Who is eligible for Medicaid? Health and Human Services. https://www.hhs.gov/answers/medicare-and-medicaid/who-is-eligible-for-medicaid/index.html.

Hodges, R. D. (2010). Medical treatment for foreign nationals: Another coin of the realm. *Army Lawyer*, 2010(5), 52–58.

Hodgetts, T. J., Mahoney, P. F., Mozumder, A., and Mclennan, J. (2005). Care of civilians during military operations. *International Journal of Disaster Medicine*, 3(1-4), 3–24.

Hodgetts, T. J. (2014). A roadmap for innovation. *BMJ Military Health*, 160, 86–91.

Hoffman, D. H., Carter, D. J., Viglucci Lopez, C. R., Benzmiller, H. L., Guo, A. X., Latifi, Y., and Craig, D. C. (2015). *Report to the special committee of the board of directors of the American Psychological Association: Independent review relating to APA ethics guidelines, national security interrogations, and torture.* July 2. https://www.apa.org/independent-review/revised-report.pdf.

Holcomb, J. B., and Hoyt, D. B. (2015). Comprehensive injury research. *JAMA: The Journal of the American Medical Association*, 313(14), 1463–1464.

Holewinski, S. (2012). Making amends, a new expectation for civilian losses in armed conflict. In D. Rothbart, K. V. Korostelina, and M. D. Cherkaoui (Eds.), *Civilians and modern war: Armed conflict and the ideology of violence* (pp. 317–333). New York: Routledge.

Holman, V. (2008). Transition of the detainee healthcare system to a correctional model: An interagency approach. *United States Military Medical Department Journal*, October–December 2008, 29–34.

Horne, S. T., and Vassallo, J. (2015). Triage in the defence medical services. *Journal of the Royal Army Medical Corps*, 161(2), 90–93.

House of Commons Defence Committee. (2018). Mental health and the armed forces, Part One: The scale of mental health issues. London: House of Commons. https://publications.parliament.uk/pa/cm201719/cmselect/cmdfence/813/813.pdf

Howe, E. G. (2003a). Point/Counterpoint: A response to Drs. Sidel and Levy. In T. E. Beam and L. R. Spracino (Eds.), *Military medical ethics* (pp. 312–320). Falls Church, VA: Office of the Surgeon General, Department of the Army.

Howe, E. G. (2003b). Mixed agency in military medicine: Ethical roles in conflict. In T. E. Beam and L. R. Spracino (Eds.), *Military medical ethics* (pp. 331–365). Falls Church, VA: Office of the Surgeon General, Department of the Army.

Howe, E. G., Kosaraju, A., Laraby, P. R., and Casscells, S. W. (2009). Guantanamo: Ethics, interrogation, and force feeding. *Military Medicine*, 174(1), iv–xiii.

Hoyt, T. (2013). Limits to confidentiality in US Army treatment settings. *Military Psychology*, 25(1), 46–56.

Human Rights Watch (HRW). 2003. Off target: The conduct of the war and civilian casualties in Iraq. https://www.hrw.org/report/2003/12/11/target/conduct-war-and-civilian-casualties-iraq

HUD. (2019). *PIT veteran counts by state 2011–2019*. US Department of Housing and Urban Development. https://files.hudexchange.info/resources/documents/2011-2019-PIT-Veteran-Counts-by-State.xlsx.

Hynes, D. M., Koelling, K., Stroupe, K., Arnold, N., Mallin, K., Sohn, M., Weaver, F. M., Manheim, L., and Kok, L. (2007). Veterans' access to and use of Medicare and Veterans Affairs health care. *Medical Care*, 45(3), 214–223.

Iacopino, V., and Waldman, R. J. (1999). War and health from Solferino to Kosovo—The evolving role of physicians. *JAMA: The Journal of the American Medical Association*, 285(5), 479–481.

icasualties. (2019). *Casualties in Iraq and Afghanistan by year and country*. http://icasualties.org/.

ICISS. (2001). *The responsibility to protect. Report of the international commission on intervention and state sovereignty*. Ottawa: International Development Research Centre.

IDF. (1958). *IDF Military Advocate v Major Melinky and others, Verdict 3/57*. Israel Defense Forces, District Military Court, Central Command.

International Committee of the Red Cross (ICRC). (1949a). Geneva Convention (I) for the amelioration of the condition of the wounded and sick in armed forces in the field. Geneva: International Committee of the Red Cross.

International Committee of the Red Cross (ICRC). (1949b). Geneva Convention (IV) relative to the protection of civilian persons in time of war. Geneva: International Committee of the Red Cross.

International Committee of the Red Cross (ICRC). (1952). Commentary, Convention (I) for the amelioration of the condition of the wounded and sick in armed forces in the field. Geneva: International Committee of the Red Cross.

International Committee of the Red Cross (ICRC). (1958). Commentary, Convention (IV) relative to the protection of civilian persons in time of war. Geneva: International Committee of the Red Cross.

International Committee of the Red Cross (ICRC). (1977a). Protocol additional to the Geneva Conventions of 12 August 1949, and relating to the protection of victims of international armed conflicts (Protocol I), June 8, 1977. Geneva: International Committee of the Red Cross.

International Committee of the Red Cross (ICRC). (1977b). Protocol additional to the Geneva Conventions of 12 August 1949, and relating to the protection of victims of non-international armed conflicts (Protocol II), June 8, 1977. Geneva: International Committee of the Red Cross.

International Committee of the Red Cross (ICRC). (1987). Commentary on the Additional Protocols of 8 June 1977 to the Geneva Conventions of 12 August 1949. Geneva: International Committee of the Red Cross.

International Committee of the Red Cross (ICRC). (2006). Iraq: First ICRC visit to detainees at newly opened facility in Baghdad 03-10-2006. News Release 06/112. https://www.icrc.org/en/doc/resources/documents/news-release/2009-and-earlier/iraq-news-031006.htm

International Committee of the Red Cross (ICRC). (2007a). ICRC report on the treatment of fourteen "high value detainees" in CIA custody. https://file.wikileaks.org/file/icrc-report-2007.pdf

International Committee of the Red Cross (ICRC). (2007b). Iraq: ICRC activities, April to July 2007. https://www.icrc.org/en/doc/resources/documents/update/iraq-update-300607.htm

International Committee of the Red Cross (ICRC). (2009a). Iraq: ICRC activities in June 2009. https://www.icrc.org/en/doc/resources/documents/update/iraq-update-150709.htm

International Committee of the Red Cross (ICRC). (2010). Prisoners of war and detainees protected under international humanitarian law. https://www.icrc.org/en/document/protected-persons/prisoners-war

International Committee of the Red Cross (ICRC). (2013). Hunger strikers in prisons: the ICRC's position. http://www.icrc.org/eng/resources/documents/faq/hunger-strike-icrc-position.htm

International Committee of the Red Cross (ICRC). (2016). Commentary, Convention (I) for the amelioration of the condition of the wounded and sick in armed forces in the field. Geneva: International Committee of the Red Cross.

International Committee of the Red Cross (ICRC). (2020). Customary IHL database. https://ihl-databases.icrc.org/customary-ihl/eng/docs/v1_rul

Ignatieff, M. (2004). The lesser evil: Political ethics in an age of terror. Princeton, NJ: Princeton University Press.

IHME. (2020). Financing global health: Flows of global health financing. Seattle: University of Washington, Institute for Health Metrics and Evaluation. https://vizhub.healthdata.org/fgh/

Iraq MOH. (2004). Health in Iraq. Iraq Ministry of Health. https://www.who.int/hac/crises/irq/background/Iraq_Health_in_Iraq_second_edition.pdf?ua=1

Iraq MOH. (2009). A basic health services package for Iraq. Iraq Ministry of Health and World Health Organization. https://www.ecoi.net/en/file/local/1325478/1788_1315486906_basic-health-service-package-en.pdf

Iraq MOH. (2014). National health policy. Iraq Ministry of Health. https://extranet.who.int/countryplanningcycles/sites/default/files/planning_cycle_repository/iraq/iraqs_national_health_policy_2014-2023.pdf

Irmak, N. (2015). Professional ethics in extreme circumstances: Responsibilities of attending physicians and healthcare providers in hunger strikes. *Theoretical Medicine and Bioethics*, 36(4), 249–263.

Isaac, L., Main, K. L., Soman, S., Gotlib, I. H., Furst, A. J., Kinoshita, L. M., Fairchild, K. J., Yesavage, J. A., Ashford, J. W, Bayley, P. J., and Adamson, M. M. (2015). The impact of depression on veterans with PTSD and traumatic brain injury: A diffusion tensor imaging study. *Biological Psychology*, 105, 20–28.

ISAF. (2009). *ISAF provincial reconstruction team (PRT) handbook* (4th ed.). https://publicintelligence.net/isaf-provincial-reconstruction-team-prt-handbook/

Israel Law Review. (1989). Symposium on the report of the commission of inquiry into the methods of investigation of the general security service regarding hostile terrorist activity. *Israel Law Review* 23(1-2), 141–406.

Israel MFA. (2009). *The operation in Gaza: Factual and legal aspects.* Jerusalem: Israel Ministry of Foreign Affairs https://mfa.gov.il/MFA_Graphics/MFA%20Gallery/Documents/GazaOperation%20w%20Links.pdf.

Israel, B. (2010). COIN operations in Afghanistan. *Afghan Culture Newsletter* 10-64, 13–21.

Jacobsen, A. (2015). Engineering humans for war: Inside the Pentagon's efforts to create a super-soldier—and change the future of the battlefield. *The Atlantic*, September 23. https://www.theatlantic.com/international/archive/2015/09/military-technology-pentagon-robots/406786/

Jaff, D., Leatherman, S., and Tomaro, J. (2019). Responsive health services and quality care in settings of extreme adversity: The case of central and northern Iraq. *Medicine, Conflict and Survival*, 35(3), 227–240.

Jalali, A. A. (2016). Afghanistan national defense and security forces. *United States Institute of Peace PEACEWORKS*, 115, May, 1–31.

JASON (2010). *The $100 Genome: Implications for the DoD.* JSR-10-100. McLean, VA: JASON, The MITRE Corporation.

Jawad, S., Mahmood, M., Al Ameri, A., and Nakano, G. (2010). Post-conflict reconstruction in the health sector: Host nation perspective. In H. R. Yarger (Ed.), *Transitions: Issues, challenges, and solutions in international assistance* (pp. 95–110). Carlisle, PA: Peacekeeping and Stability Operations Institute, US Army War College.

Jebari, K. (2013). Brain machine interface and human enhancement–an ethical review. *Neuroethics*, 6(3), 617–625.

Johnson, W. B. (2008). Top ethical challenges for military clinical psychologists. *Military Psychology*, 20(1), 49–62.

Johnson, W. B., Grasso, I., and Maslowski, K. (2010). Conflicts between ethics and law for military mental health providers. *Military Medicine*, 175(8), 548–553.

Jones, A. R., and Fay, G. R. (2004). *Executive Summary: Investigation of intelligence activities at Abu Ghraib. AR 15-6 investigation of the Abu Ghraib Prison and 205th Military Intelligence Brigade.* Washington, DC: US Army Public Affairs.

Jones, S. G, Hillborne, L. H., Anthony, C. R., Davis, L. M., and Girosi, F. (2006). *Securing health: Lessons from nation-building missions.* Santa Monica, CA: RAND Corporation.

Jones, S. G. (2008). *Counterinsurgency in Afghanistan.* Santa Monica, CA: RAND Corporation.

Jonsen, A. R. (1998). *The birth of bioethics.* New York: Oxford University Press.

Josar, D. (2003). Voices on the ground: *Stars and Stripes* surveys troops on morale in Iraq. *Stars and Stripes,* October 15.

JP 4-02. (2001). *Doctrine for health service support.* Joint Publication 4-02, US Joint Chiefs of Staff. https://www.bits.de/NRANEU/others/jp-doctrine/jp4_02%2801%29.pdf.

JP 4-02. (2006). *Health service support,* Joint Publication No. 4-02, Washington, DC: Joint Chiefs of Staff. https://www.health.mil/Reference-Center/Policies/2006/10/31/Joint-Publication-402-Health-Service-Support

JTF (2013a). Standard operating procedure #001: Medical management of detainees on hunger strike. Joint Task Force–GTMO. March 5. http://www.aele.org/law/gitmo-force-feed.pdf.

JTF. (2013b). Legal authority and policy for enteral feeding at JFT-GTMO, Joint Task Force–GTMO, June 12. https://www.scribd.com/document/254035173/Forcefeeding.

Kalshoven, F. (2007). International humanitarian law and violation of medical neutrality. In *Reflections on the Law of War* (pp. 993–1021). Leiden, The Netherlands: Brill Nijhoff.

Kass, N. E. (2001). An ethics framework for public health. *American Journal of Public Health,* 91(11), 1776–1782.

Katz, R. V., Russell, S. L., Kressin, N. R., Green, B. L., Wang, M. Q., James, S. A., and Claudio, C. (2006). The Tuskegee Legacy Project: Willingness of minorities to participate in biomedical research. *Journal of Health Care for The Poor and Underserved,* 17(4), 698–715.

Katzenstein, P. J. (1996a). *The culture of national security: Norms and identity in world politics.* New York: Columbia University Press.

Kauvar, D. S., and Drury, T. A. (2013). Forward-deployed medical assets and the COIN offensive. *Joint Force Quarterly,* 70, 15–20.

Kellet, A. (1982). *Combat motivation: The behavior of men in battle.* Dordrecht, The Netherlands: Kluwer.

Kelly, J. F., Ritenour, A. E., McLaughlin, D. F., Bagg, K. A., Apodaca, A. N., Mallak, C. T., Pearse, L., Lawnick, R. N., Champion, H. R., Wade, C. E., and Holcomb, J. B. (2008). Injury severity and causes of death from Operation Iraqi Freedom and Operation Enduring Freedom: 2003–2004 vs 2006. *The Journal of Trauma: Injury, Infection, and Critical Care,* 64(2), S21–S27.

Kennedy, J. (2017). How drone strikes and a fake vaccination program have inhibited polio eradication in Pakistan: An analysis of national level data. *International Journal of Health Services,* 47(4), 807–825.

Kevany, S. (2014). Global health diplomacy, "smart power," and the new world order. *Global Public Health,* 9(7), 787–807.

Khoury, J. (2013). Analysis: For Palestinian prisoners in Israel, hunger strikes have become a winning strategy. *Ha'aretz,* April 24.

Kilcullen, D. (2006). Twenty-eight articles fundamentals of company-level counterinsurgency. *Marine Corps Gazette,* 90(7), 29–35.

Kilcullen, D. (2010). *Counterinsurgency.* Oxford: Oxford University Press.

Kim, C., Saeed, K. M. A., Salehi, A. S., and Zeng, W. (2016). An equity analysis of utilization of health services in Afghanistan using a national household survey. *BMC Public Health*, 16, 1–11.

King, A. (2013). *The combat soldier: Infantry tactics and cohesion in the twentieth and twenty-first centuries.* Oxford: Oxford University Press.

King, A. (2016). On combat effectiveness in the infantry platoon: Beyond the primary group thesis. *Security Studies*, 25(4), 699–728.

Kirke, C. (2010). Military cohesion, culture and social psychology. *Defense and Security Analysis*, 26(2), 143–159.

Klimo, P., Ragel, B. T., Scott, W. H., and McCafferty, R. (2010). Pediatric neurosurgery during Operation Enduring Freedom. *Journal of Neurosurgery: Pediatrics*, 6(2), 107–114.

Kondro, W. (2007). Afghanistan: Outside the comfort zone in a war zone. *CMAJ*, 177(2), 131–134.

Kragh Jr., J. F., Walters, T. J., Baer, D. G., Fox, C. J., Wade, C. E., Salinas, J., and Holcomb, J. B. (2009). Survival with emergency tourniquet use to stop bleeding in major limb trauma. *Annals of Surgery*, 249(1), 1–7.

Krajeski, J. (2012). After the hunger strike. *The New Yorker*, November 29.

Krueger, C. A., Wenke, J. C., and Ficke, J. R. (2012). Ten years at war: Comprehensive analysis of amputation trends. *Journal of Trauma and Acute Care Surgery*, 73(6), S438–S444.

Kruk, M. E., Freedman, L. P., Anglin, G. A., and Waldman, R. J. (2010). Rebuilding health systems to improve health and promote statebuilding in post-conflict countries: A theoretical framework and research agenda. *Social Science and Medicine*, 70(1), 89–97.

Labarre, F. (2011). *Provincial reconstruction teams. Comparing the American, British and Canadian models* DRDC CORA CR 2011-082. Kingston, Ontario: Defence R&D Canada Centre for Operational Research & Analysis Strategic Analysis Section. https://www.academia.edu/1023707/Provincial_Reconstruction_Teams_in_Afghanistan_and_Iraq_The_American_British_and_Canadian_Approaches

Lairet, J., Bebarta, V. S., Maddry, J. K., Reeves, L., Mora, A., Blackbourne, L., and Rasmussen, T. (2019). Prehospital interventions performed in Afghanistan between November 2009 and March 2014. *Military Medicine*, 184, 133–137.

Landgericht Bonn (Bonn Regional Court). (2013). *Case number: 1O 460/11*, November 12.

Lane, I., Stockinger, Z., Sauer, S., Ervin, M., Wirt, M., Bree, S., Gross, K., Bailey, J., Hodgetts, B. T., and Mann-Salinas, E. (2017). The Afghan theater: A review of military medical doctrine from 2008 to 2014. *Military Medicine*, 182(S1), 32–40.

Langer, G. (2005). 2005 Poll: Four years after the fall of the Taliban, Afghans optimistic about the future. *ABC News*, February 4. https://abcnews.go.com/%20International/PollVault/story?id=1363276.

Langleben, D. D., and Moriarty, J. C. (2013). Using brain imaging for lie detection: Where science, law, and policy collide. *Psychology, Public Policy, and Law*, 19(2), 222.

Laurie, G. T., Harmon, S. H. E., and Porter, G. (2016). *Mason and McCall Smith's law and medical ethics.* Oxford: Oxford University Press.

Laverack, G. (2006). Improving health outcomes through community empowerment: A review of the literature. *Journal of Health, Population and Nutrition*, 24(1), 113–120.

Lederer, S. E. (2003). The Cold War and beyond: Covert and deceptive American medical experimentation. In T. E. Beam and L. R. Spracino (Eds.), *Military medical ethics* (pp. 507–531). Falls Church, VA: Office of the Surgeon General, Department of the Army.

Lederman, Z. (2018). Prisoners' competence to die: Hunger strike and cognitive competence. *Theoretical Medicine and Bioethics*, 39(4), 321–334.

Lee, J. (2012). *Detainee health care: Essential element of stability operations.* Carlisle, PA: Strategy Research Project, US Army War College. https://apps.dtic.mil/dtic/tr/fulltext/u2/a561275.pdf.

Lee, R. U., Parrish, S. C., Saeed, O., and Fiedler, J. P. (2015). Combat internist: The internal medicine experience in a combat hospital in Afghanistan. *Military Medicine*, 180(1), 12–16.

Lepora, C., and Goodin, R. E. (2013). *On complicity and compromise.* Oxford: Oxford University Press.

Lepora, C., and Millum, J. (2011). The tortured patient: A medical dilemma. *Hastings Center Report*, 41(3), 38–47.

Lerner, E. B., Cone, D. C., Weinstein, E. S., Schwartz, R. B., Coule, P. L., Cronin, M., Wedmore, I. S., Bulger E. M., Mulligan, D. A., Swienton, F. E., Sasser, S. M., Shah, U. A., Weireter L. G., Sanddal, T. L., Lairet, J., Markenson, D., Romig, L., Lord, G., Salomone, J., O'Connor, R., and Hunt, R. C. (2011). Mass casualty triage: An evaluation of the science and refinement of a national guideline. *Disaster Medicine and Public Health Preparedness*, 5(2), 129–137.

Lesho, E. P., Jawad, N. K., and Hameed, H. M. (2011). Towards a better approach to medical humanitarian assistance in Iraq and future counterinsurgency operations. *Military Medicine*, 176(1), 1–3.

Levinson, S. (2003). Precommitment and postcommitment: The ban on torture in the wake of September 11. *Texas Law Review*, 81(7), 2013–2054.

Levinson, S. (2004). Torture: A collection. Oxford: Oxford University Press.

Lewis, D. A., Modirzadeh, N. K., and Blum, G. (2015). Medical care in armed conflict: International humanitarian law and state responses to terrorism. *Harvard Law School Program on International Law and Armed Conflict* (HLS PILAC). http://pilac.law.harvard.edu/research-menu/#research

Lewis, P. (2015). Senate passes torture ban despite Republican opposition. *The Guardian*, June 16.

Library of Congress. (2006). *Profile: Iraq.* Library of Congress—Federal Research Division Country http://memory.loc.gov/frd/cs/profiles/Iraq.pdf

Library of Congress. (2008). *Profile: Afghanistan,* Library of Congress—Federal Research Division Country http://lcweb2.loc.gov/frd/cs/profiles/Afghanistan.pdf

Lifton, R. J. (2004). Doctors and torture. *New England Journal of Medicine*, 351(5), 415–416.

Liivoja, R. (2017). Biomedical enhancement of warfighters and the legal protection of military medical personnel in armed conflict. *Medical Law Review*, 26(3), 421–448.

Lin, P. (2012). More than human? The ethics of biologically enhancing soldiers. *The Atlantic*, February 16.

Linton, R. (2008). Applying for ethical approval from the MoD research ethics committee. *Journal of the Royal Naval Medical Service*, 94(1), 41–46.

Lischer, S. (2007). Military intervention and the humanitarian force multiplier. *Global Governance*, 13(1), 99–118.

Litz, B. T., and Kerig, P. K. (2019). Introduction to the special issue on moral injury: Conceptual challenges, methodological issues, and clinical applications. *Journal of Traumatic Stress*, 32(3), 341–349.

Livingston, I. S., and O'Hanlo, M. (2011). Afghanistan index: Tracking variables of reconstruction & security in Post-9/11 Afghanistan. https://www.brookings.edu/wp-content/uploads/2016/07/index20111231.pdf.

London, L., Rubenstein, L. S., Baldwin-Ragaven, L., and Van Es, A. (2006). Dual loyalty among military health professionals: Human rights and ethics in times of armed conflict. *Cambridge Quarterly of Healthcare Ethics*, 15(4), 381–391.

Lougee, D. (2007). Can we build a better medical civic assistance program? Making the most of medical humanitarian civic assistance funding. *The Defense Institute of Security Assistance Management Journal*, February 2007, 68–73.

Luban, D. (2005). Liberalism, torture, and the ticking bomb. *Virginia Law Review*, 91, 1425–1461.

Lundberg, K., Kjellström, S., Jonsson, A., and Sandman, L. (2014). Experiences of Swedish military medical personnel in combat zones: Adapting to competing loyalties. *Military Medicine*, *179*(8), 821–826.

Mabry, R. L., and Kotwal, R. (2017). Prehospital casualty care: The next frontier. In A. L. Kellerman and E. Elster (Eds.), *Out of the crucible: How the US military transformed combat casualty care in Iraq and Afghanistan* (pp. 339–347). Fort Sam Houston, TX: The Army Medical Department.

MacIntyre, A. (1981). *After virtue: A study in moral theory*. London: Duckworth.

MacKay, N. J. (2015). When Lanchester met Richardson, the outcome was stalemate: A parable for mathematical models of insurgency. *Journal of the Operational Research Society*, 66(2), 191–201.

MacQueen, G., and Santa-Barbara, J. (2000). Peace building through health initiatives. *British Medical Journal*, 321, 293–296.

Malet, D. (2015). Captain America in international relations: The biotech revolution in military affairs. *Defence Studies,* 15(4), 1–21.

Malish, R., Scott, J. S., and Rasheed, B. O. (2006). Military-civic action: Lessons learned from a brigade-level aid project in the 2003 war with Iraq. *Prehospital and Disaster Medicine*,21(3), 135–138.

Malsby, R. F. (2008). *Which end does the thermometer go? Application of military medicine in counterinsurgency*. Unpublished MA thesis. Fort Leavenworth, KS: Army Command and General Staff College.

Malsby, R. F., and Territo, B. M. (2007). Medical civilian-assistance programs (MEDCAP) in direct support of kinetic operations: A template for integration of civil medical operations as a force multiplier during combat operations. *Journal of Special Operations Medicine*, 7(1), 39–43.

Manning, F. J. (1994). Morale and cohesion in military psychiatry. In F. D. Jones, L. R. Sparacino, V. L. Wilcox, and J. M. Rothberg (Eds.), *Military psychology preparing in peace and war* (pp. 1–18). Washington, DC: Office of the Surgeon General, Department of the Army.

Martin, J. E., Teff, R. J., and Spinella, P. C. (2010). Care of pediatric neurosurgical patients in Iraq in 2007: Clinical and ethical experience of a field hospital. *Journal of Neurosurgery: Pediatrics*, 6(3), 250–256.

Mason, A. (1997). Special obligations to compatriots. *Ethics*, 107(3), 427–447.

Mayo Clinic. (2019). *Patient rights and responsibilities*. https://www.mayoclinic.org/es-es/documents/mcj6256-pdf/doc-20079310.

McCafferty, R. R., Neal, C. J., Marshall, S. A., Pamplin, J. C., Rivet, D., Hood, B. J., Cooper, P. B., and Stockinger, Z. (2018). Neurosurgery and medical management of severe head injury. *Military Medicine*, 183(suppl. 2), 67–72.

McColl, H., Bhui, K., and Jones, E. (2012). The role of doctors in investigation, prevention and treatment of torture. *Journal of the Royal Society of Medicine*, 105(11), 464–471.

McCoy, A. W. (2007). Science in Dachau's shadow: Hebb, Beecher, and the development of CIA psychological torture and modern medical ethics. *Journal of the History of the Behavioral Sciences*, 43(4), 401–417.

Mcinnes, C., and Rushton, S. (2014). Health for health's sake, winning for God's sake: US global health diplomacy and smart power in Iraq and Afghanistan. *Review of International Studies*, 40(5), 835–857.

McIntyre. A. (2019). Doctrine of double effect. *The Stanford Encyclopedia of Philosophy*. https://plato.stanford.edu/archives/spr2019/entries/double-effect/.

McManus J., McClinton, A., Gerhardt, R., and Morris, M. (2007). Performance of ethical military research is possible: On and off the battlefield. *Science and Engineering Ethics*, 13(3), 297–303.

McManus, J., Mehta, S. G., McClinton, A. R., De Lorenzo, R. A., and Baskin, T. W. (2005). Informed consent and ethical issues in military medical research. *Academic Emergency Medicine*, 12(11), 1120–1126.

McMaster University. (2019). The Hippocratic oath and others. Health Sciences Library, Guides & Tutorials, McMaster University, April 26. https://hslmcmaster.libguides.com/c.php?g=306726&p=2044095.

Mehlman, M. J. (2013). Enhanced warfighters: Risk, ethics, and policy. *Case Legal Studies Research Paper, 2013-2*. https://papers.ssrn.com/sol3/papers.cfm?abstract_id=2202982.

Mehlman, M. J. (2019). Bioethics of military performance enhancement. *Journal of the Royal Army Medical Corps*, 165(4), 226–231.

Mehlman, M. J., and Corley, R. (2014). A framework for military bioethics. *Journal of Military Ethics*, 13(4), 331–349.

Mehlman, M. J., and Li, T. Y. (2014). Ethical, legal, social, and policy issues in the use of genomic technology by the U.S. military. *Journal of Law and The Biosciences*, 1(3), 244–280.

Mehring, S. (2015). *First do no harm: Medical ethics in international humanitarian law*. Leiden: Brill.

Meisels, T. (2014). Assassination: Targeting nuclear scientists. *Law and Philosophy*, 33(2), 207–234.

Meissner, C. A., Surmon-Böhr, F., Oleszkiewicz, S., and Alison, L. J. (2017). Developing an evidence-based perspective on interrogation: A review of the US government's high-value detainee interrogation group research program. *Psychology, Public Policy, and Law*, 23(4), 438–457.

Melzer, N. (2009). *Interpretive guidance on the notion of direct participation in hostilities under international humanitarian law*. Geneva: International Committee of the Red Cross.

Melzer, N. (2020). Foreword. In J. B. Barela, M. Fallon, G. Gagioli, and J. D. Ohlin (Eds.), *Interrogation and torture: Integrating efficacy with law and morality* (pp. ix–x). Oxford: Oxford University Press.

Messelken, D. (2018). The "peace role" of healthcare during war: Understanding the importance of medical impartiality. *Journal of the Royal Army Medical Corps*, 165(4), 232–235.

METRC. (2019). *Major Extremity Trauma and Rehabilitation Consortium (METRC)*. Johns Hopkins University, Bloomberg School of Public Health. https://www.jhsph.edu/faculty/research/map/US/1413/8051

Micah, A. E., and Dieleman, J. (2018). *Financing global health 2018: Countries and programs in transition*. Seattle: University of Washington, Institute for Health Metrics and Evaluation.

Michael, M., Pavignani, E., and Hill, P. S. (2013). Too good to be true? An assessment of health system progress in Afghanistan, 2002–2012. *Medicine, Conflict and Survival*, 29(4), 322–345.

Miles, S. H., Alencar, T., and Crock, B. N. (2010). Punishing physicians who torture: A work in progress. *Torture*, 20(1), 23–31.

Miles, S. H. (2004). Abu Ghraib: Its legacy for military medicine. *The Lancet*, 364(9435), 725–729.

Miles, S. H. (2006). *Oath betrayed: Torture, medical complicity, and the war on terror*. New York: Random House.

Miles, S. H. (2020). *The torture doctors: Human rights crimes and the road to justice*. Washington, DC: Georgetown University Press.

Miller, D. (2005). Reasonable partiality towards compatriots. *Ethical Theory and Moral Practice*, 8(1-2), 63–81.

Miller, J. P. (2017). A care ethics approach to medical eligibility in armed conflict. *The American Journal of Bioethics*, 17(10), 61–63.

Miller, F. G., and Brody, H. (2003). A critique of clinical equipoise: Therapeutic misconception in the ethics of clinical trials. *Hastings Center Report*, 33(3), 19–28.

Miller, F. G., & Brody, H. (2007). Clinical equipoise and the incoherence of research ethics. *The Journal of Medicine And Philosophy*, 32(2), 151–165.

Miranda, R. A., Casebeer, W. D., Hein, A. M., Judy, J. W., Krotkov, E. P., Laabs, T. L., Manzo, J. L., Pankratz, K. G., Pratt, G. A., Sanchez, J. C., Weber, D. J., Wheeler G. L., and Ling, G. S. F. (2015). DARPA-funded efforts in the development of novel brain–computer interface technologies. *Journal of Neuroscience Methods*, 244, 52–67.

Mitchell, D. F. (2015). Blurred lines? Provincial reconstruction teams and NGO insecurity in Afghanistan, 2010–2011. *Stability: International Journal of Security and Development*, 4(1), 1–18.

MNC-I. (2009). *Money as a weapon system (MAAWS)*. MNC-I cJ8 SOP, Multinational Corps–Iraq. https://info.publicintelligence.net/MAAWS%20Jan%2009.pdf

Moreno, J. D., Schmidt, U., and Joffe, S. (2017). The Nuremberg Code 70 years later. *JAMA: The Journal of the American Medical Association*, 318(9), 795–796.

Moreno, J. D. (2013). *Undue risk: Secret state experiments on humans*. New York: Routledge.

Morton, M. J., and Burnham, G. M. (2010). Dilemmas and controversies within civilian and military organizations in the execution of humanitarian aid in Iraq: A review. *American Journal of Disaster Medicine*, 5(6), 385–391.

MOU. (2012). *Memorandum of understanding between The Islamic Republic of Afghanistan and the United States of America on transfer of U.S. detention facilities in Afghan territory to Afghanistan*. https://www.afghanistan-analysts.org/en/reports/rights-freedom/the-bagram-memorandum-handing-over-the-other-guantanamo/

Mount, M. (2009). Study: Army morale down in Afghanistan, up in Iraq. *CNN*, November 14.

Mumford, A. (2012). Veteran care in the United Kingdom and the sustainability of the "military covenant." *The Political Quarterly*, 83(4), 820–826.

Murphym D., Marteau, T., Hotopf, M., Rona, R., and Wessely, S. (2008). Why do UK military personnel refuse the anthrax vaccination? *Biosecurity and Bioterrorism: Biodefense Strategy, Practice, and Science*, 6(3), 237–242.

Murray, C. K., Roop, S. A., and Hospenthal, D. R. (2005). Medical problems of detainees after the conclusion of major ground combat during Operation Iraqi Freedom. *Military Medicine*, 170(6), 501–504.

Naland, J. K. (2011). Lessons from embedded provincial reconstruction teams in Iraq, special report. Washington, DC: US Institute of Peace. Special Report 290.

Nass, M. (2002). The anthrax vaccine program: An analysis of the CDC's recommendations for vaccine use. *American Journal of Public Health*, 92(5), 715–721.

NATO. (2010). Medical civil-military interaction—A report by NATO's Joint Analysis and Lessons Learned Centre, JALLC/CG/10/152. http://www.jallc.nato.int/products/docs/medical_civil-military_interaction.pdf.

NATO. (2011). International security assistance force (ISAF): Key facts and figures. https://www.nato.int/isaf/placemats_archive/2011-07-26-ISAF-Placemat.pdf.

NATO. (2019). Allied joint doctrine for medical support, edition C, version 1. September. https://assets.publishing.service.gov.uk/government/uploads/system/uploads/attachment_data/file/841686/doctrine_nato_med_spt_ajp_4_10.pdf

NCII and Oxfam. (2007). *Rising to the humanitarian challenge in Iraq 2007: Briefing Paper 105*. NGO Coordination Committee in Iraq and Oxfam. https://www.oxfam.org.hk/tc/f/news_and_publication/1429/content_3574tc.pdf.

Neel, S. (1991). *Medical support of the U.S. army in Vietnam 1965–1970*. Washington, DC: Department of the Army.

Neff, L. P., Spinella, P. C., Azarow, K. S., and Jafri, M. A. (2017). The pediatric patient in wartime. In M. J. Martin, A. Beekley, and M. Eckert (Eds.), *Front line surgery* (pp. 543–562). New York: Springer International Publishing.

Nessen S., Lounsbury, D. E., and Hetz, S. P. (2008). *War surgery in Afghanistan and Iraq: A series of cases, 2003-2007*. Washington, DC: Dept. of the Army, Office of the Surgeon General, Department of the Army.

Nessen, S. C. (2005). *The mobile modular surgical hospital: The army medical department's future unit of action*. MA thesis. Fort Leavenworth, KS: Army Command and General Staff College.

Neuhauser, J. A. (2010). Lives of quiet desperation: The conflict between military necessity and confidentiality. *Creighton Law Review*, 44(4), 1003–1044.

Newbrander, W., Ickx, P., Feroz, F., and Stanekzai, H. (2014). Afghanistan's basic package of health services: Its development and effects on rebuilding the health system. *Global Public Health*, 9(sup1), S6–S28.

National Health Service (NHS). (2015). NHS Constitution. https://assets.publishing.service.gov.uk/government/uploads/system/uploads/attachment_data/file/480482/NHS_Constitution_WEB.pdf.

National Health Service (NHS). (2019). Guide to NHS waiting times in England. https://www.nhs.uk/using-the-nhs/nhs-services/hospitals/guide-to-nhs-waiting-times-in-england/.

National Health Service (NHS). (2020). Veterans: Priority NHS treatment. https://www.nhs.uk/using-the-nhs/military-healthcare/priority-nhs-treatment-for-veterans/.

Nightingale, S. L., Prasher, J. M., and Simonson, S. (2007). Emergency use authorization (EUA) to enable use of needed products in civilian and military emergencies, United States. *Emerging Infectious Diseases*, 13(7), 1046–1051.

NIH. (2019). NCI dictionary of cancer terms: Investigational drug. National Institute of Health, National Cancer Institute. https://www.cancer.gov/publications/dictionaries/cancer-terms/def/investigational-drug

Nordmann G., Woolley T., Doughty H. J., Dalle L., Hutchings S., and Kirkman E. (2014). Deployed research. *British Military Journal of Military Health*, 160(2), 92–98.

NRC. (2009). *Opportunities in neuroscience for future army applications. Committee on Opportunities in Neuroscience for Future Army Applications*. Board on Army Science and Technology Division on Engineering and Physical Sciences. National Research Council.Washington, DC: The National Academies Press.

Nussbaum, M. (2007). Human rights and human capabilities. *Harvard Human Rights Journal*, 20, 21–24.

NWP 1-14M. (2007). *The commander's handbook on the law of naval operations, NWP 1-14M*. Naval Warfare Publication, Quantico, VA: Department of the Navy. https://www.marines.mil/Portals/1/Publications/MCTP%2011-10B%20(%20Formerly%20MCWP%205-12.1).pdf?ver=2017-07-11-151548-683

Nye, J. (2008). Public diplomacy and soft power. *The ANNALS of the American Academy of Political and Social Science*, 616(1), 94–109.

O'Hanlon, C., Huang, C., Sloss, E., Anhang Price, R., Hussey, P., Farmer, C., and Gidengil, C. (2017). Comparing VA and non-VA quality of care: A systematic review. *Journal of General Internal Medicine*, 32(1), 105–121.

Obama, B. (2009). *Statement of President Barack Obama on release of OLC memos*. The White House, Office of the Press Secretary. https://obamawhitehouse.archives.gov/the-press-office/statement-president-barack-obama-release-olc-memos.

Obama, B. (2014). *Paying tribute to our fallen heroes this Memorial Day*. The White House, Office of the Press Secretary. https://obamawhitehouse.archives.gov/the-press-office/2014/05/24/weekly-address-paying-tribute-our-fallen-heroes-memorial-day

O'Connell, K. M., Littleton-Kearney, M. T., Bridges, E., and Bibb, S. C. (2012). Evaluating the joint theater trauma registry as a data source to benchmark casualty care. *Military Medicine*, 177(5), 546–552.

O'Connor, M. (2009). Can we prevent doctors being complicit in torture? Breaking the serpent's egg. *Journal of Law and Medicine*, 17(3), 426–438.

Organisation for Economic Co-Operation and Development (OECD). (2006). The United States Development Assistance Committee (DAC) peer review. Organisation for Economic Co-Operation and Development. http://www.oecd.org/governance/pcsd/37885999.pdf.

Organisation for Economic Co-Operation and Development (OECD). (2011). The United States Development Assistance Committee (DAC) peer review. http://www.oecd.org/development/peer-reviews/48434536.pdf.

Organisation for Economic Co-Operation and Development (OECD). (2019). States of fragility report. https://www.oecd.org/dac/conflict-fragility-resilience/states-of-fragility-report-series.htm

Office of the Veterans Ombudsman. (2013). A review of the support provided by veterans affairs Canada through its long-term care program. Ottawa, Canada: Office of the Veterans Ombudsman. https://www.ombudsman-veterans.gc.ca/pdfs/reports/rep-rap-02-2013-eng.pdf.

Oliker O., Kauzlarich, R., Dobbins, J., Basseuner, K. W., Sampler, D. L., McGinn, J. G., Dziedzic, M. J., Grissom, A. R., Prinie, B. R., Bensahel, N., and Guven, A. I. (2004). *Aid during conflict: Interaction between military and civilian assistance providers in Afghanistan, September 2001–June 2002.* Santa Monica, CA: RAND Corporation.

Olson, L. (2006). Fighting for humanitarian space: NGOs in Afghanistan. *Journal of Military and Strategic Studies,* 9(1), 1–28.

Olsthoorn, O., Bollen, M., and Beeres, R. (2013). Dual loyalties in military medical care –Between ethics and effectiveness. In H. Amersfoort, R. Moelker, J. Soeters, and D. Verweij (Eds.), *Moral responsibility & military effectiveness* (pp. 76–96). The Hague, Netherlands: T.M.C Asser Press.

Olsthoorn, P. (2011). *Military ethics and virtues: An interdisciplinary approach for the 21st century.* London: Routledge.

O'Mara, S. (2015). *Why torture doesn't work: The neuroscience of interrogation.* Cambridge, MA: Harvard University Press.

O'Reilly, D. (2011). Proceedings of the DMS Medical Ethics Symposium. *BMJ Military Health,* 157(4), 405–410.

Orend, B. (2006). *The morality of war.* Toronto: Broadview Press.

Orend, B. (2014). Post-intervention: Permissions and prohibitions. In D. E. Scheid (Ed.), *The ethics of armed humanitarian intervention* (pp. 224–242). Cambridge: Cambridge University Press.

Osborne, L., Knudson, M. M., and Holcomb, J. B. (2017). In-Theater research: Optimizing the combat environment to continue to advance the state of the science. In A. L. Kellerman, and E. Elster (Eds.), *Out of the crucible: How the US military transformed combat casualty care in Iraq and Afghanistan* (pp. 395–400). Fort Sam Houston, TX: Army Medical Department.

Özgül v. Turkey. (2007). European Court of Human Rights. 7715/02. March 6. https:// www.echr.coe.int/Documents/FS_Hunger_strikes_detention_ENG.pdf.

Pagaard, S. A. (1986). Disease and the British army in South Africa, 1899–1900. *Military Affairs,* 50(2), 71–76.

Paine, G. F., Bonnema, C. L., Stambaugh, T. A., Capacchione, J. F., and Sipe, P. S. (2005). Anesthesia services aboard USNS *Comfort* (T-AH-20) during Operation Iraqi Freedom. *Military Medicine,* 170(6), 476–482.

Pannell, C. D., Poynter, J., Wales, P. W., Tien, C. H., Nathens, A. B., and Shellington, D. (2015). Factors affecting mortality of pediatric trauma patients encountered in Kandahar, Afghanistan. *Canadian Journal of Surgery,* 58(3), S141–S145.

Parasidis, E. (2012). Justice and beneficence in military medicine and research. *Ohio State Law Journal,* 73(4), 723–794.

Parasidis, E. (2015). Emerging military technologies: Balancing medical ethics and national security. *Case Western Reserve Journal of International Law,* 47(1), 168–181.

Parasidis, E. (2016). The military biomedical complex: Are service members a vulnerable population. *Houston Journal of Health Law and Policy,* 16, 113–161.

Paré, A. (1968). *The apologie and treatise of Ambroise Paré: Containing the voyages made into divers places with many of his writings upon surgery.* New York: Dover Publications.

Paré, A. (1968). *The apologie and treatise.* New York: Dover Publications.

Pattison, J. (2015). Jus post bellum and the responsibility to rebuild. *British Journal of Political Science,* 45(3), 635–661.

Patton, B. D. (2009). Detainee healthcare as part of information operations. *Military Review,* 89(4), 52–58.

Paul, C., Clarke, C. P., and Grill, B. (2010). *Victory has a thousand fathers: Sources of success in counterinsurgency*. Santa Monica, CA: RAND Corporation.

Pazdan, R., Lattimore, T., Whitt, E., and Grimes, J. (2019). Traumatic brain injury in the military. In F. G. O'Connor, E. B. Schoomaker, and D. C. Smith (Eds.), *Fundamentals of military medicine* (pp. 585–601). Fort Sam Houston, TX: Army Medical Department.

Pellerin, C. (2017). DARPA funds brain-stimulation research to speed learning. *DoD News*, April 27.

Penn, M., Bhatnagar, S., Kuy, S., Lieberman, S., Elnahal, S., Clancy, C., and Shulkin, D. (2019). Comparison of wait times for new patients between the private sector and United States Department of Veterans Affairs medical centers. *JAMA Network Open*, 2(1), e187096–e187096.

Penn-Barwell, J. G., Roberts, S. A., Midwinter, M. J., and Bishop, J. R. (2015). Improved survival in UK combat casualties from Iraq and Afghanistan: 2003–2012. *Journal of Trauma and Acute Care Surgery*, 78(5), 1014–10120.

Perito, R. M. (2005). *The U.S. experience with teams in Afghanistan provincial reconstruction: Lessons identified. United States Institute of Peace Special Report, 152*. Washington, DC: USIP.

Perkins, J. G., and Beekley, A. C. (2012). Damage control resuscitation. In E. Savitsky, and B. Eastridge (Eds.), *Combat casualty care, lessons learned from OEF and OIF* (pp. 121–164). Washington, DC: Office of the Surgeon General, Department of the Army.

Perkins, J. G., Brosch, L. R., Beekley, A. C., Warfield, K. L., Wade, C. E., and Holcomb, J. B. (2012). Research and analytics in combat trauma care: Converting data and experience to practical guidelines. *Surgical Clinics*, 92(4), 1041–1054.

Perlin, J. B., Kolodner, R. M., and Roswell, R. H. (2004). The veterans health administration: Quality, value, accountability, and information as transforming strategies for patient-centered care. *The American Journal of Managed Care*, 10(11), 828–836.

Perry, D. C., Griffin, X. L., Parsons, N. and Costa, M. L. (2014). Designing clinical trials in trauma surgery: Overcoming research barriers. *Bone & Joint Research*, 3(4), 123–129.

Philips, M., and Derderian, K. (2015). Health in the service of state-building in fragile and conflict affected contexts: An additional challenge in the medical-humanitarian environment. *Conflict and Health*, 9(1), 1–8.

Physicians for Human Rights (PHR). (2002). Dual loyalty & human rights: In health professional practice: Proposed guidelines & institutional mechanisms. https://s3.amazonaws.com/PHR_Reports/dualloyalties-2002-report.pdf.

Plata v. Brown. (2013). United States District Court, Northern District of California, C01-1351 THE, 19-Aug.-13.

Pogge, T. (2009). World poverty and human rights. In J. Rosenthal and C. Barry (Eds.), *Ethics and international affairs: A reader* (pp. 307–316). Washington, DC: Georgetown University Press.

Pollack, K. M. (2006). *The seven deadly sins of failure in Iraq: A retrospective analysis of the reconstruction*. Brookings. https://www.brookings.edu/articles/the-seven-deadly-sins-of-failure-in-iraq-a-retrospective-analysis-of-the-reconstruction/.

Pope, K. S. (2011). Are the American Psychological Association's detainee interrogation policies ethical and effective? Key claims, documents, and results. *Journal of Psychology*, 219(3), 150–158.

Porch, D. (2013). *Counterinsurgency: Exposing the myths of the new way of war*. Cambridge: Cambridge University Press.

Porta, C. R. (2018). Personal communication. February 6, 2018.

Porta, C. R., Robins, R., Eastridge, B., Holcomb, J., Schreiber, M., and Martin, M. (2014). The hidden war: Humanitarian surgery in a combat zone. *The American Journal of Surgery*, 207(5), 766–772.

Posner, R. (2006). *Not a suicide pact: The Constitution in time of national emergency*. Oxford: Oxford University Press.

Powell, C. L. (2001). Remarks to the national foreign policy conference for leaders of nongovernmental organizations. October 26. https://2001-2009.state.gov/secretary/former/powell/remarks/2001/5762.htm.

Price, R. A., Sloss, E. M., Cefalu, M., Farmer, C. M., and Hussey, P. S. (2018). Comparing quality of care in Veterans Affairs and non-Veterans Affairs settings. *Journal of General Internal Medicine*, 33(10), 1631–1638.

Pugh, M. (2001). The challenge of civil-military relations in international peace operations. *Disasters*, 25(4), 345–357.

RAND Corporation. (2017). Strengthening health care in the Kurdistan region of Iraq. Research Brief. https://www.rand.org/content/dam/rand/pubs/research_briefs/RB9900/RB9990/RAND_RB9990.pdf

Rasmussen, T. E., Baer, D. G., Cap, A. P., and Lein, B. C. (2015). Ahead of the curve: Sustained innovation for future combat casualty care. *Journal of Trauma and Acute Care Surgery*, 79(4), S61–S64.

Rasmussen, T. E., Rauch, T. M., and Hack, D. C. (2014). Military trauma research: Answering the call. *Journal of Trauma and Acute Care Surgery*, 77(3), S55–S56.

Rasmussen, T. E., and Baer, D. G. (2014). No drift. *JAMA Surgery*, 149(3), 221–222.

Rasmussen, T. E., and Kellermann, A. L. (2016). Wartime lessons—Shaping a national trauma action plan. *New England Journal of Medicine*, 375(17), 1612–1615.

Rawls, J. (1971). *A theory of justice*. Cambridge, MA: Belknap Press of Harvard University Press.

Recchia, S. (2009). Just and unjust postwar reconstruction: How much external interference can be justified? *Ethics & International Affairs*, 23(2), 165–187.

Rescher, N. (1969). The allocation of exotic medical lifesaving therapy. *Ethics*, 79(3), 173–186.

Rettig, R. A. (1999). *Military use of drugs not yet approved by the FDA for CW/BW defense: Lessons from the Gulf War*. Santa Monica, CA: RAND Corporation.

Reus-Smit, C. (2001). Human rights and the social construction of sovereignty. *Review of International Studies*, 27(4), 519–538.

Reyes, H., Annas, G. J., and Allen, S. A. (2013). Physicians and hunger strikes in prison: Confrontation, manipulation, medicalization and medical ethics. *World Medicine Journal*, 59(1), 27–36.

Rice, M. S., and Jones, O. J. (2010). Medical operations counterinsurgency warfare: Desired effects and unintended consequences. *Military Review*, 90(3), 47–57.

Richardson, M. C. (2008). The complexity of moving patients in today's maturing counterinsurgency environment: Whom, when, and how. *US Army Medical Department Journal*, October, 41–51.

Ricks, T. E. (2006). *Fiasco: The American military adventure in Iraq, 2003 to 2005*. London: Penguin Publishing Group.

Riley, J., & Gambone, M. (2020). The new veterans. *Journal of Military Ethics*, 19(3), 201–219.

Rinat Z. (2015). Leading Israeli experts: Hunger-striking prisoners should be force-fed. *Ha'aretz*, August 23. https://www.haaretz.com/.premium-leading-experts-endorse-force-feeding-1.5390353.

Risdall, J. E., and Menon, D. K. (2011). Traumatic brain injury. Philosophical Transactions of the Royal Society B. *Biological Sciences*, 366(1562), 241–250.

Risse, M. (2009). Do we owe the global poor assistance or rectification? In J., Rosenthal and C., Barry (Eds.), *Ethics and international affairs: A reader* (pp. 317–328). Washington, DC: Georgetown University Press.

Risse, T. (2000). Let's argue! Communicative action in world politics. *International Organization*, 54(1), 1–39.

Robbins, L. R. (2013). Refusing to be all that you can be: Regulating against forced cognitive enhancement in the military. In D. Carrick and M. L. Gross (Eds.), *Military ethics for the 21st century* (pp. 127–138). New York: Routledge.

Rodin, D. (2011). Justifying harm. *Ethics*, 122(1), 74–110.

Rubenstein, L. and Thomson, G. (2013). *Ethics abandoned: Medical professionalism and detainee abuse in the "war on terror."* New York: Institute on Medicine as a Profession, Columbia University.

Rush, R. M., Stockmaster, N. R., Stinger, H. K., Arrington, E. D., Devine, J. G., Atteberry, L., Starnes, B. W., and Place, R. J. (2005). Supporting the global war on terror: A tale of two campaigns featuring the 250th forward surgical team (airborne). *American Journal of Surgery*, 189(5), 564–570.

Rush, R. S. (2001). *Hell in the Hürtgen Forest: The ordeal and triumph of an American infantry regiment*. Lawrence: University of Kansas Press.

Rush, R. M., Martin, M. J., and Cocanour, C. S. (2017). Expectant and end-of-life care in a combat zone. In M. J. Martin, A. Beekley, and M. Eckert (Eds.), *Front line surgery* (pp. 749–760). New York: Springer International Publishing.

Rutherford, S., and Saleh, S. (2019). Rebuilding health post-conflict: Case studies, reflections and a revised framework. *Health Policy and Planning*, 34(3), 230–245.

Sargent, P. D. (2008). Task force 62 medical brigade combat healthcare support system in the mature Iraq theater of operations. *US Army Medical Department Journal*, October, 5–10.

Sasahara, K. H. (2008). Successful ICRC visit to Camp Bucca. Cable no. 08BAGHDAD298_a. 1 February. Wikileaks, https://wikileaks.org/plusd/cables/08BAGHDAD298_a.html

Scheffler, S. (2002). Families, nations, and strangers. In S. Scheffler (Ed.), *Boundaries and allegiances: Problems of justice and responsibility in liberal thought* (pp. 48–68). Oxford: Oxford University Press.

Schermer M., Bolt I., De Jongh R., and Olivier B. (2009). The future of psychopharmacological enhancements: Expectations and policies. *Neuroethics*, 2(2), 75–87.

Schlesinger, J. R., Brown, H., Fowler, T. K., and Homer, C. A. (2004). *Final Report of the Independent Panel to Review DoD Detention Operations*, Arlington, VA: Independent Panel to Review DoD Detention Operations.

Schmidt, U. (2015). *Secret science: A century of poison warfare and human experiments*. Oxford: Oxford University Press.

Schmitt, E. (2003). Army chief raises estimate of G.I.'s needed in postwar Iraq. *New York Times*, February 25. https://www.nytimes.com/2003/02/25/international/middleeast/army-chief-raises-stimate-of-gis-needed-in-postwar.html

Schoenfeld, A. J. (2012). The combat experience of military surgical assets in Iraq and Afghanistan: A historical review. *The American Journal of Surgery*, 204(3), 377–383.

Schulz, C., Kunz, U. and Mauer, U. M. (2012). Three years of neurosurgical experience in a multinational field hospital in northern Afghanistan. *Acta Neurochirurgica*, 154(1), 135–140.

Sen, A. (2000). A decade of human development. *Journal of Human Development*, 1(1), 17–23.

Sen, A. (2005). Human rights and capabilities. *Journal of Human Development*, 6(2), 151–166.

SENLIS Council. (2007). *War zone hospitals in Afghanistan: A symbol of willful neglect.* London: MF Publishing.

Shabila, N. P., Al-Tawil, N. G., Al-Hadithi, T. S., and Sondorp, E. (2012a). A qualitative assessment of the Iraqi primary healthcare system. *World Health & Population*, 13(3), 18–27.

Shabila, N. P., Al-Tawil, N. G., Al-Hadithi, T. S., Sondorp, E., and Vaughan, K. (2012b). Iraqi primary care system in Kurdistan region: Providers' perspectives on problems and opportunities for improvement. *BMC International Health and Human Rights*, 12(1), 21–30.

Shachtman, N. (2011). The secret history of Iraq's invisible war. *Wired*, April 11.

Shafran, S. N. (2007). Kabul MEDCAP treats more than 600. *ISAF Mirror.*, 36(January), 9.

Sheaffer, M. A. (2007). Detainee medical operations during Operation Iraqi Freedom: Determination of a transition plan. Unpublished MA thesis. Fort Leavenworth, KS: Army Command and General Staff College. https://apps.dtic.mil/sti/citations/ADA471445.

Sheehan, J. C. (1982). *The enchanted ring: The untold story of penicillin.* Cambridge, MA: MIT Press.

Shukor, A. R., Klazinga, N. S., and Kringos, D. S. (2017). Primary care in an unstable security, humanitarian, economic and political context: The Kurdistan Region of Iraq. *BMC Health Services Research*, 17(1), 592–610.

Sidel, V. W., and Levy, B. (2003). Physician-Soldier: A moral dilemma? In T. E. Beam and L. R. Spracino (Eds.), *Military medical ethics* (pp. 293–312). Falls Church, VA: Office of the Surgeon General, Department of the Army.

Siebold, G. L. (1999). The evolution of the measurement of cohesion. *Military Psychology*, 11(1), 5–26.

Siebold, G. L. (2007). The essence of military group cohesion. *Armed Forces and Society*, 33(2), 286–295.

SIGAR. (2017). Afghanistan's health care sector: USAID's use of unreliable data presents challenges in assessing program performance and the extent of progress, Special Inspector General for Afghanistan Reconstruction, SIGAR 17-22-AR. https://www.sigar.mil/pdf/audits/SIGAR-17-22-AR.pdf.

SIGIR. (2013). Learning from Iraq. A final report from SIGIR. Special Inspector General for Afghanistan Reconstruction, http://cybercemetery.unt.edu/archive/sigir/20131001080029/http:/www.sigir.mil/files/learningfromiraq/Report_-_March_2013.pdf.

Simmons, A. J. (1996). Associative political obligations. *Ethics*, 106(2), 247–273.

Simpson, R. G., Wilson, D., and Tuck, J. J. (2014). Medical management of captured persons. *BMJ Military Health*, 60(1), 4–8.

Singer, P. (1972). Famine, affluence, and morality. *Philosophy & Public Affairs*, 1(3), 229–243.

Slack D., and Estes A. (2018). Secret VA nursing home ratings hide poor quality care from the public. *USA Today*, June 17.

Slim, H. (2015). *Humanitarian ethics: A guide to the morality of aid in war and disaster.* Oxford: Oxford University Press.

SOFA. (2008). Status of Forces Agreement. http://en.wikisource.org/wiki/Status_of_ Forces_Agreement,_2008.

Sokol, D. K. (2011). The medical ethics of the battlefield. *British Medical Journal*, 343(7816), d3877.

Song, J. W., and Chung, K. C. (2010). Observational studies: Cohort and case-control studies. *Plastic and Reconstructive Surgery*, 126(6), 2234–2242.

Sox, H. C., Liverman, C. T., and Fulco, C. E. (Eds.). (2000). *Gulf War and health: Volume 1: Depleted uranium, sarin, pyridostigmine bromide, and vaccines*. Washington, DC: National Academies Press.

Spence, D. L. (2007). Ensuring respect for persons when recruiting junior enlisted personnel for research. *Military Medicine*, 173(3), 250–253.

Spinella, P. C., Martin, J., and Azarow, K. S. (2012). Pediatric trauma. In E. Savitsky and B. Eastridge (Eds.), *Combat casualty care: Lessons from OEF and OIF* (pp. 529–592). Falls Church, VA: Office of the Surgeon General, Department of the Army.

SSCI. (2014). Senate Select Committee on Intelligence, Committee study of the Central Intelligence Agency's detention and interrogation program (approved December 13, 2012; released with redactions December 3, 2014). https://www.intelligence.senate. gov/sites/default/files/publications/CRPT-113srpt288.pdf

Stanton, E. A. (2007). *The Human Development Index: A history*. Working Papers, Number 127. Medford, MA: Global Development and Environment Institute, Tufts University.

Statman, D. (1997). The absoluteness of the prohibition against torture. *Law and Government in Israel*, 4, 161–198.

Stein, J. (2018). Obama banned torture years ago but its replacement is still brutal. *Newsweek*, November 29. https://www.newsweek.com/2018/12/07/obama-banned-torture-interrogators-still-cant-agree-replacement-1233717.html

Steinhardt, L. C., Rao, K. D., Hansen, P. M., Alam, S., and Peters, D. H. (2013). The effects of user fees on quality and utilization of primary health-care services in Afghanistan: A quasi-experimental health financing pilot study in a post-conflict setting. *The International Journal of Health Planning and Management*, 28(4), e280–e297.

Stewart, A. M. (2009). Mandatory vaccination of health care workers. *New England Journal of Medicine*, 361(21), 2015–2017.

Swerdlow, J. (2016). *Medical Diplomacy and Soft Power*. Unpublished MA thesis, The University of Haifa.

Tanielian, T. L., Jaycox, L., and RAND Corporation. (2008). *Invisible wounds of war: Psychological and cognitive injuries, their consequences, and services to assist recovery*. Santa Monica, CA: RAND Corporation.

Tapp, C., Burkle, F. M., Wilson, K., Takaro, T., Guyatt, G. H., Amad, H., and Mills, E. J. (2008). Iraq war mortality estimates: A systematic review. *Conflict and Health*, 2(1), http://web.mit.edu/humancostiraq.

Tennison, M. N., and Moreno, J. D. (2012). Neuroscience, ethics, and national security: The state of the art. *PLoS Biology*, 10(3), e1001289.

Terry, F. (2002). *Condemned to repeat: The paradox of humanitarian intervention*. Ithaca, NY: Cornell University Press.

Terry, F. (2013). Violence against health care: Insights from Afghanistan, Somalia, and the Democratic Republic of the Congo. *International Review of the Red Cross*, 95(889), 23–39.

Thach, A. B., Johnson, A. J., Carroll, R. B., Huchun, A., Ainbinder, D. J., Stutzman, R. D., Blaydon, S. M., Demartelaere, S. L., Mader, T. H., Slade, C. S., George, R. K., Ritchey,

J. P., Barnes, S. D., and Fannin, L. A. (2008). Severe eye injuries in the war in Iraq, 2003–2005. *Ophthalmology*, 115(2), 377–382.

Thompson, D. F. (2008). The role of medical diplomacy in stabilizing Afghanistan. *Center for Technology and National Security Policy, National Defense University*, 63, 1–9.

Tilghman, A. (2014). America's military: A force adrift. *Military Times*, December 7.

Tracy, J. (2007). Responsibility to pay: Compensating civilian casualties of war. *Human Rights Brief*, 15(1), 16–19.

Tuck, J. J. H. (2005). Medical management of Iraqi enemy prisoners of war during Operation Telic. *Military Medicine*, 170(3), 177–182.

Tyson, A. (2017). Americans divided in views of use of torture in U.S. anti-terror efforts. *The Pew Research Center*. http://www.pewresearch.org/fact-tank/2017/01/26/americans-divided-in-views-of-use-of-torture-in-u-s-anti-terror-efforts/.

UCSF. (2019). The kidney project, statistics. University of California, San Francisco. https://pharm.ucsf.edu/kidney/need/statistics

United Kingdom Ministry of Defence (UK MoD). (2011). *The armed forces covenant: Today and tomorrow*. London: United Kingdom Ministry of Defence. https://assets.publishing.service.gov.uk/government/uploads/system/uploads/attachment_data/file/49470/the_armed_forces_covenant_today_and_tomorrow.pdf

United Kingdom Ministry of Defence (UK MoD). (2013). *£11 Million funding boost to improve NHS care for war veterans*. https://www.gov.uk/government/news/11-million-funding-boost-to-improve-nhs-care-for-war-veterans

United Kingdom Ministry of Defence (UK MoD). (2014). *The military medical contribution to security and stabilization*. JDN 3/14, https://www.gov.uk/government/uploads/system/uploads/attachment_data/file/324637/20140616-JDN_3_14_Med_contr_DCDC.pdf

United Kingdom Ministry of Defence (UK MoD). (2015). *FOI 2015 01104*. Defence Statistics. https://assets.publishing.service.gov.uk/government/uploads/system/uploads/attachment_data/file/412959/PUBLIC_1425293223.pdf

United Kingdom Ministry of Defence (UK MoD). (2019a). British fatalities: Operations in Iraq. https://www.gov.uk/government/fields-of-operation/ir

United Kingdom Ministry of Defence (UK MoD). (2019b). British fatalities: Operations in Afghanistan. https://www.gov.uk/government/fields-of-operation/afghanistan

United Kingdom Ministry of Defence (UK MoD). (2020a). JSP 536. Governance of research involving human, participants, Part 1: Directive. https://assets.publishing.service.gov.uk/government/uploads/system/uploads/attachment_data/file/872936/20200312-JSP536_Part_1_Governance_Research_Human_v3_1_FINAL.pdf

United Kingdom Ministry of Defence (UK MoD). (2020b). Armed forces compensation: What you need to know. https://www.gov.uk/guidance/armed-forces-compensation-scheme-afcs#armed-forces-compensation-scheme-afcs-an-overview

United Nations. (2015). The Millennium development goals report 2015. United Nations https://www.un.org/millenniumgoals/2015_MDG_Report/pdf/MDG%202015%20rev%20(July%201).pdf

United Nations Development Programme (UNDP). (2010). *Human Development Report, 2010. The real wealth of nations: Pathways to human development*. New York: United Nations Development Programme.

United Nations Development Programme (UNDP). (2017). *Human Development Report. Human development index trends, 1990–2017*. http://hdr.undp.org/en/composite/trends

United Nations Development Programme (UNDP). (2018). Human development indices and indicators, 2018 update. http://hdr.undp.org/sites/default/files/2018_human_development_statistical_update.pdf

United Nations Development Programme (UNDP). (2020). Multidimensional Poverty Index 2019 FAQs. http://hdr.undp.org/en/mpi-2019-faq

United Nations Office for the Coordination of Humanitarian Affairs (UNOCHA). What are humanitarian principles? http://www.unocha.org/sites/dms/Documents/OOM-humanitarianprinciples_eng_June12.pdf

UNICEF. (2019). UNICEF Data: Monitoring the situation of children and women. United Nations Children's Fund. https://data.unicef.org/

Upshur, R. E. G. (2002). Principles for the justification of public health intervention. *Canadian Journal of Public Health, 93*(2), 101–103.

US Army. (2016). Army medicine vision: Premier expeditionary and globally integrated medical force. US Army Medical Command. https://armymedicine.health.mil/~/media/60F95AE36CCF4588ACBC4C800DABEA46.ashx

US Army. (2017). *Information for investigators.* Headquarters, U. S. Army Medical Research and Materiel Command (USAMRMC) Office of Research Protections (ORP) Human Research Protections Regulatory Requirements ORP Human Research Protection Office (HRPO). https://mrdc.amedd.army.mil/assets/docs/orp/HRPO_Information_for_Investigators.docx

US Department of Justice. (2002). Memorandum for Alberto R. Gonzales, Counsel to the President: Re: Standards of conduct for interrogation under 18 USC §§ 2340-2340A' (1 August 2002) 2-13. Office of Legal Counsel. https://www.justice.gov/olc/file/886061/download

USCC. (2016). Summary of the airstrike on the MSF Trauma Center in Kunduz, Afghanistan on October 3, 2015. US Central Command. http://www.humanrightsvoices.org/assets/attachments/documents/Oct-3-2015-Kunduz-Trauma-Center-Strike.-CENTCOM-Summary-Memo.pdf

Van Burken, C. G., and De Vries, M. J. (2012). Extending the theory of normative practices: An application to two cases of networked military operations. *Philosophia Reformata, 77*(2), 135–154.

Veterans Health Administration (VA). (2019a). Providing health care for veterans. US Department of Veterans Affairs. https://www.va.gov/health/

Veterans Health Administration (VA). (2019b). VA priority groups. https://www.va.gov/health-care/eligibility/priority-groups/

Veterans Health Administration (VA). (2019c). PTSD treatment. https://www.va.gov/health-care/health-needs-conditions/mental-health/ptsd/

Veterans Health Administration (VA). (2020a). Annual income limits–Health benefits. https://www.va.gov/healthbenefits/apps/explorer/AnnualIncomeLimits/LegacyVAThresholds?FiscalYear=2020

Veterans Health Administration (VA). (2020b). Education and training: Post – 9/11 GI Bill. https://www.benefits.va.gov/gibill/post911_gibill.asp

Veterans Health Administration (VA). (2020c). Compensation. https://www.benefits.va.gov/compensation/rates-index.asp

Veteran Affairs Canada (VAC). (2019). 4.0 disability benefits. https://www.veterans.gc.ca/eng/about-vac/news-media/facts-figures/4-0

Vassallo, D. (2015). A short history of Camp Bastion Hospital: The two hospitals and unit deployments. *BMJ Military Health, 161*(1), 78–83.

Vizzard, J. W., and Capron, T. A. (2010). Exporting general Petraeus's counterinsurgency doctrine: An assessment of the adequacy of field manual 3-24 and the US government's implementation. *Public Administration Review*, 70(3), 485–493.

Vuving, A. L. (2009). *How soft power works*. Paper presented at the American Political Science Association Annual Meeting, Toronto. September 3.

Waldron, J. (2005). Torture and positive law: Jurisprudence for the White House. *Columbia Law Review*, 105(1681), 1714–1715.

Walerstein, J. (2009). Coping with combat claims: An analysis of the Foreign Claims Act's combat exclusion. *Cardozo Journal of Conflict Resolution*, 11, 319–352.

Walter Reed National Military Medical Center. (2019). Patient rights and responsibilities. https://tricare.mil/mtf/WalterReed/Getting-Care/Patient-Rights-and-Responsibilities (archived with author).

Waltz, E. (2017). DARPA to use electrical stimulation to enhance military training. *IEEE Spectrum*. April 26. https://spectrum.ieee.org/the-human-os/biomedical/devices/darpa-to-use-electrical-stimulation-to-improve-military-training

Walzer, M. (1970). The obligation to die for the state. In M. Walzer. *Obligations: Essays on disobedience, war and citizenship* (pp. 77–98). New York: Simon and Shuster.

Walzer, M. (1977). *Just and unjust wars*. New York: Basic Books.

Warden, D. (2006). Military TBI during the Iraq and Afghanistan war. *Journal of Head Trauma Rehabilitation*, 21(5), 398–402.

Watson Institute. (2015). US veterans & military families. Watson Institute, Brown University, The Costs of War. https://watson.brown.edu/costsofwar/costs/human/veterans

Watson Institute. (2019). Civilians killed and wounded. Watson Institute, Brown University, The Costs of War. https://watson.brown.edu/costsofwar/costs/human/civilians

Webster, P. C. (2016). Under severe duress: Health care in Iraq. *The Lancet*, 388(10041), 226–227.

Weeks, S. R., Oh, J. S., Elster, E. A., and Learn, P. A. (2018). Humanitarian surgical care in the US military treatment facilities in Afghanistan from 2002 to 2013. *JAMA Surgery*, 153(1), 84–86.

Wegrzyn, R. (nd). Safe genes. *DARPA Program Information*. https://www.darpa.mil/program/safe-genes.

Weijer, C., and Miller, P. B. (2004). When are research risks reasonable in relation to anticipated benefits? *Nature Medicine*, 10(6), 570–573.

Weingarten, M. (2017). Force-feeding political prisoners on hunger strike. *Clinical Ethics*, 12(2), 86–94.

WHO and The World Bank. (2017). Tracking universal health coverage: 2017 global monitoring report. World Health Organization and International Bank for Reconstruction and Development / The World Bank. http://pubdocs.worldbank.org/en/193371513169798347/2017-global-monitoring-report.pdf

World Health Organization (WHO). (2007). Everybody's business—Strengthening health systems to improve health outcomes: WHO's framework for action. https://apps.who.int/iris/bitstream/handle/10665/43918/9789241596077_eng.pdf

World Health Organization (WHO). (2008). Essential health packages: What are they for? What do they change? Draft Technical Brief No. 2, July 3, 2008. https://www.who.int/healthsystems/topics/delivery/technical_brief_ehp.pdf

World Health Organization (WHO). (2011). Civil-military coordination during humanitarian health action. https://www.who.int/hac/global_health_cluster/about/ghc_annex5_civil_military_coordination_february2011.pdf?ua=1

World Health Organization (WHO). (2014). Making fair choices on the path to universal health coverage: Final report of the WHO Consultative Group on Equity and Universal Health Coverage. https://apps.who.int/iris/bitstream/handle/10665/112671/9789241507158_eng.pdf;jsessionid=FB34CECFAD92E9A1BC2636D2E4151570?sequence=1

World Health Organization (WHO). (2016). WHO condemns multiple attacks on health facilities in the Syrian Arab Republic. http://www.emro.who.int/media/news/who-condemns-multiple-attacks-on-health-facilities-in-the-syrian-arab-republic.html

World Health Organization (WHO). (2018). *Delivering quality health services: A global imperative for universal health coverage.* Geneva: World Health Organization, Organisation for Economic Co-operation and Development and The World Bank.

World Health Organization (WHO). (2019). Primary Health Care Iraq. http://www.emro.who.int/irq/programmes/primary-health-care.html

World Health Organization (WHO). (2020). Global health expenditures database. http://apps.who.int/nha/database/ViewData/Indicators/en

Wike, R. (2016). Global opinion varies widely on use of torture against suspected terrorists. *The Pew Research Center.* February 9. https://www.pewresearch.org/fact-tank/2016/02/09/global-opinion-use-of-torture/

Wilensky, R. J. (2004). *Military medicine to win hearts and minds: Aid to civilians in the Vietnam War.* Lubbock: Texas Tech University Press.

Wilks, M. (2005). A stain on medical ethics. *The Lancet,* 366(9484), 429–431.

Williams, E. (2008). *Human performance.* McLean, VA: JASON, The MITRE Corporation.

Willy, C., Hauer, T., Huschitt, N., & Palm, H. G. (2011). "Einsatzchirurgie"—experiences of German military surgeons in Afghanistan. *Langenbeck's Archives of surgery, 396*(4), 507–522.

Wilson, C. (2007). Improvised explosive devices (IEDs) in Iraq and Afghanistan: Effects and countermeasures. Congressional Research Report, No. RS22330. https://fas.org/sgp/crs/weapons/RS22330.pdf

Wilton Park Conference. (2010). WP1022, *Winning hearts and minds in Afghanistan: Assessing the effectiveness of development and operations.* Wilton Park Conference, March 11–14, 2010. https://www.wiltonpark.org.uk/wp-content/uploads/wp1022-report.pdf.

Wise, P. H. (2017). The epidemiologic challenge to the conduct of just war: Confronting indirect civilian casualties of war. *Daedalus, 146*(1), 139–154.

World Medical Association (WMA). (2017a). WMA regulations in times of armed conflict and other situations of violence. https://www.wma.net/policies-post/wma-regulations-in-times-of-armed-conflict-and-other-situations-of-violence/

World Medical Association (WMA). (2017b). WMA Declaration of Malta on Hunger Strikers. https://www.wma.net/policies-post/wma-declaration-of-malta-on-hunger-strikers/.

Wolfendale, J. (2008). Performance-enhancing technologies and moral responsibility in the military. *The American Journal of Bioethics,* 8(2), 28–38.

Woll, M., and Brisson, P. (2013). Humanitarian care by a forward surgical team in Afghanistan. *Military Medicine,* 178(4), 385–388.

Wolpe, P. R., Foster, K. R., and Langleben, D. D. (2005). Emerging neurotechnologies for lie detection: Promise or peril. *American Journal of Bioethics*, 5(2), 39–49.

Wong, L., Kolditz, T. A., Millen, R. A., and Potter, T. M. (2003). *Why they fight: Combat motivation in the Iraq war*. Carlisle, PA: US Army War College.

World Bank. (2018). Progress in the face of insecurity improving health outcomes in Afghanistan. http://documents.worldbank.org/curated/en/330491520002103598/pdf/123809-WP-PUBLIC-MARCH6-530AM-14846-WB-Afghanistan-Policy-Brief-WEB.pdf

World Bank. (2020). World Bank open data, health. https://data.worldbank.org/indicator/

World Summit. (2005). *Resolution adopted by the General Assembly on 16 September 2005, A/RES/60/1, World Summit Outcome*, United Nations General Assembly. https://www.un.org/en/development/desa/population/migration/generalassembly/docs/globalcompact/A_RES_60_1.pdf

Yamin, A. E., and Norheim, O. F. (2014). Taking equality seriously: Applying human rights frameworks to priority setting in health. *Human Rights Quarterly*, 36(2), 296–324.

Yarvis, J. S. (2011). Operation Iraqi Freedom 05-07 Medical civil – military operations: Lessons learned in humanitarian assistance. In E. C. Ritche (Ed.), *Combat and operational behavioral health textbooks of military medicine* (pp. 609–618). Falls Church, VA: Department of the Army.

Zajtchuk, J. T. (2003). Military medicine in humanitarian missions. In T. E. Beam and L. R. Sparacino (Eds.), *Military medical ethics* (Vol. 2, pp. 773–804). Falls Church VA: Office of the Surgeon General, Department of the Army.

Index

For the benefit of digital users, indexed terms that span two pages (e.g., 52–53) may, on occasion, appear on only one of those pages.

Tables and figures are indicated by *t* and *f* following the page number.